KEY TOPICS IN
GENERAL SURGERY

The KEY TOPICS Series

Advisors:

T.M. Craft *Department of Anaesthesia and Intensive Care, Royal United Hospital, Bath, UK*
C.S. Garrard *Intensive Therapy Unit, John Radcliffe Hospital, Oxford, UK*
P.M. Upton *Department of Anaesthetics, Treliske Hospital, Truro, UK*

Anaesthesia, Second Edition

Obstetrics and Gynaecology, Second Edition

Accident and Emergency Medicine

Paediatrics, Second Edition

Orthopaedic Surgery

Otolaryngology and Head and Neck Surgery

Ophthalmology

Psychiatry

General Surgery

Renal Medicine

Trauma

Chronic Pain

Oral and Maxillofacial Surgery

Oncology

Cardiovascular Medicine

Neurology

Forthcoming titles include:

Neonatology

Gastroenterology

Respiratory Medicine

Thoracic Surgery

Critical Care

Orthopaedic Trauma Surgery

KEY TOPICS IN
GENERAL SURGERY

C.R. LATTIMER
FRCS
Royal Sussex County Hospital, Brighton, UK

N.M. WILSON
FRCS
Royal Hampshire County Hospital, Winchester, UK

N.R.F. LAGATTOLLA
FRCS
Eastbourne District General Hospital, Eastbourne, UK

Consultant Editors

J. COLLIN
MA, MD, FRCS
*Consultant Surgeon and Reader in Surgery, John Radcliffe Hospital,
Oxford, UK*

N.E. DUDLEY
FRCS
Consultant Surgeon, John Radcliffe Hospital, Oxford, UK

βIOS
SCIENTIFIC
PUBLISHERS

© BIOS Scientific Publishers Limited, 1996

First published 1996
First reprinted 1998
Second reprint 2000

A CIP catalogue record for this book is available from the British Library.

ISBN 1 872748 02 3

BIOS Scientific Publishers Ltd
9 Newtec Place, Magdalen Road, Oxford OX4 1RE, UK
Tel. +44 (0)1865 726286. Fax +44 (0)1865 246823
World Wide Web home page: http://www.bios.co.uk/

Important Note from the Publisher
The information contained within this book was obtained by BIOS Scientific Publishers Ltd from sources believed by us to be reliable. However, while every effort has been made to ensure its accuracy, no responsibility for loss or injury whatsoever occasioned to any person acting or refraining from action as a result of information contained herein can be accepted by the authors or publishers.

The reader should remember that medicine is a constantly evolving science and while the authors and publishers have ensured that all dosages, applications and practices are based on current indications, there may be specific practices which differ between communities. You should always follow the guidelines laid down by the manufacturers of specific products and the relevant authorities in the country in which you are practising.

Typeset by Chandos Electronic Publishing, Stanton Harcourt, UK
Printed by Print in Black, Midsomer Norton, Bath, UK

CONTENTS

a Contributed by S. Dorudi, The Royal London Hospital, London, UK.

ABBREVIATIONS

5-ASA	5-aminosalicylic acid
5-HT	5-hydroxytryptamine
AAA	abdominal aortic aneurysm
ABPI	ankle–brachial pressure index
ACPO	acute colonic pseudo-obstruction
ACTH	adrenocorticotrophic hormone
ADH	antidiuretic hormone
AIDS	acquired immunodeficiency syndrome
APTT	activated partial thromboplastin time
ARDS	adult respiratory distress syndrome
ATLS	advanced trauma life support
AV	atrioventricular
AXR	abdominal X-ray
b.d.	two times per day
BCC	basal cell carcinoma
BCG	Bacillus Calmette Guérin
BXO	balanitis xerotica obliterans
CDC	Centers for Disease Control
CEPOD	Confidential Enquiry into Perioperative Deaths
CMV	cytomegalovirus
CNS	central nervous system
CPP	cerebral perfusion pressure
CSF	cerebrospinal fluid
CT	computerized tomography
CVP	central venous pressure
CXR	chest X-ray
DIC	disseminated intravascular coagulation
DSA	digital subtraction arteriography
DU	duodenal ulcer
DVT	deep vein thrombosis
EAS	external anal sphincter
ECG	electrocardiogram
EMG	electromyography
ENT	ear, nose and throat
ERCP	endoscopic retrograde cholangiopancreatography
ESR	erythrocyte sedimentation rate
ESWL	extracorporeal shock wave lithotripsy
FBC	full blood count
FFP	fresh frozen plasma
FiO_2	fractional inspired oxygen tension
FNAC	fine needle aspiration cytology
GCS	Glasgow Coma Scale

GP	general practitioner
GU	gastric ulcer
HBsAg	hepatitis B surface antigen
HIDA	diethylacetanilido-iminodiacetic acid
HIV	human immunodeficiency virus
HPV	human papilloma virus
HRT	hormone replacement therapy
HSV	herpes simplex virus
i.a.	intra-arterial
i.v.	intravenous
IAS	internal anal sphincter
IBD	inflammatory bowel disease
ICP	intracranial pressure
ICU	intensive care unit
IL	interleukin
INR	international normalized ratio
ISS	injury severity store
IU	international units
IVC	inferior vena cava
IVU	intravenous urography
KUB	penetrated plain abdominal X-ray ('kidneys, ureters, bladder')
LD	latissimus dorsi flap
LFT	liver function test
LHRH	luteinizing hormone–releasing hormone
MDA	manual dilatation of the anus
MEN	multiple endocrine neoplasia
MIBG	metaiodobenzylguanidine
MOF	multiple organ failure
MRI	magnetic resonance imaging
MSU	mid-stream urine
NSAID	non-steroidal anti-inflammatory drug
OPSI	overwhelming post-splenectomy infection
$PaCO_2$	carbon dioxide tension in arterial blood
PAN	polyarteritis nodosa
PaO_2	oxygen tension in arterial blood
PAP	prostatic acid phosphatase
PCN	percutaneous nephrolithotomy
PDS	polydioxanone synthetic
PE	pulmonary embolism
PEEP	positive end expiratory pressure
PEG	percutaneous endoscopic gastrostomy
PET	positron emission tomography
PG	prostaglandin
PSA	prostatic specific antigen
PTC	percutaneous transhepatic cholangiography

PTFE	polytetrafluoroethylene
PTLA	percutaneous transluminal angioplasty
PTS	paediatric trauma score
qds	four times per day
RBL	rubber band ligation
RTS	revised trauma score
s.c.	subcutaneous
SCC	squamous cell carcinoma
SAP	systemic arterial pressure
SIRS	systemic inflammatory response syndrome
SLE	systemic lupus erythematosus
T_3	tri-iodothyronine
T_4	thyroxine
TBG	thyroid-binding globulin
TCC	transitional cell carcinoma
tds	three times per day
TIPS	transjugular intrahepatic portasystemic anastomosis
TNF-α	tumour necrosis factor α
TPHA	treponema pallidum huemagglutination antigen
TPN	total parenteral nutrition
TRAM	transverse rectus abdomonis myocutaneous flap
TRUS	transrectal ultrasound probe
TS	trauma score
TSH	thyroid-stimulating hormone
TURP	transurethral resection of prostate
U&E	urea and electrolytes
UTI	urinary tract infection
VDRL	venereal disease reference laboratory
VMA	vanillyl mandelic acid
WBC	white blood count
YAG	yttrium aluminium garnet

PREFACE

This book is primarily directed at trainees preparing for the Membership and Fellowship examinations of the various Royal Colleges of Surgeons. We feel that the format will remain pertinent throughout the forthcoming changes to these examinations. The book should be used in conjunction with larger texts, but will be particularly useful in the run-up to an examination when key facts need to be crystallized out from the larger pool of information assimilated from other sources. We hope that medical students preparing for finals will also find this book informative and easy to use. Nursing staff managing surgical patients may find it useful as a basic source of reference.

We have attempted to provide a contemporary review of the key topics in general surgery. Each chapter is limited to several pages of concise information presented in a 'short notes' style. Long lists are generally avoided because they are difficult to remember and superfluous information has been omitted to aid concentration.

We are grateful to the many consultants under whose guidance we have learned and practised much that is contained within this book. We thank Jonathan Ray and Priscilla Goldby of BIOS for their help and patience in its preparation, and are grateful to our friends and families for their encouragement and hard work in checking the manuscript.

C.R. Lattimer
N.M. Wilson
N.R.F. Lagattolla

ABDOMINAL TRAUMA

The majority of abdominal injuries sustained in mainland Britain follow road traffic accidents. Recognition of the presence of an intra-abdominal injury requiring surgery is far more important than its precise definition. A high index of suspicion is necessary, based on the history, especially the mechanism of injury and associated injuries, as physical signs can be misleading initially.

Mechanism of injury

1. Blunt. Direct blow, compression, shearing and tearing forces.

2. Penetrating. Stab wounds – 30% chance of visceral injury. Projectiles – low and high velocity – 95% chance of visceral injury. Laparotomy is mandatory if the projectile has breached peritoneum.

Management

A rapid primary assessment and resuscitation should be performed (see Trauma management – principles, p. 301). It is vital to recognize co-existing cervical and spinal injuries.

1. History
- Mechanism of injury, associated injuries.
- Site and nature of pain.
- Alcohol.

2. Physical signs
- Pulse, blood pressure, central venous pressure, postural hypotension and urine output – hypovolaemia.
- Seat-belt abrasions, bruising and penetrating wounds.
- Generalized or localized abdominal distension – bleeding.
- Generalized tenderness and shoulder discomfort – free intestinal contents or blood.
- Localized tenderness – damage to a particular organ.
- Bowel sounds – unhelpful initially.
- Rectal examination – sphincter tone, blood in rectum, high riding prostate.
- Peripheral pulses. Auscultate for bruits – arterial compression or AV fistula.
- Regular reassessment – initial signs are often misleading.

3. Special investigations
- FBC, U&E, amylase, cross-match blood.
- CXR, plain AXR – of limited value.
- Peritoneal lavage, CT in children.
- CT scan.

- IVU – non-function indicates severe renal disruption or vascular injury.
- If shock and clinical condition indicate need for laparotomy – do not waste time with lavage or CT.

Specific visceral injuries

Do not remove implements embedded in the abdomen until laparotomy. A long midline incision gives good access for most injuries. After opening the abdomen, control bleeding with sucker, clot evacuation and packs in each quadrant. Once blood volume restored, remove packs one by one to determine source of bleeding.

1. Spleen. In patients presenting with shock and extensive splenic injury, splenectomy should be performed immediately. In stable patients (particularly children) with less extensive splenic damage, splenic repair may be attempted but is time-consuming and requires an experienced surgeon. Pneumococcal vaccination and prophylactic antibiotic cover should be given.

2. Liver. Blunt, macerating injuries are more hazardous than sharp penetrating injuries. No action is required if bleeding from the wound has stopped. Subcapsular haematomas should be explored and bleeding points controlled. Massive bleeding should be controlled by pressure, Pringle's manoeuvre and packs. Devitalized liver tissue should be removed. Heavy bleeding from the hepatic veins may require caval bypass to gain control. Gall bladder and bile duct injuries should be sought. The common bile duct can be repaired over a T-tube, but a damaged common hepatic duct requires drainage into a Roux loop.

3. Duodenum and pancreas. These injuries are easily missed. A midline haematoma in the lesser sac must be explored and Kocher's manoeuvre performed. Small duodenal lacerations may be repaired, but larger injuries are best treated by gastroenterostomy, closure of the pylorus and drainage. Distal pancreatectomy should be performed for transection of the pancreatic neck.

4. Stomach. Most stomach injuries can be treated by wound excision and suture. For severe distal injuries, Polya gastrectomy may be necessary. Injuries to the cardia and the posterior wall are easily missed.

5. *Intestines*. Sharp penetrating injuries of both small and large bowel can usually be excised and primary suture or anastomosis performed. Left colon projectile injuries may require excision, anastomosis and defunctioning or Hartmann's operation. Blunt injuries produce bowel lacerations, transections (which can usually be excised and anastomosed) and mesenteric haematomas. Tears at the ileocaecal junction, the splenic flexure and rectosigmoid junction are easily overlooked.

6. *Kidneys and ureter*. Haematuria and loin swelling indicate renal injury and IVU may show parenchymal damage and confirm the presence of a normal contralateral kidney. Angiography may be required if a vascular injury is suspected. Lateral haematomas overlying the kidneys found at laparotomy need not be explored providing they are not expanding and there is no hypotension. Partial nephrectomy and/or repair of renal vessels should be performed from the front and the renal pedicle controlled before opening the haematoma. Ureteric injuries are rare but often missed. Reanastomosis with stenting and drainage should be performed for upper injuries and reimplantation for lower injuries. Nephrostomy and late reconstruction may be necessary in extensive injuries.

7. *Bladder and urethra*. Blunt or penetrating injury may rupture a full bladder. Operative repair with catheter drainage is necessary. Blood at the urethral meatus implies urethral injury requiring suprapubic catheterization and subsequent urethral repair.

8. *Major blood vessels*. A midline haematoma should be explored and any underlying aortic, iliac or caval injury sutured, patched or excised and grafted as appropriate. Contained pelvic haematomas are not explored for fear of uncontrollable venous haemorrhage. Pelvic stabilization with an external fixator is usually required.

Complications

1. *General*
- Pulmonary dysfunction – atelectasis, infection, ARDS.
- DVT, PE. Appropriate thromboembolic precautions should be taken.
- Shock.
- Ileus.
- Duodenal stress ulceration. Prophylactic measures reduce incidence.

- Peritonitis.
- Intra-abdominal abscess.
- Fistula.
- Nutritional problems.

2. *Local*
- Wound – infection, dehiscence, necrotizing fasciitis.
- Liver and biliary tree – continued bleeding, bile leak.
- Spleen – subphrenic abscess, thrombocytosis, OPSI.
- Pancreas – cysts, pseudocysts, abscess.
- Bladder and kidneys – urine leak.

Further reading

ATLS Core Handbook. Chicago: American College of Surgeons, 1993.
Flint L. Assessment of abdominal trauma. *Current Practice in Surgery*, 1994; **6**: 65–9.

Related topics of interest

ACUTE COLONIC PSEUDO-OBSTRUCTION

Acute colonic pseudo-obstruction (ACPO) is a condition that closely mimics acute large bowel obstruction, both clinically and radiologically, but for which there is no apparent mechanical cause. Despite the accurate description of this syndrome, diagnosis is often delayed and patients are still managed inappropriately. This leads to increased morbidity and mortality, as early diagnosis and correct management of these patients is essential in reducing complications. It is also known as Ogilvie's syndrome. Chronic colonic pseudo-obstruction also occurs.

Pathogenesis

The pathogenesis of this condition remains unclear but ACPO occurs in two broad groups of patients. In 80% of cases it appears to be a complication of other clinical conditions and these can be local or systemic. Common local factors include postpartum, Caesarean section, pelvic surgery or trauma but ACPO has been documented after a very wide range of abdominal or remote surgery, intra-abdominal sepsis/inflammation and retroperitoneal malignancy. Many systemic conditions (metabolic, sepsis, drugs) are also associated with ACPO. In a minority of patients no specific underlying disorder can be found (idiopathic). The list of conditions associated with ACPO is extremely diverse, however, colonic dysmotility is probably the final common pathway, although it may be produced by a variety of biochemical and physiological disturbances.

Clinical features

Many of these patients are already in hospital and have a concomitant systemic illness or are recovering from surgery or pelvic/spinal injury. Colicky abdominal pain and constipation are common. Fever may occur and is more frequent in patients with ischaemic or perforated bowel. Enormous abdominal distension is the most dramatic physical finding. Abdominal tenderness is often less than expected but its presence (especially in the right iliac fossa) can indicate incipient caecal perforation. Bowel sounds are rarely absent and digital examination usually reveals an empty ballooned rectum.

Investigations

There are no diagnostic laboratory investigations but electrolyte abnormalities or uraemia may indicate a cause for the pseudo-obstruction. Plain abdominal radiography is the single most useful investigation and often reveals distal colonic obstruction with dilatation of the proximal large bowel. Distended small bowel is rarely seen. The colonic gas pattern has a clear cut-off, most commonly at the splenic flexure but also at the rectosigmoid and hepatic flexure. Perforation normally occurs in the caecum. It is unlikely with caecal diameters of less than 12 cm but the risk increases significantly with measurements of 14 cm or greater. Appropriate radiographs will detect a pneumoperitoneum (an erect chest film) if perforation has occurred.

Management

1. Diagnosis. Prompt diagnosis of this condition is essential before any inappropriate measures are undertaken. The clinical picture can be difficult to differentiate from malignant large colonic obstruction, particularly with idiopathic ACPO. Large bowel obstruction is rarely a surgical emergency and only requires urgent intervention when the patient displays peritoneal signs. An accurate diagnosis can usually be made by a contrast enema or if this is equivocal, colonoscopy. An urgent limited contrast enema has a well established place in the management of patients with acute large bowel obstruction. It will confirm functional obstruction in approximately 20% of patients and also reveal the site of a mechanical obstruction. Emergency colonoscopy has also been used to establish the diagnosis of ACPO but in such a situation it is a difficult and hazardous procedure as the bowel is unprepared.

2. Conservative treatment. The initial management is essentially conservative: nasogastric decompression, minimal oral intake, correction of fluid and electrolyte abnormalities and treatment of any associated conditions or infections. Opiates (and anticholinergic drugs) should be stopped. If there is distal colonic distension, then passage of a flatus tube or regular proctoscopy may aid decompression. Pharmacological treatment with combined sympathetic/ parasympathetic blockade or motility enhancing drugs (e.g. cisapride) have both been used with some success. Such stimulation is contraindicated if there is gross caecal distension. Repeated clinical assessment (preferably by the same observer) is essential as the caecum can dilate to the point of rupture. Plain abdominal films, every 12–24 hours, should be taken to monitor the caecal diameter. This conservative regimen can be continued for 48–72 hours as long as the patient does not develop right iliac fossa signs or progressive caecal distension. Absence of resolution or progressive caecal dilatation are both indications for prompt colonic decompression to avoid the risk of caecal ishaemia and perforation. Laparotomy should be performed without delay if caecal tenderness develops.

3. Colonoscopy. Successful decompression is achieved in approximately 80% of patients after the initial colonoscopy. Recurrence can occur in up to 15% of cases but the procedure can be repeated in such cases. Colonoscopy has also been used to aid placement of vented transanal tubes in the caecum, which can be left to prevent or treat recurrent distension. If the distension remains refractory, a decompressive caecostomy should be performed without delay.

4. Surgery. Failure of conservative treatment and colonoscopy or clinical signs indicating caecal ischaemia or perforation are the indications for surgery in patients with ACPO. In the absence of ischaemic or perforated bowel. caecostomy is the decompressive procedure of choice. This can be performed as either a tube or a formal caecostomy and considerable debate exists as to merits and drawbacks of both. What is clear is that caecostomy rather than any form of colostomy is essential as the latter invariably results in very poor decompression. In the presence of peritoneal signs a laparotomy should be performed. The state of the caecum will dictate the choice of procedure. Extensive caecal necrosis will necessitate formal resection. The rest of the colon should also be carefully examined. A well localized area of caecal ischaemia or a small perforation can both be treated adequately by excision and exteriorization or intubation as a caecostomy.

Outcome

ACPO carries a significant mortality rate even when adequate colonic decompression is achieved as patients are often already sick from an underlying illness. The overall mortality rate in patients undergoing surgery is 30% compared to 14% for conservative treatment. In the presence of a faecal peritonitis from caecal perforation the mortality rate rises to over 90%. Early diagnosis of ACPO is one of the most important aspects of the management of this condition, before inappropriate action is taken.

Further reading

Dorudi S, Berry AR, Kettlewell MGW. Acute colonic pseudo-obstruction. *British Journal of Surgery*, 1992; **79**: 99–103.

Related topics of interest

ACUTE MESENTERIC ISCHAEMIA

Acute mesenteric ischaemia refers to a condition whereby major portions of the intestine become ischaemic due to vascular insufficiency. The ischaemia may be focal or diffuse. Focal ischaemia frequently results from mechanical intestinal obstruction, for example bowel strangulation caused by hernia, adhesive bands or volvulus. Rarely, focal ischaemia may result from an embolus lodging distally in a mesenteric artery. Diffuse ischaemia results from thrombosis or embolism in a major artery supplying the bowel or thrombosis of a mesenteric vein, and rarely occurs as a result of hypotension. This leads to multifocal or generalized ischaemic bowel damage. As an indication for urgent laparotomy, this diagnosis will account for less than 5% of operations but diffuse ischaemia continues to carry a very high mortality — between 80 and 90% depending on the underlying cause.

Focal ischaemia

This is far more common than diffuse ischaemia. The wall of obstructed bowel is relatively ischaemic compared to normal bowel, and thus perforation readily occurs. Perforation follows the development of necrosis as a result of the ischaemia, and this will occur at the site of any obstruction, due to a pressure necrosis, or at the site of the bowel most distal from the point at which the arterial supply is obstructed; for example, in a strangulated femoral hernia, the bowel may necrose and perforate at the neck of the hernia, or at the apex of the herniated bowel loop.

Clinical signs suggesting there are ischaemic changes in bowel are a change in the nature of the pain from colicky to constant, and the presence of signs of peritonism, if not frank peritonitis. These signs warrant surgery, and if any ischaemic bowel is encountered that fails to recover after envelopment in warm packs, then it should be excised. Telltale signs that bowel is no longer viable include the loss of the usual serosal lustre, lack of peristalsis, and absence of mesenteric arterial pulsation.

Diffuse ischaemia
Aetiology

Non-occlusive infarction (i.e. where no arterial or venous occlusion is apparent) accounts for approximately one third of all cases. The most common type of non-mesenteric ischaemia is that caused by a critical reduction of intestinal perfusion due to extramesenteric factors, including cardiac failure and septic/hypovolaemic shock. Splanchnic vasoconstriction is a predictable secondary response in this setting. Many of these patients are either digitalized for cardiac failure or receiving vasopressor therapy.

Next in frequency is superior mesenteric artery occlusion, with thrombosis being more common than embolism.

Embolism usually results from either a mural thrombus postmyocardial infarction or atrial fibrillation. Rarer causes include venous occlusion and infarction and focal vasculitides like rheumatoid disease and polyarteritis nodosa.

Clinical course

The clinical picture will depend on the extent and severity of the initial problem. Pain is almost always present and is the earliest symptom. Next vomiting, diarrhoea, ileus and rectal urgency occur and reflect the frequent disturbance in intestinal function. Blood is lost into the lumen as the infarction progresses resulting in occult or frank blood in the faeces. Extensive infarction eventually produces systemic effects including hypovolaemia, metabolic acidosis and endotoxic shock. Perforation and ensuing peritonism ensue as the final stages of the condition.

Diagnosis and treatment

1. At presentation. The early diagnosis of acute mesenteric ischaemia remains elusive. The only consistent symptom is abdominal pain but this is a vague general pain. Additional clinical information that should raise the index of suspicion includes the presence of peripheral vascular disease, recent myocardial infarction or a recent aortic catheterization. There is a paucity of physical findings before the onset of gangrenous bowel and perforation. Laboratory investigations are not diagnostic but may be useful in excluding other diagnoses such as acute pancreatitis. However, acute mesenteric ischaemia is one of many causes of the acute abdomen that can cause an elevated serum amylase. There is often a very high leucocytosis. Plain abdominal radiography may reveal an ileus. Intramural or intraportal gas occurs only in late stages. Angiography remains the definitive investigation but it is indicated only in the management of patients with chronic intestinal ischaemia. Angiography can reveal the site of occlusion or stenosis of a major artery and is useful in planning revascularization.

2. At operation. Adequate resuscitation prior to surgery is essential, as in all acute abdominal cases. The principles here are accurate assessment of bowel viability, revascularization if indicated and/or resection. Clinical assessment relies on colour, contractility and bleeding, all of which are highly subjective criteria. The use of a Doppler ultrasound probe and systemic fluoroscein dye perfusion are more objective but are either seldom available or rarely used. Appropriate treatment will be dictated by the cause of the original insult. In occlusive ischaemia embolus or thrombus formation in the superior mesenteric artery should be treated by embolectomy and thrombo-endarterectomy/bypass grafting respectively. As much as 70% of the small intestine can be resected without long-term nutritional consequences, but a careful record of the length and type of remaining bowel should be made. More small bowel can be resected, but the patient is likely to require permanent parenteral nutrition. If after resection the viability of remaining bowel is in doubt, then anastomosis should be deferred until a second-look laparotomy (24 hours later) when further resections can be performed and/or intestinal continuity restored. In acute colonic ischaemia, the general condition of the patient and local factors such as peritoneal contamination will dictate whether an immediate anastomosis is performed or a stoma is constructed in a staged resection. These patients require careful postoperative monitoring, preferably in a high-dependency unit. Continued fluid depletion and the release of toxic vasoactive mediators into the circulation following resection or successful vascular reconstruction can cause circulatory collapse.

3. Non-operative measures. With non-mesenteric causes of reduced intestinal perfusion, management clearly is directed at correction of the primary problem. Transthoracic/Transoesophageal echocardiography may determine the source of emboli requiring long-term anticoagulation. Atrial fibrillation and other cardiac dysrhythmias require treatment, and referral to a cardiologist. The use of vasopressor agents that increase mesenteric vascular resistance should be avoided. However, such measures will generally supplement surgery, as infarcted bowel will need to be resected.

Prognosis

In occlusive cases, thrombosis carries a higher mortality than embolism (50–80%). Non-occlusive ischaemia has a uniformly high mortality rate (80%), reflecting that intestinal ischaemia is often a pre-terminal event in the course of a serious illness.

Related topic of interest

Assessment of the acute abdomen (p. 42)

ACUTE PANCREATITIS

The incidence of acute pancreatitis appears to have increased over the last 40 years. In the UK the condition is a common cause of hospital admission with an acute abdomen and the overall mortality has remained unchanged at 10%. In approximately 75% of patients complete recovery occurs after a few days of bed rest and intravenous fluids, however in the remainder the attack is severe and in these patients the mortality rises to 25–30%. There is thus a clear need for the early identification of this group of patients.

Epidemiology

Clinical series will under-report the incidence as they will omit the cases diagnosed at autopsy. The overall worldwide and, indeed nationwide, incidence will vary in relation to alcohol consumption (the main cause in the young) and the prevalence of gallstones (the predominant cause in the elderly). In may cases, no cause is evident, and these so-called idiopathic cases are often grouped as the third common 'cause' of acute pancreatitis.

Aetiology

The common predisposing conditions are well documented: gallstones and alcohol. In Britain gallstones account for 50–60% of cases. Other causes of acute pancreatitis include:

- Trauma (blunt, penetrating, iatrogenic, post-aortography, post endoscopic retrograde cholangiopancreatography (ERCP) or post cardiopulmonary bypass).
- Obstruction (neoplasm, pancreas divisum).
- Hypercalcaemia.
- Hyperlipidaemia.
- Drugs (thiazides, corticosteroids, oestrogens).
- Renal failure.
- Viral infections (mumps).

The precise mechanisms by which the above factors induce acinar rupture and release of activated enzymes within the parenchyma of the gland are still not understood.

Diagnosis

Typically the patient complains of sudden-onset, severe upper abdominal pain which can radiate into the back. Repeated vomiting is very characteristic. Abdominal findings range from mild tenderness to generalized peritonism. Intradermal staining by extravasated blood in the flank (Grey Turner's sign) or at the umbilicus (Cullen's sign) heralds a severe attack with high mortality. The diagnosis is usually confirmed by an elevated serum amylase > 1200 i.u./l. Urinary amylase can also be estimated rapidly by reagent strips. It is essential to exclude hyperamylasaemia in every acute abdomen. False positives (i.e. acute abdominal pain with serum amylase > 1000) can occur in:

- Perforated peptic ulcer.
- Perforation of the gall bladder.
- Afferent loop obstruction following gastrectomy.
- Ruptured aortic aneurysms.
- Mesenteric infarction.
- Ruptured ectopic pregnancy.

False negatives can occur if presentation is very early (within the first 3–4 hours) or late in the episode. In alcohol abusers, previous destruction of the gland parenchyma accounts for slowly rising levels.

Determination of severity

Unless the serum amylase is very high, the degree of hyperamylasaemia does not correlate with the severity of the disease. Early identification of the 25% of patients with a severe, life-threatening attack is desirable, as this will allow much closer monitoring of these patients. Clinical assessment is unreliable in the crucial first 48 hours of an attack though certain signs (shock, abdominal mass and tetany) are informative.

A number of scoring systems using multiple laboratory criteria have been proposed of which Imrie's is widely accepted.

- Age > 55 years.
- WBC > 15 x 10⁹/l.
- Glucose > 10 mmol/l.
- Albumin < 32 g/l.
- Urea > 16 mmol/l.
- P_aO_2 < 8 kPa (60 mmHg).
- LDH > 600 i.u./l.
- AST > 200 i.u./l.

The presence of three or more of the above criteria within the first 48 hours indicates a severe attack. A quicker assessment of severity can be made by abdominal paracentesis and examination of the fluid. A severe attack may be indicated by aspiration of more than 20 ml of free fluid irrespective of colour, dark free fluid or a dark lavage return. The combination of clinical assessment, multiple laboratory criteria and abdominal paracentesis will be accurate in identifying 75% of severe attacks.

Non-operative management

Repeated and careful clinical assessment of all patients during the first 24 hours is essential as the course of the disease is unpredictable during this time. A chest radiograph is mandatory as is estimation of arterial blood gases daily for the first 48 hours and oxygen should be administered by mask if there is hypoxaemia. Plain abdominal radiographs may show a sentinel loop, pancreatic calcification or gallstones. Vital signs and urine output should be monitored hourly. Oral intake is withheld, so adequate fluid replacement, especially of colloid, is necessary. Energetic fluid replacement is the single most important therapeutic measure, since a large volume of protein-rich fluid can be sequestered in the retroperitoneum. Volume replacement should be guided by central venous pressure measurement at the first sign of hypovolaemia (hypotension or low urine output). In a severe attack, parenteral nutrition will be necessary. Adequate pain control is important — an intravenous infusion of morphine or patient-controlled analgesia are both preferable to repeated intramuscular boluses. At present there are no specific non-operative measures that have been shown to improve the outcome in acute pancreatitis (e.g. antiproteases or peritoneal lavage). All patients require an abdominal ultrasound, and a CT scan if the attack is severe.

Complications

1. Systemic. The systemic response can vary from a mild fever to MOF in an episode of fulminant pancreatitis. The pathophysiological basis of this response is probably due to the release of cytokines and other inflammatory mediators that cause endothelial damage and capillary leakage in many organ systems. This can lead to refractory shock, where maintenance of the circulating volume can only be achieved by measurement of left atrial pressures (pulmonary capillary wedge pressures) to allow appropriate fluid replacement and inotrope administration. The lungs are commonly affected and respiratory failure occurs because capillary leak results in interstitial oedema. This is exacerbated by the presence of pain or an abdominal mass, both of which will promote sputum retention, atelectasis and pneumonia. Metabolic problems include hyperglycaemia and hypocalcaemia. Hypocalcaemia largely reflects the hypo-albuminaemia but calcium may be sequestered within intra-abdominal soaps. Calcium administration is only necessary if tetany occurs.

2. Abdominal
(a) *Pseudocyst.* Peripancreatic effusions occur in up to 20% of cases but the majority of these resolve within 4–6

weeks. Pseudocysts are enzyme-rich fluid collections which arise due to disruption of a pancreatic duct and persist after 6 weeks. They have no epithelial lining but are surrounded by granulation tissue. They are generally detected by ultrasound or CT scanning but can present as an abdominal mass. Pseudocysts are more common in alcoholic pancreatitis than in gallstone pancreatitis (15% versus 3%). Complications of pseudocysts include infection, haemorrhage (from a splenic artery branch or vein tributary), rupture and obstruction of the duodenum or rarely the common bile duct. Haemorrhage and sepsis occur more frequently in gallstone-associated cysts and the incidence of these complications increases with the passage of time.

(b) *Pancreatic abscess/necrosis.* Many terms have been applied to the destructive process that accompanies severe pancreatitis. Pancreatic phlegmon is a CT diagnosis and describes a non-infected inflammatory mass. Infected pancreatic necrosis should be distinguished from pancreatic abscess. The former carries a poor prognosis despite surgical intervention, while for the latter the prognosis is good with simple drainage. Infected necrosis becomes apparent early during the course of the attack (within two weeks) and produces a dramatic clinical picture with hectic fever, deteriorating respiratory and renal function, abdominal mass and a leucocytosis. Pancreatic abscess usually occurs after the acute episode has resolved and rarely produces progressive system failure. Both of these conditions are readily diagnosed by CT, however, infected necrosis will only be imaged satisfactorily by contrast-enhanced CT. Percutaneous CT-guided needle or tube drainage of a pancreatic abscess allows microbiological examination of the pus and can also be therapeutic.

(c) *Colonic infarction.* This can occur if the blood supply is interrupted by extension of the extrapancreatic necrosis and may follow drainage of a pancreatic abscess.

(d) *Pancreatic fistula.* This results from external drainage of a pancreatic abscess but spontaneous closure is the rule. Somatostatin or its synthetic analogues have been used with some success to aid closure.

Surgery

There are two indications for surgery in patients during the course of an emergency admission.

1. To aid resolution of the acute attack. In a small proportion of patients a severe episode is evident from the outset or there is clinical deterioration despite full supportive measures. Early ERCP and endoscopic sphincterotomy in patients with gallstone pancreatitis (and a predicted severe attack) results in significantly fewer major complications, however the urgent diagnosis of gallstones in acute pancreatitis can be difficult. The major determinant of outcome in the early stages of acute pancreatitis is the recognition of pancreatic necrosis. In these patients surgery is necessary despite intensive supportive therapy as there is continued clinical deterioration with sequential organ failure and sepsis. If possible, surgery should be delayed for 7–10 days as this results in demarcation of necrotic tissue and allows for safe digital debridement at laparotomy. Following this the abdomen can be closed with large silicone tubes left in the cavity that can be irrigated postoperatively (closed drainage). Alternatively the abdomen is left open (laparostomy) but covered by moist packs and can be re-explored repeatedly in the intensive care unit (ICU) with intravenous sedation as most of these patients are ventilated (open drainage).

2. To prevent another attack. The most effective method of preventing recurrent episodes is to perform early cholecystectomy in patients with gallstones. The presence of these should be energetically sought in all patients with acute pancreatitis, including those with alcohol-induced disease. This can be achieved by gall bladder ultrasonography in the majority of patients but ERCP is indicated after an attack of 'idiopathic' pancreatitis. Early cholecystectomy refers to surgery undertaken during the same admission (i.e. some 5–15 days after onset of symptoms). Immediate surgery is associated with an increased incidence of postoperative complications, while deferring operation to a subsequent admission means there is a 30–40% risk of another attack.

Further reading

Poston GJ, Williamson RCN. Surgical management of acute pancreatitis. *British Journal of Surgery*, 1990; **77**: 5–12.

Related topic of interest

Chronic pancreatitis (p. 89)

ADRENAL TUMOURS

Adrenal tumours are rare. The commoner tumours include adrenal carcinoma or adenoma, phaeochromocytoma, lipoma, myelolipoma, metastatic deposit, or a simple cyst.

Presentation

Adrenal tumours present in a number of diverse ways:

1. Hormonal. The hormonal effects include Cushingoid or virilizing features. The latter condition may occur with an adrenocortical tumour of the zona reticularis producing an excess of sex hormones. Conn's syndrome (weakness, attributable to potassium deficiency, with hypertension, polyuria and polydipsia) occurs when an adrenal adenoma secretes excessive amounts of the mineralocorticoid, aldosterone, from the zona glomerulosa of the adrenal cortex.

2. Incidentaloma. This is usually discovered by a CT scan performed during the course of investigations for other pathology. The majority are not functional tumours.

3. Intragland haemorrhage. If haemorrhage occurs into the tumour the presentation is often dramatic, mimicking abdominal aortic aneurysm rupture with sudden onset back pain, hypotension and a retroperitoneal haematoma.

4. Hypertension. Unexplained hypertension in a child or young adult should always raise suspicion.

5. Non-specific. Back pains, weight loss and an abdominal mass.

Hormone profile

A full hormonal profile is very expensive, frequently normal, beloved by physicians and should be undertaken selectively. It is indicated if there are suspicious clinical or biochemical features or there is a family history of hormone derangement. Urinary VMA and catecholamine and metanephrine concentrations should, however, be determined in every patient because the intraoperative diagnosis of a phaeochromocytoma or a needle biopsy of such lesions can have disastrous consequences. A low potassium in a hypertensive, especially if the patient is not receiving diuretic medication, may indicate an aldosterone-secreting adenoma.

CT and MRI

The complementary nature of CT and MRI allows a 'histological' diagnosis to be made for the majority of lesions. This specificity is increased to over 90% if MRI gradient-echo sequences are combined with gadolinium diethylenetriamine-pentacetic acid (Gd-DTPA) perfusion enhancement. The signal intensity of the spin-echo images of the tumour are compared with the liver and fat. Adenomas demonstrate low intensity. Phaeochromocytomas are extremely bright with high signal intensity; a useful fact which identifies the absolute contraindication to fine needle biopsy, since this can precipitate a massive catecholamine crisis. Adrenocortical carcinomas and metastases have intermediate intensities but metastases usually retain the same image characteristics as the primary. If doubt arises a needle biopsy can confirm the diagnosis. Cystic lesions are usually found within adenomas or phaeochromocytomas. Functional discrimination is sometimes possible with T_2 weighted images.

Surgery

The preferred surgical approach to the adrenal gland is transabdominal. This will allow inspection of the contralateral adrenal (small lesions can be missed on CT or MRI) and extra-adrenal sites such as the organ of Zuckerkandyl (found, if present, just below the inferior mesenteric artery). The retroperitoneal loin approach over a broken table however gives a better exposure in the obese patient with a large tumour. The adrenal is located within Gerota's fascia and on the right a portion is usually situated behind the inferior vena cava. A short central adrenal vein drains directly into the cava where it can easily be traumatized. Right adrenal gland exposure is optimized by pulling down on the kidney and rolling the vena cava carefully to the left. In principle, the patient should be dissected away from the adrenal gland to avoid the sudden hormone surges which may occur during tumour handling. Other gland approaches include the posterior approach, or a thoraco-abdominal incision for large tumours. Laparoscopic adrenalectomy is under evaluation.

Adrenocortical carcinoma

1. Diagnosis. Adrenocortical carcinomas are usually large at clinical presentation with a median diameter of 13 cm. Half metastasize and half exhibit evidence of endocrine dysfunction, commonly with Cushingoid or virilizing features. The majority of tumours have abnormal biochemical hormone profiles which do not manifest clinically but are of some value in detecting recurrent disease.

2. Treatment. Surgical excision should be aggressive with removal of adjacent organs even when metastatic disease is present. Only half of these tumours are, however, resectable. Steroid cover is essential during the perioperative period to avoid an Addisonian crisis because the opposite adrenal gland is usually suppressed. Spironolactone may be given as a poor alternative to surgery in patients with Conn's syndrome.

3. Prognosis. Prognosis depends upon the clinical features of the disease and the technique of surgery rather than the tumour size or histology. Tumour disruption during dissection can spill cells that implant, which is associated with a poorer prognosis. The chemotherapeutic agent Mitotane (1,1 dichlorodiphenyldichloroethane) is still the only drug which has been shown to produce regression of pulmonary metastasis and increase survival.

Phaeochromocytoma

1. Presentation. Phaeochromocytomas present clinically with the characteristic symptoms of headache, sweating, palpitations, tremor and weight loss. Although hypertension is a feature, this tumour occurs in less than 0.1% of all adult hypertensives. Unexplained hypertension in a child or young adult should alert one to the diagnosis. Ten per cent are malignant, 10% are multiple and 10% are familial (including the MEN II syndrome).

2. Investigations. Urinary VMA, catecholamine and metanephrine concentrations are usually elevated. A gamma camera will identify [131I]metaiodobenzylguanidine (MIBG), which is actively taken up by tumour cells, and its occasional extra-adrenal and metastatic locations. MRI and CT scanning both increase the diagnostic accuracy. Needle biopsy is absolutely contraindicated.

3. Surgery. The specific perioperative problems include a massive hypertensive surge during tumour handling, hypotensive shock following tumour devascularization and hypoglycaemia which reaches a peak 3 hours after removal. A week's pre-operative treatment with the long acting alpha-blocker phenoxybenzamine combined with a beta-blocker, if tachycardia develops, has reduced the operative mortality by controlling the catecholamine surges. Metyrosine inhibits catecholamine synthesis by antagonizing the enzyme tyrosine hydroxylase. It is occasionally added to the pre-operative regime. Adequate pre-operative catecholamine blockade and generous vascular compartment filling dampens the hypotensive shock inevitable following tumour removal. Plasma glucose levels should be monitored hourly for the first 7 hours after surgery to pre-empt the problem of hypoglycaemia.

4. Follow up. Recurrence can occur many years after removal which underlines the importance of life-long follow up with urinary catecholamine estimations. Neuropeptide Y and neurone-specific enolase can be used as serum markers for malignancy but their exact clinical role has yet to be established.

Metastasis

Carcinoma of the breast and bronchus and malignant melanoma all occasionally metastasize to the adrenals. If destruction of adrenal tissue occurs bilaterally, an acute Addisonian crisis can be precipitated. Miliary tuberculosis, though rare, frequently destroys adrenal tissue bilaterally.

Incidentaloma

The incidentaloma occurs in about 9% of all patients undergoing a CT scan. Evaluation is based on tumour size and CT appearance. A mass larger than 6 cm is usually malignant, requiring removal, and masses smaller than 3 cm are usually benign, requiring regular CT assessment. Opinion is divided with regard to lesions between 3 and 6 cm as to which line of management to follow.

Further reading

Farndon JR, Dunn JM. Adrenal tumours. *Recent Advances in Surgery*, 1992; **15**: 55–68.

Related topic of interest

Renal tumours (p. 258)

AIDS

Aquired immunodeficiency syndrome is becoming an increasing problem to the general surgeon. It is caused by infection with the human immunodeficiency virus (HIV) which suppresses cellular immunity and allows the development of malignancies (Kaposi's sarcoma, lymphoma) and opportunistic infections (*Pneumocystis carinii* pneumonia, cryptosporidium, CMV, HSV). HIV has been isolated from every body fluid including blood, urine, tears, saliva, semen and cervical secretions. There is no cure but anti-retroviral drugs such as Zidovudine (AZT) prolong survival in some patients. Surgical presentation is with anorectal complaints (40%), requests for venous access (20%), cutaneous manifestations (20%), abdominal pain, requests for biopsy and other (20%).

Anal warts

Anal warts in AIDS patients tend to be aggressive, dysplastic and harder to eradicate. Topical podophyllin or 5% 5-fluorouracil cream applied through a proctoscope is time consuming, tedious and often of little benefit. Diathermy is satisfactory for isolated warts but precise scissor excision on a bleb of raised skin is preferable for extensive warts to preserve the intervening skin bridges. Females should undergo regular cervical colposcopic screening because of the associated risk of cervical cancer. There is good evidence that severe dysplasia may progress to carcinoma-*in-situ* and thence to squamous cell carcinoma. Human papilloma virus (HPV) subtyping and biopsy helps to predict those lesions likely to develop into invasive carcinoma. HPV subtype 16 is often associated with severe dysplasia.

Anorectal disorders

Perianal sepsis and anal ulceration in AIDS patients have a long duration of onset and an extensive differential diagnosis which necessitates the need for histological analysis, and bacterial and viral cultures. Sphincter preservation is of the utmost importance during all anal operations because male homosexuals have a tendency towards incontinence and the diarrhoea associated with opportunistic colonic infections is often severe. Setons are recommended for most fistulae. Kaposi's sarcoma may resemble an ulcerated haemorrhoid, non-Hodgkin's lymphoma may resemble a perianal abcess and squamous cell carcinoma may be mistaken for a small benign ulcer. Long-term cultures from an ulcer base may reveal *Mycobacterium avium intracellulare*. Viral cultures can detect CMV or acyclovir-resistant strains of HSV which can both cause extensive anal ulceration. Diarrhoea also encourages anal ulceration. Stool cultures for *Salmonella*,

Shigella, Campylobacter and *Cryptosporidium* with microscopy for *Giardia*, ova cysts and amoebae are mandatory. CMV can also be detected on rectal biopsy. Anal ulcers can be iatrogenic occurring in the region of a previous lateral sphincterotomy initially performed for an ulcer which was mistaken for a fissure. Inappropriate anal instrumentation or 'fisting' injuries can result in the most horrendous sphincter injuries which usually require permanent faecal diversion.

Abdominal pain

Abdominal pain is common and is caused by gastrointestinal malignancies and opportunistic infections. CMV is the commonest cause resulting in a wide range of conditions: oesophagitis, acalculous cholecystitis, sclerosing cholangitis, small bowel perforation, toxic megacolon, colonic perforation and haemorrhage, and spontaneous rupture of the spleen. Gastrointestinal Kaposi's sarcoma or lymphoma may present with unremitting haemorrhage, small bowel obstruction, intussusception, perforation or mesenteric infiltration. Lymphadenopathy from *Mycobacterium avium intracellulare* or lymphoma can result in appendicitis or jaundice by obstructing the appendiceal ostium or porta hepatis, respectively. Appendicectomy and colectomy are the commonest abdominal operations. The decision to raise a colostomy should not be undertaken lightly since they are rarely reversed. A platelet count is mandatory prior to any surgery since thrombocytopenia is common.

Surgery

Operative mortality for emergency and elective surgery is high (30% for a routine open cholecystectomy). General anaesthesia results in depression of cell-mediated immunity and AIDS progression. The poor nutritional state contributes to impaired wound healing and susceptibility to infection. Negative laparotomy is not too infrequent an event for a patient with undiagnosed abdominal pain. These factors lead to an increased indication for diagnostic laparoscopy. Care should be taken during laparoscopy by insisting upon using disposable ports with a vestibular flange to prevent splashback, and by deflating the abdomen prior to port withdrawl because any aerosol emanating from the port entry wound will harbour HIV. The decision to undertake surgery is aided by staging patients according to their level of general immunity (CDC stages I-IV). A CD4 level of greater than 500 indicates mild disease and implies that appropriate operative treatment should not be withheld. A CD4 level of less than 500 indicates advanced disease and an exceedingly poor outcome.

Venous access

Venous access with a Hickman line or an implantable injection port (Portacath) is often requested for the administration of antiviral agents to treat CMV retinitis.

Lymphadenopathy

Lymphadenopathy can be generalized (during sero-conversion or in the persistent generalized lymphadenopathy (PGL) state) or discrete (infection or tumour). Open biopsy is rarely necessary since AIDS lymphadenopathy demonstrates non-specific reactive follicular hyperplasia and the diagnosis is better established by a good clinical examination and a familiarity with the disease.

Cutaneous manifestations

Lymphoepithelial cysts are fluid-filled cutaneous lesions which are diagnosed on ultrasound and are best obliterated by aspiration and tetracycline instillation. Cutaneous malignancies are treated in their own right.

Precautions

1. High risk groups. The cost would be immense if universal precautionary procedures were undertaken for everyone. Homosexual males, intravenous drug abusers, haemophiliacs, sexual partners and children of the above, and residents of Central Africa constitute the high risk groups where strict precautions should be employed. Moreover, people not belonging to these groups are very unlikely to have AIDS.

2. Surgeon protection. Precautions involve wearing gloves and eye protection for sigmoidoscopy, fibre-optic endoscopy and surgical procedures, placing specimens in double plastic bags labelled 'risk of infection', avoiding hand needles and using staples for skin closure, placing all sharp objects into a receiver, excluding anyone with abrasions or wounds from theatre, and wearing double gloves to reduce the risk of skin exposure to the patient's blood. If a needlestick injury occurs (the risk of seroconversion from a patient with HIV is estimated at 1 in 200) advice should be sought from the Centers for Disease Control (CDC) guidelines for the prophylactic administration of AZT and the implications of serological testing. Kevlar gloves are manufactured with a chain-mail arrangement of strong fibre which protects against cuts and some of the lighter needlestick injuries. Double latex gloves afford no protection from anything sharp.

3. Patient protection. Surgeons, unless suspected of harbouring HIV, are under no obligation to take an AIDS test. Just having an AIDS test would invalidate most insurances and mortgage agreements, and if it was positive it would ruin a surgical career. Surgeons catch HIV from patients and only under exceptional circumstances is the converse true. A good case can be made for insisting that all patients are HIV tested before any pressure is placed upon the surgeon to have one.

Further reading

Miles AJG, Wastell C. AIDS and the general surgeon. *Recent Advances in Surgery*, 1991; **14**: 85–98.

Related topics of interest

Anorectal investigation (p. 35)
Assessment of the acute abdomen (p. 42)

AMPUTATIONS

Most amputations are performed for lower limb ischaemia. Modern techniques of lower limb revascularization reduce the incidence of major amputation together with its attendant social and financial burdens and increase the ratio of below-knee to above-knee amputations. Where major amputation is unavoidable, the below-knee level is almost always preferable to the above-knee procedure, as subsequent mobility and prosthetic limb use are far superior. For most patients undergoing major amputation, the procedure itself is merely the beginning of a long process of rehabilitation, limb fitting and return to partial mobility. In those patients unlikely to walk again, the longest stump possible (commensurate with successful wound healing) will aid stability in a chair or bed and will facilitate transferring. Even after successful revascularization for critical ischaemia, some patients require minor amputations of a digit or possibly the forefoot. Wound healing may be delayed, but most patients attain a high level of mobility with minimal difficulty.

Indications
- End-stage unreconstructable atherosclerotic disease. Approximately 80–90% of all amputations are performed for ischaemic arterial disease.
- Buerger's disease.
- Diabetic microangiopathy and infection.
- Emboli.
- Trauma.
- Infection (gas gangrene, necrotizing fasciitis, septic arthritis, osteomyelitis).
- Soft tissue or bony malignancy.
- Malformations, deformities.
- Intractable ulceration.
- Painful paralysed limbs.

The ideal amputation stump
- Primary wound healing.
- No redundant tissue.
- Cylindrical stump.
- No pressure on suture line.
- Painless.
- Full extension and flexion in adjacent joint.

Complications
- Wound infection.
- Breakdown of suture line.
- Stump too long or too short.
- Bony spurs.
- Stump neuroma.
- Phantom pain.
- Causalgia.

Postoperative wound care, physiotherapy and limb fitting

A firm stump bandage should be applied after wound closure and this should be left undisturbed for five days unless there are indications of wound infection or breakdown. Fitting of a temporary prosthesis in theatre with early weight-bearing has been abandoned by most surgeons. Weight-bearing in a PAMaid (pneumatic postamputation mobility aid) may start at 5–7 days, providing the stump is satisfactory. Physiotherapy to strengthen the upper and lower limb musculature should begin as early as possible. Care should be taken to prevent or improve flexion contractures in the hip and knee joints. Early referral to the regional limb-fitting centre should be made for measurement and fitting of a prosthetic limb. Many elderly patients, particularly those with above-knee amputations, will not use an artificial limb and are unsuitable for walking rehabilitation.

Specific amputations

1. Toe and foot amputations. A good blood supply is required to allow wound healing and patients most suitable for these distal amputations are those who have distal ischaemia following successful revascularization, diabetic patients with small vessel disease or localized infection and patients with small/medium artery disease (e.g. Buerger's disease). Toe amputations are usually performed through racket-shaped incisions, the 'handle' being used to divide bone and tendons proximal to the skin incision. A more extensive ray amputation may be indicated in diabetic patients to remove a toe with most or all of its metatarsal bone where there is deep infection.

Where all or most of the toes are non-viable, transmetatarsal amputation is indicated. Bone division is through the middle of the metatarsal shafts leaving a long plantar flap which is rolled up to leave a non-weight-bearing dorsal suture line.

Diabetic infection frequently calls for *ad hoc* foot amputations where non-viable tissue is excised and deep infection is drained. The heel and other weight-bearing areas are retained if possible and once the infection has resolved the wound may be closed with primary suture or skin grafting.

2. Below-knee amputation. Where major amputation is required, this level is preferable to through- or above-knee procedures in patients who are likely to use a prosthetic limb. Many investigations (transcutaneous oxymetry, thermography, Doppler pressures, arteriography, plethysmography) have been assessed to predict the success of wound healing at this level, but none matches experience and the presence of bleeding from the skin flaps. The two techniques used are the long posterior flap (Burgess) and the Robinson skew flap, employing equal anteromedial and posterolateral flaps. Both techniques result in similar rates of wound healing and mobilization.

3. Through-knee and Gritti-Stokes amputation. Through-knee amputation is easy and quick to perform with equal lateral flaps and a posterior scar but leaves a large bulbous stump which causes difficulties with limb fitting. Wound healing is frequently delayed in ischaemic disease. The Gritti-Stokes procedure is performed at the supracondylar level, leaving a longer stump than an above-knee amputation which provides good stability for the amputee in a chair or in bed. The fitting of an internal knee mechanism is difficult. The knee joint is disarticulated and the femur transected just above the condyles. The patella is cut to leave a flat posterior surface which is laid over the transected femur and may be wired in position. The patellar tendon is sutured to the hamstrings.

4. Above-knee amputation. Equal anterior and posterior flaps are fashioned, with their upper ends at the level of bone section (12–14 cm above the knee joint line). Vastus lateralis is sutured to the adductors and the quadriceps are sutured to the hamstrings. This amputation is quick to perform and usually results in satisfactory wound healing, but many elderly patients fail to walk despite provision of carefully measured prostheses.

5. Disarticulation at the hip. This is used for malignant disease and infection and is rarely necessary for ischaemia. An anterior approach is made to the hip and the joint disarticulated. A long posterior gluteal flap is fashioned to cover the defect leaving an anterior suture line.

6. Hindquarter amputation. This amputation was performed for soft tissue and bony tumours of the pelvis, but is occasionally indicated for pelvic trauma. It is rarely used now.

7. Amputations of the upper limb. Most of these amputations are performed for trauma, infection or tumour. Below the elbow, a stump of 15 cm allows the fitting of a prosthesis, as does a stump of 19 cm from the shoulder above the elbow. Disarticulation at the shoulder joint or forequarter amputation are sometimes indicated for malignant disease.

Further reading

Green RM, Rob CG. Amputations of the lower extremities. In: Jamieson CW, Yao JST (eds) *Rob and Smith's Operative Surgery – Vascular Surgery.* London: Chapman and Hall, 1994.

Related topics of interest

Critical leg ischaemia (p. 102)
Vascular trauma (p. 341)
Wounds: healing and closure (p. 349)

ANAL FISSURE

An anal fissure is a longitudinal tear of the anoderm, the area between the dentate line and verge. It occurs in young adults with equal sex incidence, is almost always midline, and 90% are posterior in men but a higher proportion, 20%, anterior in women. Lateral ulcers arouse suspicion and should be biopsied.

Aetiology

Fissures are associated with hard stools and high anal pressures, and indeed recurrence is less likely if patients are maintained with softer stools. It is unclear if the constipation results from a fear of defecation, and it is also unclear if the increase in anal tone is just sphincter spasm from the presence of the fissure. The aetiology is probably that the anoderm, supported by a tight internal sphincter, undergoes a shearing force and tear from a descending hard stool. A fissure can complicate a bout of diarrhoea and can arise during anal intercourse. Trauma from vigorous anal wiping or anal instrumentation can also cause fissures. A fissure is also the commonest anal lesion in Crohn's disease and ulcerative colitis.

Presentation

Pain, immediately after defecation and lasting 1 or 2 hours, is typical. Bright red blood, seen on the toilet paper, and a stinging sensation often accompany wiping. Half of patients suffer with pruritis probably due to the highly irritant endopeptidases produced by the anal flora.

Examination

On abdominal examination a loaded sigmoid colon and distention implies constipation. Anal inspection, however, provides the most useful information. Rectal examination and instrumentation is contrindicated in the presence of a fissure and is often unnecessary because a full anorectal examination should be undertaken at the time of surgery.

Evaluation

Anal examination requires separating the anal verge carefully and widely until either the fissure becomes visible or just before the patient starts to feel discomfort, whichever is the sooner. Fissure chronicity is recognized if a thickened, undermined edge surrounds a granulating base. The circular fibres of the internal sphincter are often recognizable. A papilla (fibroepithelial polyp) can form at the upper limit with a skin tag (sentinal pile) at the distal end. If the centre part heals a subcutaneous fistula may be identified.

Differential diagnosis

Fissures are commonly misdiagnosed as piles. Although aetiological associations are similar, fissures usually sting rather than throb, blood presents on the paper and rarely spatters into the pan, and anal lumps occur less commonly. Non-midline fissures, especially in the presence of an exudate, arouse suspicion and should be biopsied. A proctoscopy and sigmoidoscopy, are carried out to exclude proctitis from ulcerative colitis, Crohns or infection and, if present, biopsy with stool and ulcer exudate culture are performed. Differential diagnosis is from other ulcerative conditions like carcinoma, HIV, leukaemic ulcer and anorectal tuberculosis. A syphilitic ulcer is painless and often produces an exudate.

Conservative treatment

Stool softeners and analgesic jelly can heal acute fissures in 50% of patients. Most fissures in childhood and pregnancy respond in this way. By the time a fissure presents to a surgeon it is often chronic and most require surgical treatment. Care should be taken with anaesthetic jelly as the intense anal pain is converted into an itch which encourages nocturnal excoriation and thereby prevents fissure healing. There is no evidence that anal dilators promote healing.

Surgery

Disabling pain, failure of conservative treatment and chronicity are indications for operative treatment by manual dilatation of the anus (MDA) or sphincterotomy. An MDA produces healing in 80–90% of patients and involves placement of a maximum of four fingers into the anal canal. Popularity is swinging away from MDA because 39% of patients who had undergone MDA reported temporary post-operative soiling. Furthermore, endoanal ultrasonography has demonstrated internal sphincter and external sphincter damage following MDA whereas after a sphincterotomy only the lower half of the internal sphincter is divided. In patients who rely on their internal sphincter for continence (mothers with puborectalis or external sphincter damage from childbirth) an MDA can cause permanent incontinence.

Sphincterotomy

If a lateral sphincterotomy is the treatment of choice it can be achieved by the open or closed technique. Healing after a sphincterotomy occurs in 96% of patients within 3 weeks. Outpatient sphincterotomy with local anaesthetic is performed in the USA but has not gained popularity here. A posterior sphincterotomy is harder to perform and disturbances of continence occur in up to 25% of cases. A lateral sphincterotomy is the preferred method and is performed in the lithotomy position. After a full anorectal examination an Eisenhammer retractor is used to open the anal canal. The intersphincteric plane is identified by palpation and in the open procedure a short incision is placed over this plane and the internal sphincter is dissected away from the anoderm and external sphincter. The fibres are divided with scissors to a level just above the apex of the fissure. Confirmation of complete division is made by palpation when a characteristic 'gap' is felt. Any papilla or tag is removed at the same time. In the closed procedure sphincter division is carried out through a stab incision using a tenotomy knife.

Crohn's disease   A Crohn's fissure should be treated conservatively. The majority heal spontaneously.

Further reading

McDonald P. Haemorrhoids and anal fissures. *Recent Advances in Surgery*, 1992; **15**: 107–18.

Related topics of interest

Anorectal investigation (p. 35)
Crohn's disease (p. 106)
Haemorrhoids (p. 158)
Ulcerative colitis (p. 305)

ANEURYSMS

An aneurysm is a localized dilatation of a blood vessel. Cardiac and venous aneurysms will not be discussed. The significance of aneurysms lies in their tendency to rupture, thrombose or give rise to emboli.

Terminology

A true aneurysm involves all layers of the arterial wall and may be fusiform or saccular, whilst a false aneurysm comprises clot which has leaked from the true lumen and surrounding connective tissue. Dissection of an aneurysm occurs when blood enters a tear in the diseased intima tracking down the wall splitting the media. A mycotic aneurysm develops when a bacterial (rarely fungal) focus locally infects an artery, weakening the wall. Alternatively, an established aneurysm may become infected. Periaortitis with thickening and dilatation of the aortic wall and a glistening white outer coat is known as an inflammatory aneurysm. The aetiology is unknown, but there is an association with retroperitoneal fibrosis.

Pathology

1. Degenerative. Most true aneurysms are degenerative (affecting the intima and media). Atherosclerotic aneurysms contain a core of organized thrombus with a lumen through the middle. There may be an abnormality of collagen and elastin synthesis.

2. Syphilis. Now an uncommon cause of aneurysm. The ascending aorta is affected and the adventitia and media are infiltrated by plasma cells and lymphocytes. Aortic valvular regurgitation and coronary osteal narrowing may also occur.

3. Collagen diseases. Marfan's syndrome, Ehlers–Danlos syndrome and pseudoxanthoma elasticum are rare conditions associated with the development of saccular or dissecting aneurysms.

4. Congenital aneurysm. Berry aneurysms occurring on the circle of Willis are caused by a congenital weakness of the arterial wall.

Abdominal aortic aneurysm

Aneurysms (aortic diameter $\geq$ 3 cm) occur most frequently in the abdominal aorta affecting 7% of males and 2% of females aged 65–80 years. The prevalence is greatest among male hypertensives who smoke and appears to be increasing in Western countries. Approximately 20% of affected males have a first degree relative with an abdominal aortic aneurysm (AAA). Extension above the renal arteries occurs in only 2%, but aneurysms of other vessels are commonly associated. Over 50% of people with an AAA remain asymptomatic and die of other causes with their AAA intact. A pulsating abdominal mass may be found by the patient or on routine medical examination. Rapid expansion or leaking of the aneurysm usually gives rise to severe back or abdominal pain.

Rupture is the principal complication of AAA, but thrombosis, distal embolization, and aorto-enteric and aortocaval fistula occur rarely. Treatment of AAA is currently by surgical inlay prosthetic grafting. Elective surgery is associated with a 30-day mortality of 5%, complications usually arising as a result of concomitant cardiovascular disease. Following this period, however, life expectancy is returned to that of a healthy, age-matched population. Aortic rupture is fatal in approximately 80% of cases, surgery for rupture having a mortality of 45–65%. Small aneurysms (3–4 cm maximum diameter) are unlikely to rupture, whereas the probability of rupture in an aneurysm measuring 5.5 cm or more is 10–15% per year and these should be repaired electively.

Ultrasound is the usual method of imaging following clinical aneurysm detection, but CT scanning and/or digital subtraction angiography are frequently required to determine the relationship with the iliac and renal arteries. Ultrasound screening programmes to detect asymptomatic aneurysms (the majority) are currently being evaluated. Recently, endovascular methods of AAA repair have been described involving the transfemoral introduction of an aortic prosthesis.

Thoracic and thoraco-abdominal aortic aneurysm

These aneurysms are much less common than AAA and may present incidentally or with back pain and dyspnoea if expanding rapidly or dissecting. Repair should be considered if symptoms occur or if expansion occurs in an asymptomatic, fit patient. Surgery is associated with a considerable operative mortality and morbidity (particularly paraplegia and renal failure). Cardiopulmonary bypass is required for thoracic arch aneurysm repair.

Iliac artery aneurysms

The common iliac (90%), internal iliac (9–10%) and (rarely) the external iliac (1%) arteries may be affected. These aneurysms may occur in isolation or in conjunction with an AAA. They are rarer than AAA and are usually degenerative. Some can be detected on rectal examination. False aneurysms can arise where there has been previous aorto-iliac surgery. They usually go undetected, but may give rise to symptoms attributable to pelvic organs or present as a pulsating pelvic mass. CT scanning is the most reliable imaging technique. Rupture is often the first indication and surgery for this complication has a higher mortality than that for AAA rupture. Common and external iliac artery aneurysms require exclusion and grafting, whereas internal iliac artery aneurysms can usually be ligated or possibly embolized if unilateral.

Femoral artery aneurysms

Femoral artery aneurysms may be true or false. True aneurysms often occur in conjunction with aneurysms at other sites (they affect 3–7% of patients with AAA). The common and profunda femoral arteries are usually affected. False femoral aneurysms affect 3% of groin anastomoses. Many femoral aneurysms are symptomless, but the presence of a pulsatile mass is common. Lower limb ischaemia caused by thrombosis, embolism or, less commonly, rupture occurs in about one third of patients.

Popliteal artery aneurysms

These are bilateral in 50% of patients and account for 70% of peripheral aneurysms. In over half of patients affected these aneurysms present with distal leg ischaemia caused by thrombosis or embolism. Less than 10% of presentations are for rupture. Thromboembolic distal ischaemia is ideally treated using thrombolysis, followed by aneurysm ligation and bypass. Large, asymptomatic aneurysms in fit patients should be repaired.

Axillosubclavian aneurysms

These aneurysms usually present as a mass in the supraclavicular fossa. Post-stenotic dilatation caused by a cervical rib may occur with symptoms of thoracic outlet syndrome. Distal embolization or thrombosis may occur, resulting in digital ischaemia or dense ischaemia of the forearm and hand. Treatment is by ligation and bypass with or without excision of cervical rib.

Carotid aneurysms

These account for less than 5% of peripheral aneurysms and are situated at the carotid bifurcation. They must be distinguished from tortuous and ectatic arteries. Patients may present with neurological symptoms as a result of embolization and treatment is by resection and replacement.

Visceral aneurysms

1. Splenic artery. These are the second commonest abdominal aneurysm comprising two thirds of all visceral aneurysms. They are four times commoner in women than in men and occur during childbearing years and in old age. They are usually symptomless, unless they rupture. Rupture is most likely during the third trimester of pregnancy. Treatment is by aneurysm excision and interposition grafting, ligation or splenectomy, and should be considered if the aneurysm exceeds 3 cm diameter or during pregnancy.

2. *Hepatic artery.* These are one third as common as splenic artery aneurysms. They usually present with rupture into the biliary system causing biliary colic, obstructive jaundice and upper gastrointestinal haemorrhage. Treatment is by aneurysm excision and grafting if possible.

3. *Coeliac and mesenteric arteries.* These are rare and usually present with non-specific abdominal pain. Sometimes, a mobile pulsatile mass is present. They are frequently mycotic. Resection and reconstruction should ideally be performed, but the collateral circulation will sometimes allow simple ligation.

4. *Renal artery.* These aneurysms are rare and are usually associated with hypertension. Rupture is unusual and most can be ignored.

Further reading

Collin J, Scott RAP, O'Donnell T, *et al.* Mini-symposium on aortic aneurysms. *Current Practice in Surgery*, 1990; **2**: 65–98.
Greenhalgh RM, Mannick JA. *The Cause and Management of Aneurysms.* London: WB Saunders, 1990.
MacSweeney STR, Powell JT, Greenhalgh RM. Pathogenesis of abdominal aortic aneurysm. *British Journal of Surgery*, 1994; **81**: 935–41.

Related topics of interest

ANORECTAL INVESTIGATION

Anorectal investigation comprises the objective measurement of the various components of anorectal function and their contribution to the normal continent state. These results can be applied to the diagnosis of anorectal disease and their subsequent response to appropriate treatment.

Maintenance of continence

This is dependent upon a combination of factors.

1. Anal sphincters. The internal anal sphincter (IAS) is a major determinant of faecal continence, providing as much as 80% of the pressure within the anal canal through tonic contraction. The IAS is under autonomic control with the parasympathetic system inhibiting, and sympathetic fibres stimulating contraction. The external anal sphincter (EAS) is comprised of voluntary/striated muscle innervated by branches of the pudendal nerve. This sphincter complex (i.e. both IAS and EAS) constitutes an effective muscular barrier to the outflow of faeces.

2. Puborectalis and the anorectal angle. The puborectalis muscle also plays an important role in faecal continence. This striated muscle, supplied by branches of the pudendal nerve, maintains an acute angle between the rectum and upper anal canal and damage to it uniformly results in incontinence. The anorectal angel may function as a flap valve so that an increase in intra-abdominal pressure results in compression of the anterior rectal wall into the upper anal canal, thus occluding its lumen.

3. Intact rectal and anal sensation. Distension of the rectum with faeces results in a sensation of filling which is an additional factor in continence. The receptors for this reflex are located in the musculature of the pelvic floor and also probably in the rectal wall itself. The existence of sensory receptors in the mucosa of the lower anal canal allows fine discrimination between flatus and faeces, which again contributes to the maintenance of faecal continence.

4. Other factors. These include the capacious and compliant nature of the rectal reservoir and also the formation of bulky and solid faeces.

Clinical investigations

1. Anal manometry. Pressure measurements are taken from within the anal canal. The maximum squeeze pressure

(MSP) refers to the highest recorded pressure at any site within the anal canal during maximal contraction of the pelvic floor, and reflects the activity of the EAS and thus of voluntary continence. The maximum resting anal pressure (MRP) is mainly an indicator of IAS activity. Anal manometry is a useful technique in studying continence and its disturbance, particularly after pelvic colorectal surgery (low anterior resections, ileo-anal pouch formation and sphincter repair procedures).

2. Rectal sensation. This is the subjective response of the patient as known volumes of air or water are introduced into a balloon that has been placed in the rectum, while rectal compliance is an objective measure of the response during rectal distension. Compliance is measured in units of volume/pressure over volumes up to a litre, depending on patient tolerance.

3. Electromyography (EMG). This technique allows an objective and physiological measurement of muscle denervation by recording the electrical activity in the puborectalis, EAS and IAS through appropriate placement of fine wire electrodes. Thus EMG can map sphincter deficiencies, or, alternatively, locate the position of an ectopic sphincter.

4. Endo-anal ultrasound. This is a new technique that has emerged from modification of the endorectal ultrasound probe. The investigation is performed with the patient in the left lateral position and is relatively comfortable as compared to EMG. Images are taken from the upper, middle and lower anal canal and thus the entire sphincter complex is examined. Defects in the puborectalis, EAS and even IAS can be clearly visualized and localized. Additionally, the integrity of sphincter reconstruction procedures can be assessed.

5. Defecating proctography. This technique can reveal anatomical abnormalities such as rectal and anal intussusception, rectocele and megarectum, but its main application lies in the observation of the sequence of events in incontinence and rectal prolapse. Videoproctography and still radiographs are taken during rest, maximal contraction of the pelvic floor and defecation of a known volume of radio-opaque stool substitute introduced into the rectum.

Anorectal angle, perineal and pelvic floor descent can be calculated from the still radiographs during videoproctography. The investigation can be integrated with puborectalis, EAS and IAS EMG together with anal manometry (dynamic integrated videoproctography).

6. *Colonic transit time.* Colonic transit is assessed by asking the patient to swallow radio-opaque markers of three different shapes on three consecutive mornings while fully active and off all laxatives. Plain abdominal radiographs are taken on the fourth and seventh days to assess the progress of the markers and hence calculate the transit time. The use of such studies is normally confined to the investigation of patients with intractable constipation in whom total colectomy is being considered.

Related topics of interest

Acute colonic pseudo-obstruction (p. 5)
Fistula-in-ano (p. 133)

APPENDICITIS

Acute appendicitis is the most common surgical emergency in developed countries. Its incidence has fallen over the last three decades. About one in six of the population undergo appendicectomy. It is rare before the age of 2 years, reaches maximal incidence in childhood and declines thereafter with increasing age.

Pathogenesis

Inflammation is initiated by luminal obstruction, secondary to either lymphoid hyperplasia in response to a viral infection or obliteration of the lumen by a faecolith. Obstructive appendicitis can also be caused by tumours of the appendix or caecal pole. The extent of inflammation varies from a mild catarrhal response with resolution, to mural necrosis and perforation. Faecoliths are found in 30–40% of appendicectomies and in these appendices gangrene is twice as common (75–80%).

Course of the disease

Progression of inflammation to perforation and peritonitis is more likely if the appendix is not removed, but is not inevitable. Perforation occurs in 25% of patients with a history of pain of less than 24 hours and in 35% with a history exceeding 48 hours.

Clinical features

Typically a patient presents with gradual onset of colicky, central abdominal pain with anorexia and slight vomiting. Within several hours this visceral peri-umbilical pain localizes to the right iliac fossa as transmural inflammation causes peritoneal irritation. Only 50% of patients give such a classical history. In 30% the history exceeds 24 hours and the pain starts in the right iliac fossa. The systemic response (tachycardia, fever, dehydration) is variable and can be absent in early cases. The abdominal examination is pivotal in diagnosis of the condition. The point of maximal tenderness may be far removed from the right iliac fossa, depending on the position of the appendix. With a high retrocaecal appendix tenderness may be felt in the loin, while in a pelvic appendix tenderness may only become apparent on rectal examination. Diffuse peritonism due to perforation of the appendix occurs most commonly in very young and elderly patients and can be indistinguishable from other causes of peritonitis. A tender mass in the right iliac fossa is suggestive of an inflammatory mass around the appendix (consisting of adherent omentum and adjacent viscera) or, more rarely, an abscess. In an elderly patient this finding suggests a caecal carcinoma.

Differential diagnosis

Diagnosis is difficult in young children, women of child-bearing age and the elderly. Among young men the negative appendicectomy rate is relatively low (5–20%). The figure rises to in excess of 30% in young women and children. The difficulty of diagnosing appendicitis in the elderly is reflected by the high incidence of perforation (>50%), rather than by a high negative appendicectomy rate. There are numerous conditions which have been mistaken for acute appendicitis. In children the most common differential diagnosis is mesenteric adenitis (sore throat and high fever), while in young women it is important to distinguish appendicitis from pelvic inflammatory disease. Pain of immediate onset without prior warning is rarely due to appendicitis. The more common differential diagnoses are listed below.

- Mesenteric adenitis.
- Urinary tract infection/pyelonephritis.
- Salpingitis.
- Ectopic pregnancy.
- Ruptured ovarian follicle (Mittelschmerz).
- Torsion/ruptured ovarian cyst.
- Acute cholecystitis.
- Inflammatory bowel disease.
- Caecal carcinoma.

Aids in diagnosis

The morbidity and mortality of appendicitis greatly increases when perforation occurs. It is clear that the surgeon should aim to prevent perforation at all costs but a high rate of negative appendicectomy is also unacceptable. Removal of a normal appendix is associated with the familiar spectrum of immediate complications. Additionally, patients can suffer late complications such as adhesive intestinal obstruction. Considerable efforts are now being made to improve diagnostic accuracy and prevent unnecessary appendicectomies by using techniques some of which are listed below.

1. White cell count. High sensitivity for appendicitis (only 4% of patients with appendicitis have normal counts) but of limited value as it is raised in many other conditions (i.e. low specificity).

2. Urine analysis. Useful in excluding significant urinary tract infection, particularly in children and young women. A positive pregnancy test strongly infers an ectopic pregnancy.

3. Barium enema examination. Highly accurate in the diagnosis of appendicitis (as revealed by non-filling of the appendix, deformity, spasm and colonic displacement) but technical failure is common and false positives do occur.

4. Ultrasound. Visualization of the appendix by ultrasonography is diagnostic for acute appendicitis (in the hands of an expert). The sensitivity of the technique is reduced in early appendicitis and in retrocaecal appendix. Ultrasound, besides being highly specific for appendicitis, can accurately diagnose other conditions that do not require surgery (mesenteric adenitis, gynaecological disorders), as well as diagnosing disorders where surgical intervention is indicated (ectopic pregnancy).

5. Laparoscopy. Appendicitis can be excluded if a normal appendix is seen or another cause of intra-abdominal pathology revealed that explains the clinical signs (particularly in young women with gynaecological disorders not requiring surgery). It is an invasive procedure (requiring general anaesthesia) with well recognized complications.

6. Catheter peritoneal aspiration. This technique does not distinguish between appendicitis, salpingitis and mesenteric adenitis as all can cause an abnormal number of leucocytes on a smear but negative cytology will exclude all three conditions.

7. Active observation. This is safe in patients with an equivocal clinical picture. Repeated examinations are performed and appendicectomy undertaken if definitive signs develop. There is no evidence that such a policy increases the incidence of perforation.

8. Computer aided diagnosis. In conjunction with structured patient interview, this technique is highly accurate in diagnosing acute appendicitis and reduces the negative exploration rate.

Management

Appendicectomy is the treatment for acute appendicitis, performed as soon as the patient's condition allows, and normally by open operation although there is an emerging trend for laparoscopic removal. The technique is still under evaluation. There are a number of problem areas.

1. Palpable mass pre-operatively. Appendicectomy during the first admission is the correct management for both the likely aetiologies (inflammatory mass or abscess). In experienced hands this is safe, expeditious and prevents the serious consequences of missing a carcinoma in an elderly patient.

2. Normal appendix. The terminal ileum (60 cm) should be inspected to exclude a Meckel's diverticulum, mesenteric adenitis or terminal ileitis. The right tube and ovary must be visualized and the left ovary palpated. In terminal ileitis, if the caecal pole is healthy, the appendix should be removed.

3. Tumour in the appendix. This is normally a carcinoid tumour found incidentally on histology. Appendicectomy is adequate treatment if the tumour is less than 2 cm in diameter. If greater than 2 cm or incompletely excised, right hemicolectomy is necessary.

Complications

Overall mortality for appendicitis is less than 1% but rises to over 5% in the presence of perforation, especially in the elderly. The most widespread complication is wound sepsis. With appropriate perioperative antibiotic prophylaxis the prevalence, even in cases of perforation, can be reduced to 5%. Inadequate peritoneal toilet can lead to subsequent intra-abdominal or pelvic abscess formation.

Further reading

Hoffmann J, Rasmussen OO. Aids in the diagnosis of acute appendicitis. *British Journal of Surgery*, 1989; **76**: 774–9.
Paterson-Brown S, Vipond M. Modern aids to clinical decision-making in the acute abdomen. *British Journal of Surgery*, 1990; **77**: 13–18.

Related topic of interest

Non-specific abdominal pain (p. 211)

ASSESSMENT OF THE ACUTE ABDOMEN

The acute abdomen may be considered as abdominal pain of recent onset. Most causes reside within the abdomen, however there are exceptions. Pain may result from epigastric pain in inferior myocardial infarction or basal pneumonia. Conversely, abdominal pathology may present outside the abdomen, for example shoulder tip pain from subdiaphragmatic irritation by free blood (Kehr's sign) or pus, or inner thigh pain from an obturator hernia (Howship–Romberg sign).

History

1. Origin of pain. It is essential to elicit a history from patients with an acute abdomen. In many inflammatory and obstructive conditions, pain is first experienced in the midline. This reflects the embryological origin of the diseased viscus, with pain from foregut structures referred to the epigastrium, midgut structures to the umbilicus and hindgut structures to the suprapubic area. This visceral pain is often poorly localized and colicky. An inflammatory process progressing through the bowel wall to involve the serosa causes local peritonitis, and the pain becomes constant and localized to the site of the inflammation.

2. Colicky and constant pain. The obstruction of a hollow viscus causes an intermittent cramping pain. This is termed colic, and it represents overactivity of the viscus in an attempt to relieve the obstruction; for example, obstructed small bowel (a midgut structure) causes central abdominal colic.

Obstruction of the ureters by calculi results in pain that radiates from the loin to the groin. The pain has very severe colicky exacerbations, though there is also a constant background ache. A similar pain in the loin suggests renal colic. The gallbladder and pancreas are foregut structures and thus biliary colic and acute pancreatitis are usually experienced in the epigastrium. The pain often radiates to the back in pancreatitis, and to the right hypochondrium in biliary colic.

Localized sepsis or peritonitis results in a constant pain in that area. The patient will have systemic signs of sepsis. Generalized peritonitis results from the presence of free intraperitoneal irritant fluid, such as pus, gastric juice, bile or blood. This causes a constant and severe generalized pain. Retroperitoneal haemorrhage also results in a severe constant pain, though this is experienced in the back rather than in the abdomen. Retroperitoneal haemorrhage often occurs to one side or in the iliac fossa, causing pain in the loin or groin respectively. This is a source of diagnostic confusion between leaking abdominal aortic aneurysms and renal or ureteric colic.

3. Associated symptoms. Vomiting occurs early and prominently in small bowel obstruction, but may not occur at all in colonic obstruction. Distension occurs in both small and large bowel obstruction. Vomiting may occur in association with severe abdominal pain, including ureteric colic and acute pancreatitis. An alteration in bowel habit or the passage of blood per rectum suggests colonic pathology.

Gynaecological symptoms must be sought in young women with acute abdominal pain. Missed menstruation with recent vaginal bleeding points to an ectopic pregnancy. Pains that are bilateral and inguinal plus the presence of a vaginal discharge point to salpingitis. Urinary frequency and dysuria suggest a lower urinary tract infection, and if associated with rigors and loin pain then an acute pyelonephritis is likely.

4. Past medical history. Small bowel obstruction with prior abdominal surgery suggests adhesion obstruction. Previous episodes of peptic ulceration, acute diverticulitis, biliary colic, or known chronic pancreatitis may prompt the diagnosis of recurrence of that disorder.

Examination

The patient is examined for tachycardia, pyrexia and hypotension. The presence of pallor, jaundice and lymphadenopathy is noted. Tachypnoea may signify an acidosis. The patient may be dehydrated from vomiting, as assessed by inspecting the tongue or feeling the turgidity of the skin. Cool and clammy peripheries suggest hypovolaemic shock, whilst warm peripheries and hypotension suggest endotoxaemia.

1. Abdominal inspection. A rigid abdomen from underlying peritonitis fails to move with respiration. Pain from an inflamed viscus may be reproduced on coughing. Masses may be visible such as pulsating abdominal aneurysms, retroperitoneal haematomas, hernias or tumours. The groins and scrotum are inspected for strangulated hernias. Old scars are noted. The abdomen may be distended.

2. Abdominal palpation. The acute abdomen is usually associated with tenderness. An exception occurs in acute mesenteric infarction which often causes exceptional pain but few signs. Localized tenderness suggests an inflamed viscus. If the inflammation involves the serosa, localized peritonitis is present, and pain will be felt if the examining hand is quickly released from the tender area. This represents rebound tenderness. This can be very painful and the sign should not be repeatedly elicited. A gentler method for eliciting rebound is percussion of the abdomen.

If the inflammation spreads to involve the parietal peritoneum, the patient will exhibit involuntary rigidity of the abdominal wall caused by reflex muscular tensing. Diffuse rigidity occurs if there is a generalized peritonitis. The patient appears unwell, with tachycardia, fever, hypotension or endotoxaemia. In a patient with no systemic signs but apparent rigidity on palpation, the rigidity is likely to be entirely voluntary and not true reflexic rigidity. Rigidity is often termed guarding.

3. Bowel sounds. In peritonitis these are often reduced or absent. Bowel obstruction causes increased sounds. The abdomen is distended in obstruction, and if one looks carefully, peristaltic waves may be seen coursing over the abdomen, particularly in small bowel obstruction.

Radiology

Small bowel and colonic obstruction is readily differentiated, as small bowel has numerous transverse folds (valvulae conniventes) that course around the entire circumference of the bowel, while colon has wide sacculations (haustrae). Multiple air-fluid levels occur on erect abdominal films in a 'step pattern' in small bowel obstruction. Colonic obstruction with an incompetent iliocaecal valve results in small bowel dilatation. If some colon is dilated, the obstruction must be colonic.

Free intraperitoneal gas indicates a perforated gas-containing hollow viscus. This is commonly caused by perforated peptic ulcers. The gas is seen under one or both hemidiaphragms, but up to 20% of patients with perforated peptic ulcers, and most patients with colonic perforations, do not have it. Free gas may also be seen between loops of bowel, such that both sides of the bowel wall are visible on a plain X-ray. This is known as Rigler's sign and may be the only clue of a colonic perforation.

Blood tests

FBC and U&E are requested. Arterial blood gases are performed if acute pancreatitis is suspected, or in any patient with suspected metabolic disturbance or renal failure. Serum amylase must be requested to exclude acute pancreatitis. In all cases, blood must be sent for group and save if there is any possibility of the patient undergoing surgery.

Immediate management

The severely unwell patient with an acute abdomen must be resuscitated fully and later reassessed. i.v. fluids, antibiotics and analgesia will settle many patients, and allow a clearer picture to emerge. The patient ought to be catheterized, and a central venous catheter placed via the internal jugular route. The immediate 'blind' operation of such patients results in a high mortality. Patients with severe acute pancreatitis or acute diverticulitis frequently present in this fashion, and conservative treatment, rather than surgery, is required. If surgery later becomes necessary, then the additional resuscitation performed will always prove to be of benefit.

Special investigations

Peritoneal lavage with estimation of the amylase and red and white blood cell counts of the peritoneal fluid may be performed in cases where the diagnosis is in doubt. Laparoscopy is frequently performed in younger women presenting with lower abdominal pain, as the ovaries, uterine tubes or uterus are far more often the origin of lower abdominal pain than the appendix. Sometimes the cause of an acute abdomen remains obscure. If the clinical picture warrants it, the ultimate investigation for acute abdominal pain is a laparotomy.

Further reading

de Dombal FT. Acute abdominal pain. *Surgery*, 1990; **82**: 1967–71.
The acute abdomen. In: Clain A (ed.) *Hamilton Bailey's Demonstrations of Physical Signs in Clinical Surgery*. Briston Wright, 1986; 294–330.
Patterson-Brown S, Vipond MN. Modern aids to clinical decision-making in the acute abdomen. *British Journal of Surgery*, 1990; **77**: 13–8.

Related topics of interest

AUDIT

Definitions

Audit is best defined as a systematic process by which a group of professionals review a current system, identify possible weaknesses in that system, make alterations in practice and monitor whether the standard of practice has improved. The aim is to provide an efficient cost-effective service with improvement in the quality of patient care, avoidance of complications and a smooth running, well-managed department. In short, quality assurance.

Terms

Audit must be distinguished from clinical research and audit meetings from morbidity and mortality meetings. Audit is an activity carried out between individual firms and departments reviewing their own activity and setting their own standards. Clinical research involves changing current practice through a controlled prospective clinical trial for the purpose of a recommendation to other centres through publication. A morbidity and mortality meeting simply reviews deaths and complications but audit includes every aspect of clinical practice which has potential for improvement. The systems which are commonly audited will be discussed followed by the mechanisms with which they are carried out.

Medical records

Medical records are often all that is left to extract information if a retrospective analysis takes place. They are also legal documents which patients have a right to see. They must be clearly signed and dated with the time the patient was seen. Management changes, treatment changes and a record of all complications as they happen should be clearly documented. Comprehensive operation notes, completed fluid balance and temperature charts, accurate records of drug regimes, and up-to-date continuation notes with filed pathology reports are not always achieved.

Postgraduate training

Since 1989, the Royal Colleges of Surgeons and Physicians have required evidence that audit takes place in a department before renewing training posts for postgraduates. If adequate supervision and assessment of trainees, with encouragement to take study leave, does not take place the career grade post may be replaced with a staff grade post. Education by apprenticeship is no longer considered adequate for training. It should be combined with lectures, courses, research and opportunities to improve surgical skill.

Theatre utilization

Deficiencies in theatre utilization occur all too frequently, for a number of differing reasons: anaesthetic delays, patient cancellations (social, medical, administrative), autoclaving times and portering delays, as well as surgical delays. Operations can be divided into their 'hernia equivalents' with a recommendation of four hernia equivalents being performed per theatre session. This should provide adequate service commitment as well as training time for junior staff. All day lists are more efficient than half day lists. Several surgical lists running concurrently provides opportunity for the transfer of patients from an overbooked list to an under-utilized theatre.

Patients' charter

Length of time on waiting lists, patient cancellations, time spent waiting in outpatients and the recommendation of all new patients to be seen by a consultant are issues which were audited and led to the *patients' charter*. In an already overstretched NHS these criteria can be met by encouraging the General Practitioners to review more follow-up surgical patients, by referring fewer patients to the surgeon and by decreasing the number of inappropriate referrals. Surgeons themselves can reduce the number of inappropriate investigations by the process of audit to reduce further outpatient attendances. Placing fewer patients on operation waiting lists by redefining the criteria of an NHS operation, as opposed to a private operation, is another alternative. Increasing the straddling of outpatient appointment times and increasing the proportion of patients treated as day cases is also contributary to reducing waiting times and lists. Cancelling patients is extremely inefficient, expensive in patient, secretarial and GP time and should be avoided by not placing them on the admission list in the knowledge that they might be cancelled. It is a common fallacy to assume that giving a patient an admission date removes that patient from the waiting list.

Day surgery

Day case procedures are frequently audited as they fulfil an increasing role in surgical practice. Particular aspects to audit include patient satisfaction, availability of help after discharge, adequacy of postoperative instructions including suture removal and analgesia, the cost in time and resources on the GP, and patient cancellation rates for medical reasons or inappropriatenesses in selection.

CEPOD

The report of a Confidential Enquiry into Perioperative Deaths (CEPOD) in 1987 stimulated awareness that audit was a necessary activity. In particular, it recognized deficiencies in the emergency management of patients. These included inadequate resuscitation prior to laparotomy, inadequate supervision of emergency operations, the poor availability of immediate help when operative problems arose, the performance of complicated operations at night with poor facilities when they could more safely be performed during the daytime, and incorrect operative decisions (blind femoral embolectomy in progressive arterial disease, colonic defunction when a primary anastomosis would have been more appropriate).

Staff activity

Audit is also useful for the protection of departmental integrity. Much activity takes place that usually escapes audit but, if recorded, could justify demands for more resources. These include surgical operations performed on behalf of the casualty department and on patients of other firms (Hickman line insertion, AV fistula formation), as well as casualty referrals and ward consultations, and the treatment of concurrent medical illness.

Meetings

Audit should be effected by frequent chaired meetings. Time should be set aside so that all involved staff and an audit officer can attend. Points for improvement are written down and any special problems which are identified can then be specifically audited. It is intended that the meetings are not a witch hunt but an exercise for improving service quality. All meetings must be treated in a confidential manner.

Data base

Information access can be facilitated by computerizing audit. A departmental database is established for the collection of data which should be linked to the general hospital network. The integrity of the data depends entirely on the individual member of staff feeding in the information. This must be supervised at the highest level for a meaningful record. Data transfer from ward round or theatre to the computer seems to be a universal problem. A card system or dictaphone can facilitate this process. Alternatively, entry into the computer can be made on the day of patient discharge directly from the notes, or even from a personal pocket organizer.

Auditing audit

Finally, the audit process itself should be audited, to ensure that the changes identified at the meetings have been carried out effectively and each audit loop is closed. Written protocols or guidelines can then be established. Consideration must also be given to the computer cost, staff time and additional labour in administrating audit. A poor process with a good outcome is preferable to a good process with a poor outcome.

Further reading

Nicol DK, Spilby J, Dunn DC, Hay AM, Wright S. Mini-symposium: Surgical audit. *Current Practice in Surgery*, 1992; **4**: 3–19.
Secker Walker J. Audit of surgical practice. *Current Surgical Practice*; 1991; **6**: 15–31.

Related topic of interest

Day case surgery (p. 114)

BENIGN BREAST DISEASE

Benign conditions of the breast are commoner than malignant disease. They present with a lump, pain, nipple retraction or nipple discharge, and are frequently difficult to differentiate from malignant disease.

Congenital abnormalities

1. Absence of a breast. Complete absence of a breast and nipple (amastia) is accompanied by pectoral muscle aplasia or hypoplasia in 90% of cases. Breast hypoplasia (amazia) is commoner, and minor asymmetry quite normal. Breast construction, augmentation and/or reduction of the contralateral side may be required. Isolated absence of a nipple is very rare.

2. Accessory breasts and nipples. This is caused by failure of full regression of the primitive breast line. Supernumerary nipples are present in 1–5% of people, but accessory breasts are less common. Treatment is by excision.

Developmental disorders

1. Excessive breast enlargement. Minor degrees of breast enlargement frequently occur in infancy and before puberty. Uncontrolled juvenile hypertrophy usually occurs in the absence of endocrine abnormalities. There is proliferation of periductal connective tissue and ducts but not of lobules. Breast reduction may be required.

Male breast enlargement (gynaecomastia) occurs in neonates, puberty (30–70% of boys) and old age. It is benign and usually regresses spontaneously. Occasionally, subcutaneous mastectomy is necessary. Pathological gynaecomastia can be induced by hypogonadism, hormone-secreting neoplasms, hepatic and renal disease, and drugs (spironolactone, cimetidine, digoxin, metoclopramide, cytotoxics).

2. Fibroadenoma. These are probably developmental anomalies rather than benign neoplasms. They occur between the ages of 15 and 40, accounting for 15–20% of all discrete breast masses. They are firm, smooth, mobile and may be multiple. Clinical diagnosis is frequently wrong and FNAC or excision biopsy are advisable. Following diagnosis by FNAC, the fibroadenoma may be observed or removed. A few will gradually increase in size. Giant fibroadenomata (> 5 cm diameter) are usually excised. Malignant change occurs occasionally (1:1000).

Disorders of cyclical change and involution

1. Benign mammary dysplasia. This affects premenopausal women and is characterized by marked premenstrual breast nodularity and discomfort affecting the outer quadrants. There may be excessive prolactin release or abnormal sensitivity of breast tissue hormone receptors. FNAC, biopty or Tru-Cut biopsy are advisable to exclude malignancy. Histological changes include cyst formation, fibrosis, adenosis and epitheliosis. Mammography should be performed in women over 35. Reassurance, simple analgesia and a firm bra usually help. Linoleic acid (oil of evening primrose) is sometimes beneficial. Occasionally, danazol, bromocryptine or tamoxifen are required, but side effects occur in 30% of patients. Rarely, mastectomy is justified.

2. Cystic disease. Palpable cysts occur frequently in women approaching the menopause. They present as discrete, smooth breast lumps. Aspiration should be attempted. Yellow/green/brown fluid is obtained which should only be sent for cytological examination if blood-stained. Ultrasound and mammography should be performed in women over 35. Persistence of a mass following aspiration, repeated refilling of a cyst and blood-stained aspirate with cytological abnormalities are indications for excision biopsy. Cysts associated with breast cancer are commoner in postmenopausal women and should be investigated.

Infective disorders

1. Mastitis neonatorum. Neonatal breast enlargement may be complicated by infection and abscess formation. Antibiotics may help in the early stages, but if fluctuation develops, incision and drainage is necessary.

2. Lactational breast abscess. This is commonest during the first month after delivery and is caused by *Staphylococcus aureus*, *Staphylococcus epidermidis* or a *Streptococcus* entering through a cracked nipple. The breast becomes tense, inflamed and tender. Antibiotics can resolve the infection if given early. Repeated aspiration of pus with antibiotic cover may be successful but, frequently, incision and drainage is necessary. Providing no antibiotic harmful to neonates is used, lactation using both breasts may continue.

3. Non-lactational abscess. Most result as a complication of periductal mastitis, but should be distinguished from an inflammatory cancer by FNAC. Repeated aspiration with antibiotics may be attempted if the overlying skin is normal, otherwise incision and drainage are required. Mammary duct fistula may be a complication.

4. *Tuberculosis, syphilis, actinomycosis.* Rare. Tuberculosis usually spreads by lymphatics from regional lymph nodes or directly from a rib. An axillary or breast sinus is strongly suggestive. Treatment is by antituberculous chemotherapy. A syphylitic chancre may occur on the nipple with axillary lymphadenopathy. Syphilis and actinomycosis are treated with penicillin or other appropriate antibiotics.

Inflammatory disorders

1. *Periductal mastitis.* Women in their early 30s are affected. Mastalgia, nipple discharge, nipple retraction and peri-areolar inflammation are prominent. The ducts are surrounded by polymorphs, giant cells and epithelioid cells, but are not dilated. Treatment is by antibiotics, but abscess or mammary duct fistula may follow.

2. *Duct ectasia.* Duct dilatation occurs with an intermittent clear, cheesy or blood-stained discharge or nipple retraction. This affects older women. Cytology reveals benign changes only and duct thickening and coarse calcification may be seen on mammography. A persistent discharge can be treated by microdochectomy, or duct excision.

3. *Mammary duct fistula.* Most follow periductal mastitis but may result from biopsy of a peri-areolar mass or drainage of a non-lactational breast abscess. The nipple is usually indrawn. Fistulotomy or fistulectomy are frequently successful, but total duct and fistula excision may be required.

4. *Fat necrosis.* A dense fibrous scar forms causing skin tethering and retraction, mimicking a carcinoma. In the early stages, haemorrhage can usually be seen, with fat liquefaction and surrounding inflammation. A history of trauma is often lacking. FNAC or excision are required to exclude carcinoma.

Benign neoplasms

1. *Duct papilloma.* These are common and may be multiple. They present with a blood-stained nipple discharge. Treatment is by microdochectomy or total duct excision if there is multiple duct discharge.

2. *Lipoma.* These are common, but may be confused with the soft fatty mass that sometimes surrounds a carcinoma.

3. Granular cell myoblastoma, leiomyoma, chondroma, chondrolipoma, myxoma. All are rare and must be distinguished from carcinoma.

Miscellaneous

1. Non-cyclical breast pain. No cause is usually found, but malignancy, costochondritis and periductal mastitis should be excluded. A firm bra and simple analgesia provide relief. Oil of evening primrose capsules work in some patients. Others may respond to a change in hormonal environment = Pill, pregnancy, danazol, bromocryptine.

2. Fibromatosis. Benign proliferation of myelofibroblasts. Behaves like desmoid tumours. A variant, nodular fasciitis affects the pectoral fascia.

3. Haematoma. Follows FNAC, Tru-Cut biopsy, trauma or anticoagulation.

4. Amyloid. Rare.

5. Intramammary lymph node. Common. Enlarge in response to local or general causes.

6. Silicone granulomas. Silicone used in breast augmentation may escape from the silastic capsule inducing the formation of granulomata and foreign body giant cells. Evidence is lacking of an association with breast cancer. The prosthesis envelope can induce fibrous capsule formation.

7. Galactocoele. Encysted milk collection. Treated by aspiration.

8. Mondor's disease. Superficial thrombophlebitis of veins overlying the breast. Usually self-limiting.

9. Sebaceous cyst. Common on the skin overlying the breast.

10.Eczema of the nipple. A biopsy is frequently necessary to differentiate this from Paget's disease. Nipple erosion, unilateral site and an associated mass suggest Paget's disease. May signify underlying periductal mastitis or duct ectasia or may be local or part of generalized eczema.

11.Nipple adenoma. Ulceration of nipple. Remove by wide excision.

Further reading

Dixon JM, Mansel RE. The breast. In: Burnand KG, Young AE (eds) *The New Aird's Companion in Surgical Studies.* Edinburgh: Churchill Livingstone, 1992; 811–44.
Mansel RE (ed.) *Benign Breast Disease.* Carnforth: Parthenon, 1992.

Related topic of interest

Breast cancer (p. 60)

BLOOD TRANSFUSION

There are two main landmarks in blood transfusion which have allowed many major operations to be successfully performed. Firstly, the discovery of the ABO isoagglutinins in 1901 by Landsteiner marked the development of safe blood transfusion. Secondly, the addition of acid–citrate–dextrose (ACD) from 1943 provided anticoagulant activity and nutrition for red cells which resulted in a dramatic increase in the shelf life of stored blood. The main indications for the transfusion of blood and its components are to replace acute blood loss, treat anaemia and to correct any disorders of haemostasis.

Replacement

The ideal replacement fluid in rapid haemorrhage is whole blood or red cells in saline–adenine–glucose–mannitol (SAG-M). Crystalloid and colloid solutions dilute blood and its clotting factors in the circulation and encourage further bleeding. Therapy for rapid blood loss should be directed primarily toward the arrest of haemorrhage. Although compatible whole blood is best, packed red cells can be administered with replacement of the fluid volume lost in the form of colloid or thrice the volume of crystalloid. Neat packed cells have a high viscosity and are not indicated in the acute situation as the sole replacement fluid. Blood substitutes like the synthetic perfluorocarbons (PFCs) and modified haemoglobin solutions (polyhaemoglobins) are not yet in clinical use.

Anaemia

Correction of anaemia is essential prior to elective surgery, especially if ischaemic events like angina, claudication, transient ischaemic attacks and gut ischaemia are anticipated. Units of packed cells are administered over 3–4 hours each with frusemide cover to avoid heart failure. The ideal haemoglobin is around 11 g/dl because this is the level at which the benefits of a low viscosity are balanced with maximal oxygen carrying capacity.

Haemostasis

The major bleeding problems that accompany surgical disease occur in patients on warfarin, heparin or aspirin, in those patients with disseminated intravascular coagulation (DIC), and in patients with haemophilia, liver disease, thrombocytopenia and hypersplenism. Heparin is easily reversed with protamine sulphate. Warfarin is reversed by an intramuscular injection of vitamin K which takes about 2 days to work; FFP is required for emergency reversal. Regular prothrombin estimations are still required because the half-life of warfarin is much longer than that of FFP. Aspirin prolongs the bleeding time by interfering with platelet function. The aim of treating DIC is to correct the underlying surgical problem (usually sepsis). Component therapy (platelets, clotting factors) or heparin is given on the advice of a haematologist.

Infection

The following infections can be transmitted by blood transfusion:

Viral	Bacterial	Protozoal
Hepatitis B	Syphilis	Malaria
Hepatitis C	Brucellosis	Chagas' disease
Hepatitis D	Contaminants	Babesiosis
HIV		
CMV		
Epstein–Barr		

Hepatitis

1. Hepatitis B. All donors are routinely screened for HBsAg. Infection still occurs because of the undetectable concentrations of antigen present at the beginning and end of an acute infection. Ten per cent of all infected patients develop chronic hepatitis. All patients requiring multiple transfusions and all health-care workers should be vaccinated against Hepatitis B.

2. Hepatitis C. This virus was successfully cloned in 1989. It has always been responsible for the majority of cases of post-transfusion hepatitis even before routine HBsAg testing. Fifty per cent of infected patients develop chronic hepatitis and 10% of patients cirrhosis or hepatoma.

3. Hepatitis D (delta agent). This virus uses HBsAg as its coat and cannot exist without HBsAg. This is fortunate because screening for HBsAg is all that is required to exclude the virus.

Human immunodeficiency virus

HIV can be transmitted by cellular elements and by plasma. In the UK, most infection occurs in haemophiliacs treated with clotting factors but now these can be virus inactivated. One in 100,000 donors are seropositive but this increases to 1 in 25,000 for new donors. The incubation period between infection and seroconversion has resulted in the occasional HIV infection being transmitted from screened blood. The present HIV antibody detection techniques are sensitive and reliable.

Cytomegalovirus	Immature neonates, immunosuppressed patients and pregnant mothers seronegative for CMV are all susceptible to CMV infection. In these groups, blood must be filtered to remove the leucocytes which transmit the intracellular virus.
Glandular fever	The Epstein–Barr virus is not screened for because in most cases the donor's antibodies protect against infection and the majority of recipients have high levels of antibodies already in their circulation.
Malaria	In areas where malaria is endemic, a course of antiprotozoal therapy is usually prescribed along with the transfusion. In non-endemic areas, travellers who have recently resided in an endemic area are excluded from donation.
Autologous predonation	Autologous predonation of blood for elective surgery began in 1960 and is now widespread in Europe and the USA. The method avoids the cost of extensive screening used for homologous blood. It also prevents immunosuppressive and allergic reactions, and is acceptable to some Jehovah's witnesses. Donation criteria consist of:

1. Haemoglobin. This should be greater than 11 g/dl.

2. Infection. Active infection is a contraindication.

3. Blood loss. Procedures where this is expected like vascular or cardiothoracic operations.

4. Cardiorespiratory disease. If severe (unstable angina, left main coronary stenosis, myocardial infarction within the last 6 months), donation is ill advised.

The minimum accepted haemoglobin level for surgery is around 9 g/dl. A unit is taken each week, 500 ml of saline are infused to maintain the intravascular volume and 200 mg of ferrous sulphate is started. Two to four units of blood predeposited in this way, especially in the polycythaemic arteriopath, would nearly always result in a haemoglobin of greater than 10 g/dl prior to surgery. Blood is screened for HIV, hepatitis and syphilis, and grouped. 'Cross-over' for use on other patients is prohibited. The use of erythropoietin, given prior to predeposit, and the method of cryoprecipitation using hydroxyethyl starch (blood can be stored over 10 years and thawed for immediate use) can increase the amount of blood predonated. Should there be much blood loss at the time of surgery, the haemopoietic system will already be primed to function at an increased rate of manufacture.

Intraoperative autotransfusion

Intraoperative autotransfusion decreases the need for homologous transfusion and thus the risk of transmissible disease. It is indicated in cardiothoracic surgery, trauma and aortic surgery, where major blood loss is often expected, and involves the retrieval of blood shed during an operation and its subsequent reinfusion into the patient.

1. Solcotrans. This passive system of retrieval was introduced in 1980. It consists of a polycarbonate container with an inner bag attached to a low pressure suction system. When full this is inverted and any unwanted air is tapped. Reinfusion occurs by gravity through a 40 µm filter. It is insufficient to have anticoagulant only in the reservoir; the patient must be fully systemically heparinized.

2. Cell saver system. This system is an active process which involves centrifugation and cell washing. It can be used in the non-heparinized patient.

Relative contraindications to intraoperative autotransfusion include its use in putative curative cancer resection (although peritoneal–venous shunting for malignant ascites does not encourage pulmonary metastasis), contamination with faecal material and in the HIV patient (risk to health-care worker). The concurrent use of collagen haemostats is an absolute contraindication.

Transfusion immunomodulation

Modulation of immunological behaviour by perioperative transfusion was first noted in 1973 when renal allograft survival was enhanced in patients receiving over 10 units of blood. Over 70 publications exist examining the deleterious effects of blood transfusion on colonic, prostatic, breast, renal and lung cancers. With most tumours, the literature is divided but the balance of evidence points towards perioperative transfusion being detrimental to colonic and prostatic cancer patients. The data should be interpreted with caution as the biological behaviour of the tumour determining the need for tranfusion may be more aggressive and due to the observation that blood loss and blood donation are themselves immunosuppressive. The components of blood (red cells, white cells or plasma proteins) thought to be detrimental have not been fully established but studies using packed cells instead of whole blood and white cell filters are in progress.

Further reading

Greaves M, Slater NGP, Parrott NR, Kay LA, Thompson JF. Mini-symposium. Blood transfusion. *Current Practice in Surgery,* 1993; **5**: 119–41.
Lawrance RJ. Blood transfusion: indications and hazards. *Recent Advances in Surgery*, 1992; **15**: 119–35.

Related topics of interest

Fluid replacement (p. 136)
Lower gastrointestinal haemorrhage (p. 192)
Trauma management – principles (p. 301)
Upper gastrointestinal haemorrhage (p. 313)

BREAST CANCER

This is the commonest cancer amongst women, affecting 1 in 13 and resulting in 25,000 new cases and 15,000 deaths per year in the UK. Nulliparous women in developed countries are at increased risk; women who have their first child young and breast feed are protected. Predisposing factors include oestrogen exposure unopposed by progesterone, hyperoestrogenism, family history of premenopausal breast cancer, saturated dietary fats and previous benign atypical hyperplasia. The incidence rises rapidly to 200:100, 000 women per year by the age of 45 and continues to rise into old age. One per cent of breast cancers occur in men.

Pathology

1. Epithelial tumours
  (a) Non-invasive
      • Ductal carcinoma-*in-situ* (DCIS)   3–5%
      • Lobular carcinoma-*in-situ* (LCIS)   1%
  (b) Invasive
      • Invasive ductal   80–90%
      • Invasive lobular   1–2%
      • Mucinous, medullary, papillary Rare
      • Tubular, secretory, apocrine Rare
  (c) Paget's disease   2%

2. Mixed connective tissue/epithelial.

3. Miscellaneous/unclassified.

Staging

The TNM and Manchester systems are commonly used. Tumours up to T2 N1 M0 (stage 2) are termed 'early breast cancer' and are potentially curable. Tumours beyond this stage are advanced.

The TNM classification of breast cancer

Primary tumour = T		*Nodes = N*	
Tis	Carcinoma-in-situ/Paget's	N1	Ipsilateral axillary (mobile)
T1	≤ 2 cm	N2	Ipsilateral axillary (fixed)
T2	> 2 cm but < 5 cm	N3	Ipsilateral internal mammary nodes
T3	> 5 cm		
T4a	Chest wall extension (fixed)	*Metastases = M*	
T4b	Dermal extension (ulcer, peau d'orange)	M0	None
T4c	Both 4a and 4b	M1	Distant (lung, liver, other nodes)

Clinical features

- Firm, irregular, painless lump. May be fixed to skin or muscle.
- Pain (10%).
- Axillary/supraclavicular lymph node involvement.

- Recent nipple retraction and/or bloody discharge.
- Paget's disease.
- Peau d'orange.
- Signs of metastatic disease (weight loss, ascites, jaundice, CNS signs).
- Asymptomatic presentation following screening.

Investigations

1. Mammography. Used for investigating symptomatic patients and for screening; 80–95% accurate, but less accurate in young, dense breasts.

2. Ultrasound. Demonstrates cystic disease. Colour flow duplex mode may distinguish abnormal tumour circulation.

3. Fine needle aspiration cytology (FNAC). Simple and quick; 95% accurate.

4. Tru-Cut or biopty gun biopsy. For lumps larger than 2 cm diameter a tissue core can be obtained under local anaesthesia for histological examination.

5. Excision biopsy. This is performed where other investigations have failed to define the lump. Proceeding to a more extensive procedure after frozen section analysis is not recommended.

6. Wire-guided biopsy. Impalpable suspicious lesions identified at mammography are localized by insertion of a wire under screening control. A core of breast tissue around the wire is then excised surgically. A radiograph of the specimen is taken to ensure total excision of the abnormality.

7. Bone scan, CT scan, MRI scan. Helpful in defining the extent of metastatic disease.

Control of local disease

1. Surgery. In patients without systemic disease, local surgery may be curative, but most patients have occult micrometastases. A mobile tumour with or without axillary lymph nodes is generally operable. Prospective trials indicate no difference in the 5–10-year survival rate of patients undergoing mastectomy or breast conservation (lumpectomy, wide local excision, quadrantectomy) and radiotherapy, but the local recurrence rate in the latter group is slightly higher. Mastectomy with axillary clearance results in 5-year recurrence rates of 4% and 8% in node-negative and node-positive patients, respectively. It is not yet clear if there are differences in longer term survival (10–25 years) between radical surgery and conservation.

Palliative mastectomy with or without additional local treatment may be necessary to control advanced local disease.

Anxiety and depression accompany mastectomy in many women, but breast conservation does not protect against this, many women fearing the possibility of residual or recurrent disease.

2. Management of the axilla. Failure to treat the axilla does not confer a worse prognosis, node involvement being an expression of poor outcome rather than a determinant. Level III axillary clearance, however, has a long-term local recurrence rate of under 2%, provides useful prognostic information and indicates which patients will benefit from systemic adjuvant treatment. Arm swelling affects less than 5% of women providing the axilla is not irradiated. Axillary node sampling provides less reliable information regarding prognosis. Radical axillary irradiation effectively prevents node recurrence, but brachial plexus neuropathy occurs in 0.5–1.0% and no reliable information regarding node status is obtained. Level III axillary dissection is recommended in premenopausal women with a palpable primary tumour.

3. Radiotherapy. Radiotherapy is necessary after breast conserving surgery to reduce local recurrence rates. Overall survival is not improved, but aggressive radiotherapy causes excess long-term mortality from other tumours and ischaemic heart disease. Chest wall radiotherapy is unhelpful in patients undergoing modified radical mastectomy, and axillary irradiation should not be performed if level III axillary clearance has been performed. Chest wall and axillary radiotherapy is usually the treatment of choice in advanced, inoperable tumours.

4. Breast reconstruction. Reconstruction probably does not interfere with the detection of tumour recurrence and restores appearance to near normal. Latissimus dorsi (LD) and rectus abdominis myocutaneous (TRAM) flaps involve further major surgery, resulting in extensive scarring and possible complications (infection, flap necrosis, late capsule formation). Considerable asymmetry is the norm and nipple reconstruction is often unsatisfactory.

Control of systemic disease

1. Radiotherapy. Provides excellent palliation of metastases, particularly of bone.

2. Chemotherapy. Reduces the 10-year probability of death by 16% in younger, premenopausal women with axillary lymph node involvement and/or large tumours with unfavourable features (poor differentiation and lymphovascular invasion). Cyclophosphamide, methotrexate and fluorouracil (CMF) given for 6 months is a typical regimen. A short course of chemotherapy in a fit patient may temporarily control advanced or inoperable disease.

3. Hormonal treatment. Tamoxifen used for at least 2 years at a dose of 20 mg/day reduces the 10-year probability of death by 17%, together with reduced local recurrence rates. This benefit is most apparent in older women, but is independent of menopausal and oestrogen receptor status.

4. Oophorectomy, ovarian irradiation, LHRH agonists. Useful in advanced, metastatic disease to induce regression or delay spread. If no response is obtained, second-line agents (aminoglutethamide, progestogens) can be used.

Pain relief and counselling

Oral opiates, non-steroidal agents, radiotherapy and steroids (for cerebral involvement) should be used liberally when the disease advances and symptoms develop. Drainage of effusions and ascites may be beneficial. Counselling and contact with a hospice are helpful in the late stages of disease.

Breast screening

Evidence that breast screening reduces mortality from breast cancer in women in New York, Holland and Sweden has resulted in the UK breast screening programme offered to women aged 50–64. No clear survival advantage has yet been seen in the UK, although more early tumours are being detected and treated. A considerable increase in workload has resulted and women are unnecessarily alarmed when mammograms are falsely positive.

Further reading

Dixon JM, Mansel RE. The breast. In: Burnand KG, Young AE (eds) *The New Aird's Companion in Surgical Studies*. Edinburgh: Churchill Livingstone, 1992; 811–44.

Frykbeg ER, Bland KI. Early invasive carcinoma of the breast. In: Daly JM (ed.) *Current Opinion in General Surgery*. Philadelphia: Current Science, 1993; 316–24.

Sacks NPM, Baum M. Primary management of carcinoma of the breast. *Lancet*, 1993; **342**: 1402–8.

Related topic of interest

Benign breast disease (p. 50)

BURNS

Burn injuries are considered the most severe metabolic insult that a person can experience. The alcoholic, epileptic, drug addict and mentally handicapped are the most at risk together with children under six with scald injuries from bath water, hot drinks and kettle spills. Treatment requires a radical and aggressive approach to curb a mortality from fluid loss and sepsis which increases with age and the percentage surface area burnt.

Fluid replacement

A burn results in a substantial loss of fluid, protein, blood and heat. The percentage area burnt is estimated from the Wallace 'Rule of Nines' chart. One per cent of the patient's surface area is represented by the palmar surface of his hand. Adults suffering a burn greater than 15 per cent surface area or children greater than 10 per cent require admission and fluid resuscitation. The Muir and Barclay regime calculates plasma replacement during the first 36 hours. Each of the six time periods requires an equal volume of fluid replacement in addition to normal requirements.

Period	1	2	3	4	5	6
Duration (hours)	4	4	4	6	6	12

$$\frac{\text{Surface area burnt } (\%) \times \text{Weight (kg)}}{2} = \text{Requirement (ml/Period)}$$

This is only a guide which must be supplemented with regular haemoglobin, haematocrit, electrolyte and urinary output measurements. With burns greater than 30% the increase in capillary permeability becomes generalized with a tendency to shock lung (ARDS), adynamic ileus and stress ulceration. Crystalloids exacerbate these complications and should be avoided. Human Plasma Protein Fraction (albumen) and blood are commonly used replacement fluids.

Analgesia

Intravenous morphine is the most appropriate analgesia and can be administered from a patient-controlled analgesia system. Cool water (uncovered ice is harmful) is an effective analgesic for smaller burns and has been demonstrated to reverse tissue damage. Rectal paracetamol for pyrexia is useful in children.

Sepsis

Burnt surfaces are an excellent culture medium for bacteria. Colonization is rapid and the associated immunosuppression of large burns makes septicaemia inevitable. Severely burnt patients should be isolated and barrier nursed. Intravenous antibiotics are required for septicaemia, pneumonia, UTI or obvious cellulitis, but blood cultures are frequently sterile and signs of septicaemia can be subtle. Hyperthermia with an elevated white count indicates Gram +ve sepsis and the converse is often true with Gram −ve organisms. Other signs include thrombocytopenia, hyperglycaemia, delirium and, in children, toxic shock syndrome (due to a staphlococcal enterotoxin). Regular cultures of the urine, sputum, wound and blood are taken to determine the most appropriate antibiotic therapy. The injudicious use of prophylactic antibiotics allows colonization with resistant strains and provides a great problem in treating an established infection.

Inhalation injuries

Inhalation injuries are suspected from the appearance of facial oedema, singed nasal hair and oropharyngeal carbon with stridor and bronchospasm. The carbon monoxide and hydrogen cyanide gas released from the incomplete combustion of plastic furnishings are often lethal. Treatment consists of humidified oxygen, bronchodilators and occasionally intubation or tracheostomy.

Escharotomy

Deep circumferential burns of the chest or limbs require relieving incisions, escharotomies, to prevent respiratory compromise or perfusion problems. Bleeding is controlled with adrenaline packs and blood transfusion.

Nutrition

All burns require high energy dietary supplementation to facilitate healing. In addition, with larger burns, fine-bore nasogastric feeding should be used. Intravenous feeding lines present a high risk of infection and should be avoided.

Open or closed therapy?

Burns of the face and perineum and superficial burns should be treated by exposure. A dry eschar discourages bacterial colonization and often separates spontaneously after two weeks. Closed treatment involves covering the burn with vaseline gauze and leaving the inner layers undisturbed for 10 days. Burns are often covered with silver sulphadiazine which has a good spectrum of antibacterial activity. Topical antibiotics are readily absorbed into the circulation and care should be exercised when administering them. All closed treatments moisten the eschar which prevents spontaneous separation. This then requires surgical debridement under general anaesthesia.

Surgery

The surgical approach depends upon the extent and depth of the burn. A general guide to depth identification is tabulated below.

Depth	Sensation	Blistering	Colour	Healing
Superficial	Painful	Often	Pink	Regeneration
Deep dermal	Analgesic	Occasional	White/yellow	Repair
Full thickness	Anaesthetic	None	Grey/olive	Contraction

Superficial burns heal by regeneration from undamaged keratinocytes in hair follicles, sebaceous glands and sweat glands. Deep dermal burns mostly heal by repair but are capable of some regeneration from the deeper situated sweat glands. They are treated by tangential excision (shaving) using a skin graft knife between the third and fifth day to preserve the deeper dermis which would otherwise die. This is because the interface between viable and non-viable tissue deepens from the time of injury due to thrombosis of the microcirculation. Grafts take well on this prepared surface. Full thickness burns are treated by excision and skin cover. If small, the surrounding skin can be sutured directly over the defect. Defects over the face, palms and pressure areas or over denuded perichondrium, periosteum or paratenon require full thickness skin cover. Larger defects are covered with meshed split skin which is expanded to allow blood, pus and serum to escape through the interstices.

Electrical burns

Electrical burns are usually much deeper than the skin wound might suggest because current flows preferentially along nerves, muscle and blood vessels rather than the skin. They should be treated aggressively with early debridement and grafting.

Acid/alkali burns

Acid burns damage tissues by coagulative necrosis and alkaline burns (e.g. cement) damage by a slower, more prolonged colliquative necrosis. Treatment consists of immediate immersion in running water until wound pH has returned to normal. This may take several hours with alkaline burns.

Further reading

Clarke J. Current management in burns. *Current Practice in Surgery*, 1990; **2**: 227–31.

Related topics of interest

CALF PUMP FAILURE AND VENOUS ULCERATION

The calf pump failure syndrome comprises dermatological and subcutaneous changes developing after any condition impairing calf pump function (varicose veins, DVT). The prevalence of venous ulceration (the end-point of calf pump failure) is 0.1–0.25%, and 40–60% of such patients have post-thrombotic changes. Milder calf pump failure is much commoner. The annual cost of treating venous ulcers in the UK is £230–400 million.

Pathophysiology

Calf pump failure occurs because of an inability to reduce superficial venous pressure during exercise as a result of one or more of the following:

1. *Valvular incompetence*
- Deep vein reflux (post-thrombotic or non-thrombotic).
- Communicating vein reflux (post-thrombotic or non-thrombotic).
- Superficial vein reflux (varicose veins).

2. *Outflow tract obstruction*
- Post-thrombotic.

3. *Muscle pump failure*
- Primary (neuromuscular disorders, stroke).
- Secondary (ankle stiffness).

The underlying pathological events are varicose veins, post-thrombotic damage to the deep and/or communicating veins and non-thrombotic deep vein incompetence. The effects of these factors are countered by poorly understood phenomena that protect tissues against venous hypertension (the fibrinolytic capacity of the skin and subcutaneous tissues), many patients who have poor calf pump function never developing the syndrome.

Several theories have been proposed to explain the effects of calf pump failure on the microcirculation:
- Stasis (venous stasis causing desaturation and tissue hypoxia – disproven).
- Arteriovenous shunts (no evidence).
- Fibrin cuff (fibrin cuff exists but unclear if it impedes gas exchange).
- The white cell theory (activated white cells release toxic metabolites – unproven).

Clinical presentation

The clinical features are:
- Aching.
- Venous claudication.
- Swelling.
- Varicose veins.
- Incompetent communicating veins.
- Pigmentation.
- Eczema.
- Lipodermatosclerosis.
- Atrophie blanche.
- Ankle stiffness.
- Ulceration.

Ulceration is the end-point of the calf pump failure syndrome. Lipodermatosclerosis is frequently present before an ulcer develops, and local trauma is often an initiating factor. Post-thrombotic ulcers are usually intractable and even when healed often recur.

Investigation

1. Anatomical and functional assessment
- Define anatomy of any varicose veins. Varicograms/ saphenograms if necessary.
- Ascending phlebography. Demonstrate post-thrombotic damage, incompetent communicating veins. Both legs should be investigated.
- Duplex ultrasound. To detect significant deep vein reflux (30–60% of patients).
- Plethysmography or foot vein pressure measurement to determine efficiency of calf pump.
- Femoral vein pressure measurements. If bypass surgery considered for iliac vein occlusion. A rise of 10 mmHg or more indicates significant iliac vein obstruction.

2. Prothrombotic screen
- Including FBC, antithrombin III, proteins S, C, plasma fibrinogen, lupus anticoagulant.

3. Differential diagnosis of leg ulcers
- Doppler ankle pressure (arterial disease/ulcer).
- Urinalysis/blood glucose (diabetic ulcers).
- ESR/rheumatoid serology (rheumatoid or arteritic ulceration).
- VDRL (syphilitic ulceration – rare).
- Skin biopsy (malignant ulcers).
- Sickle cell test (sickle cell ulcers).
- Self-inflicted (dermatitis artefacta).

Treatment

Most treatment is palliative.

1. Compression and elevation. Prolonged elevation reduces venous pressure at rest, relieving most symptoms and healing almost all ulcers. Graduated compression reduces the transmural venous pressure by increasing the surrounding tissue pressure. Class III elastic stockings exert 30–40 mmHg pressure at the ankle and lower pressures (20–30 mmHg) at the knee. Below-knee stockings are prescribed for all patients and should be worn continuously when the patient is out of bed.

2. Superficial and communicating vein reflux. Where superficial and/or communicating vein incompetence contributes to calf pump failure, high saphenous ligation and stripping should be performed. Ligation of incompetent communicating veins is highly successful in limbs with non-thrombotic deep veins. This can now be performed laparoscopically but is unclear whether it will replace the more traditional subfascial ligation (Cockett's operation).

3. Deep vein obstruction. Bypass surgery. Anatomical and functional obstruction must be demonstrated. Only 2% of patients are suitable.

The Palma procedure is used for unilateral iliac vein obstruction, and the Warren–Thayer bypass for femoral vein occlusion. The 5-year patencies are 80% and 55%, respectively. Inferior vena caval occlusion may be bypassed with a PTFE graft if conservative methods fail. Patency rates are 70–90% up to 1 year after implantation.

4. Deep vein reflux. There must be evidence of significant deep venous reflux demonstrated by duplex ultrasound and calf pump function tests.

Direct valve repair (valvuloplasty) to tighten floppy valve cusps and indirect valvuloplasty to compress the valve sinus with a collar restoring cusp apposition (venocuff) can be used in patients with non-thrombotic deep vein reflux.

Valve transposition which employs anastomosis of incompetent superficial femoral veins to valve-bearing segments of either long saphenous or profunda femoris veins has not proved durable.

Valve autotransplantation has become the most widely practised form of valve replacement. A valve-bearing segment of the axillary vein is resected and transplanted into either the femoral or popliteal veins. Patients are encouraged to continue wearing graduated compression stockings and anticoagulants are given for a short period.

Long-term benefit of these procedures remains uncertain and their use limited.

Ulcer healing

Layered graduated compression bandaging remains the most useful treatment for healing venous ulcers, the various different bandages and topical agents available offering no demonstrable benefit. Bandages comprise a paste inner layer, elastic compression middle layer and weaker elastic protective outer layer. Bandages and dressings should ideally reduce pain, be non-allergenic, prevent ulcer desiccation, and be easy to change, whilst remaining inexpensive.

1. Pharmacological agents
- Fibrinolytic agents. Reduce lipodermatosclerosis but do not heal ulcers.
- Hydroxyrutosides. May reduce oedema and discomfort.
- Prostaglandins. Prolonged infusion may improve ulcer healing.
- Methylxanthines. Oxypentifyline may speed ulcer healing.

2. Ulcer excision and skin grafting. When ulcers fail to heal with compression bandaging, split skin grafting should be considered. The ulcer base should be tangentially excised and meshed split skin grafts applied immediately or after a few days dressing when the granulation tissue has started to form.

Further reading

Browse NL, Burnand KG, Lea Thomas M. *Diseases of the Veins: Pathology, Diagnosis and Treatment.* London: Edward Arnold, 1988.
Wilson NM, Burnand KG. The post-thrombotic syndrome. *Current Practice in Surgery,* 1994; **6**: 47–55.

Related topics of interest

CARCINOMA OF THE BLADDER

Superficial transitional cell carcinoma (TCC) of the bladder is the fifth commonest carcinoma in males and the tenth in females. Seventy per cent behave in a benign manner and are kept under control by regular cystoscopy and resection.

Superficial TCC

Risk factors

Carcinogens causally associated with bladder TCC include benzidine, coal tar pitches, and β-napthylamine, and the increased incidence in males results from their predisposition to outflow obstruction. Occupations involving printing, dyeing, rubber and coal carry an increased risk together with laboratory and leather workers and hairdressers. There is a strong association with smoking.

Presentation

Patients usually present over the age of 40 with painless terminal haematuria. This finding is more significant in men since menstrual contamination is excluded. Other presentations include recurrent UTI (the tumour bed is an excellent culture medium), a sterile pyuria and painful frequency.

Cytology

Urine cytology has been used to screen for disease in occupations of high risk and provides a rough indication of tumour advancement, since extensive tumours are more likely to exfoliate their malignant cells into the urine.

Intravenous urography

This permits imaging of the upper tracts as well as the bladder. Ureteric obstruction can occasionally be identified. A bladder carcinoma is demonstrated as a filling defect. A postmicturition film often provides increased detail of the tumour extent.

Cystoscopy

This should be performed in all patients in whom the disease is suspected. The urological dictum 'anyone with haematuria should be investigated with a cystoscopy and an IVU' still holds true. The typical cystoscopic appearance of a superficial tumour is a luxuriant fronded structure arising from a flat surface. Red patches or solid tumours are more sinister usually indicating *in situ* or invasive disease, respectively. Tumours are resected and any red areas are biopsied with four random biopsies of apparently normal endothelium. Careful bimanual palpation is mandatory before and after resection for staging purposes. A palpable mass before resection indicates at least invasion into superficial muscle. If the mass is palpable after resection it has invaded into deep muscle. Follow up is by regular flexible cystoscopy as a day case procedure.

Grade/stage

Tumour cells are graded on histology from 1 to 3 corresponding to well, moderate or poor differentiation. The extent of spread, or staging, of the local tumour is determined pathologically and clinically.

Pis	*in situ*
Pa	Papillary, non-invasive
P1	Lamina propria invasion
P2	Into superficial muscle
P3a	Deep muscle invasion
P3b	Into perivesical tissue
P4a	Prostate invasion
P4b	Extravesical (pelvic wall)

Superficial disease (Pa), which comprises 70%, falls into four behaviour patterns. A quarter never develop recurrence, a quarter develop single recurrences from time to time, a further quarter develop multiple low activity recurrences and the final quarter multiple high activity recurrences. Sixty-six per cent of patients with poorly differentiated superficial disease progress to invasive carcinoma. Despite this, superficial disease metastasizes in less than 1% of patients.

Intravesical chemotherapy

Mitomycin or adriamycin are usually used to prevent the frequent, numerous recurrences that are difficult to control cystoscopically. The regime is tailored to the patient such that the minimum effective dose is administered for the shortest time that will keep the bladder tidy.

Cystectomy

This is required for uncontrollable superficial disease. This treatment, though radical, results in a 90% cure rate.

Other therapeutic methods

These include laser coagulation (YAG laser), photodynamic therapy (the administration of a photosensitizing drug selectively taken up by the lesion followed by panvesical laser delivery) and immunotherapy with BCG. The intravesical and intradermal administration of the Montreal strain of BCG reports a response rate of 60% in 2 years. Radiotherapy has little influence on superficial disease control.

Carcinoma-*in-situ*

Carcinoma-*in-situ* is dangerous and requires prompt aggressive treatment. It exists in two separate forms.

Normal endothelium This occurs as a positive biopsy of apparently normal endothelium remote or adjacent to the presenting tumour. This finding with a P1 lesion predicts that 50% of patients will progress to invasive disease in 2 years.

Malignant cystitis This presents with pain, dysuria, frequency and haematuria. Urine cytology is nearly always positive and cystoscopy reveals areas of inflammation which on biopsy demonstrate generalized malignant change. Treatment involves intravesical mitomycin or BCG with frequent urine cytology and cystoscopic biopsy. Radical cystoprostatourethrectomy is indicated for relapse.

Invasive TCC

Invasive TCC is by far the commonest invasive bladder cancer comprising 30% of TCCs at presentation. Squamous cell carcinoma is common in schistosomiasis endemic areas (the squamous metaplasia of papillary fronds is of little significance). Adenocarcinoma is occasionally located to the urachus in which case a partial cystectomy can be curative.

Investigations Investigations should determine the presence or absence of nodal and distant disease with a CXR, bone scan and abdominal and pelvic CT. Nodes greater than 1 cm are suspicious and require biopsy. The recent advent of laparoscopic pelvic lymphadenectomy has been advocated for the determination of lymph node status.

Treatment The prognosis of all the invasive carcinomas is very poor. The aim is to control local disease which is traditionally carried out by cystoprostatourethrectomy. Pelvic lymphadenectomy, external beam radiotherapy and chemotherapy in various combinations improve the prognosis. Most patients are too frail and elderly for multimodality treatment, which is generally reserved for those under 65 years. Impotence is a common sequela of radical surgery unless the periprostatic neurovascular bundles are preserved. The standard UK management involves either radical radiotherapy followed by salvage cystectomy or pre-operative radiotherapy and elective cystectomy using an ileal conduit for diversion.

Occasionally the appendix can be mobilized on its vascular pedicle to provide a more continent diversion (the Mitrofanoff procedure).

Further reading

Woodhouse CJ. Superficial transitional cell carcinoma of the bladder. Carcinoma *in situ* and invasive disease. *Surgery*, 1992; 133–43.

Related topic of interest

Urinary outflow obstruction (p. 322)

CARCINOMA OF THE PROSTATE

The incidence of prostatic adenocarcinoma increases with age. It is rare below 50, and less common in the Japanese. The highest incidence is seen amongst blacks in the USA. Autopsy studies demonstrate evidence of the disease in about 60% of men over 80 years of age.

Presentation

Seventy per cent of patients present with symptoms of bladder outflow obstruction. Other patients may present with a prostatic nodule found incidentally during a rectal examination. Advanced local disease may cause deep peroneal pain or renal failure from chronic retention or ureteric encroachment. The remainder present with evidence of metastatic disease: bone pain (ribs, spine, pelvis), leg lymphoedema from nodal disease, deep vein thrombosis, anaemia from marrow destruction or, rarely, cord or nerve root compression.

Diagnosis

Most patients will have symptoms that justify a transurethral resection irrespective of whether carcinoma is present. This will provide tissue for histology and confirm the diagnosis. In symptomless patients a prostate biopsy is required. This is effected by a transrectal or transperineal route using a Tru-Cut biopsy needle guided either by a finger or with a transrectal ultrasound probe (TRUS).

Tumour markers

Prostatic specific antigen (PSA) is a very sensitive marker for prostatic cancer although minimal blood elevations may occur with benign prostatic hyperplasia. Levels usually fall in response to local or systemic treatment, and elevated values may predict a relapse. Prostatic acid phosphatase (PAP) is much less sensitive; however, significantly elevated levels indicate the likelihood of bone metastasis.

Staging

Local staging accuracy by rectal examination can be improved by using TRUS. Hypoechoic areas indicate malignancy. A CT scan can detect pelvic and abdominal lymphadenopathy but is poor at delineating the prostate itself. A positive bone scan is an unfavourable prognostic indicator. Care must be taken in interpretation because extensive widespread uptake can be mistaken as a normal scan. Staging is completed with chest and abdominal radiographs, and an IVU or renal ultrasound to detect possible upper tract delay.

Screening

Screening by PSA to all males over 50 years of age will identify a subpopulation suitable for TRUS. This would be extremely expensive and possibly of limited value because an effective treatment for early disease is not available. The natural history of screen-detected tumours is unknown.

Radical prostatectomy

The radical retropubic cavernous-sparing prostatectomy is popular in the USA for tumours confined to the capsule of the gland on TRUS. A preliminary open or laparoscopic pelvic lymphadenectomy is first required to determine node negative disease. The radical prostatectomy involves dividing the prostatic vessel branches close to the gland itself so that the cavernous nerves are spared because impotence is a common complication. Good results have been published but the procedure has not gained popularity in Europe. The natural history of untreated local disease is also favourable and there is no high risk of impotence or incontinence.

Radiotherapy

1. Local. External beam radiotherapy is the commonest form of local therapy for early and advanced local disease. In the aged population the prognosis of men with bone scan negative disease, as far as death is concerned, is not too bad. Consequently, a good case can be made for deferring such treatment until symptoms occur. The side effects of local radiotherapy include radiation cystitis and colovesical fistula. Interstitial radiotherapy using TRUS-placed radio-iodine-131 seeds is not often used in Europe.

2. Systemic. Bone pain from relapsing disease can be treated effectively by local irradiation. Strontium-89 can be administered as a single injection to be taken up into osteoblastic metastasis. It also provides effective palliation for bone pain.

Hormonal manipulation

Prostatic adenocarcinoma is very sensitive to hormonal manipulation. Despite this, there is no difference in survival with immediate hormone therapy compared with deferred therapy. If immediate hormone therapy is effected, a powerful tool for symptom control would be lost should the patient subsequently develop symptoms. Most urologists decide upon deferred therapy with careful monitoring for ureteric obstruction by upper tract ultrasound and serum electrolytes. Should this develop, urgent hormone treatment is indicated. Three-quarters of patients treated for symptoms develop a useful subjective response. Most patients relapse after 2 years. Endogenous androgens enhance the growth of prostatic adenocarcinoma. These can be blocked by oestrogens, orchidectomy, LHRH analogues, progestogens and anti-androgens.

1. Oestrogens. These are rarely used today. Formerly, the oestrogen diethylstilboestrol was considered so effective that it was administered on the mere suspicion of a urologist's finger. The unacceptable side effects of fluid retention are dose related, and can precipitate cardiac failure, especially in the elderly.

2. Orchidectomy. Although superceded by LHRH analogues, orchidectomy is very effective and remains a useful option. It can be performed under the same anaesthetic as a TURP. The subcapsular operation involves complete avulsion of the contents of the tunica albugenia. It partially alleviates the stigma of castration because a 'testis' of epididymis and plicated capsule is left behind.

3. LHRH analogues. Goserelin (Zoladex) is a depot synthetic analogue of LHRH which is implanted subcutaneously every month. It initially causes temporary stimulation followed by inhibition causing testosterone levels to fall into the castrate range. Patients at risk of spinal cord compression from spinal metastases should be covered with cyproterone acetate during the first few weeks in order to offset this initial period of stimulation.

4. Cyproterone acetate. The progestogen, cyproterone acetate, acts centrally by inhibiting the release of LH and peripherally as a competitive antagonist of testosterone. Its main use is as second-line therapy for relapse.

5. Total androgen blockade. Aminoglutethamide blocks all androgen production within the body including the adrenal androgens. There is no conclusive evidence yet that it is superior to LHRH analogues but further trials are awaited.

Further reading

Kirk D. The current management of prostatic adenocarcinoma. *Current Practice in Surgery*, 1991; **3**: 113–7.

Related topic of interest

Urinary outflow obstruction (p. 322)

CEREBROVASCULAR DISEASE

Stroke is the third leading cause of death in developed countries and a major cause of morbidity. Although hypertension and embolization from cardiac causes are major causes for stroke, between 17% and 24% of ischaemic strokes are due to carotid artery disease. The North American Symptomatic Carotid Endarterectomy Trial (NASCET) and the European Carotid Surgery Trial (ECST) have both demonstrated clear benefits of carotid endarterectomy in patients with severe stenosis by the prevention of stroke.

Pathology

Atherosclerosis is the most common pathology of carotid artery disease. It occurs almost exclusively within 2–3 cm of the carotid bifurcation. Transient neurological events are the main symptoms that occur in patients and these may precede a stroke. Symptoms are usually due to plaque degeneration, with the release of platelet, cholesterol or thrombotic emboli, but are occasionally due to cerebral hypoperfusion. Fibromuscular dysplasia is a rare cause that occurs predominantly in young women. Medial hyperplasia is the underlying pathology that occurs in a segmental fashion. This is observed radiologically by a beaded appearance of the vessels. Other rare causes include arteritis (temporal artery, lupus erythematosus, polyarteritis nodosa, Takayasu's disease), trauma, irradiation injury and aneurysmal disease (atherosclerotic, syphilitic, fungal or following trauma).

Clinical examination

The common carotid artery is evaluated by a carotid impulse on palpation and a bruit on auscultation. It is important to recognize that the internal carotid artery is usually not palpable in the neck and may be occluded despite the presence of a good neck pulsation. The presence of radial and superficial temporal pulses should be noted and any delay between both sides recorded. Blood pressure should be taken in both arms to evaluate any potential proximal disease. The presence of rubeosis or a reduced intraoccular pressure (occuloplethysmography) may indicate hypoperfusion secondary to a carotid stenosis or occlusion. The presence of retinal cholesterol emboli confirms an embolic cause.

Diagnosis

All patients presenting with transient ischaemic attacks should have a duplex examination of their carotid arteries. Detection of a heterogeneous plaque or a severe or critical stenosis should prompt an intravenous digital subtraction arteriogram (IVDSA) to confirm these findings. A peak systolic velocity of greater than 1.25 m/s with marked spectoral broadening indicates a significant stenosis on duplex. A reduction in diameter by 70%, or more, indicates a significant stenosis on arteriography. Intra-arterial arch studies (IADSA) give better resolution in doubtful cases. Selective catheterization of the common carotid artery origin should be avoided if possible as this can occasionally dislodge plaque-derived emboli. A cerebral CT scan is performed to exclude the presence of unsuspecting pathology and as a baseline prior to endarterectomy. The presence of lacunar infarcts is noted. Referral to a neurologist for a second opinion is desirable if an endarterectomy is considered.

Carotid endarterectomy

The most common indication for carotid endarterectomy is in recurrent transient ischaemic events or amaurosis fugax when the ipsilateral carotid artery is confirmed as being responsible. This operation is also indicated for non-stenotic atherosclerotic ulcers and in symptomless patients with a high grade stenosis, as prophylaxis against stroke prior to cardiac bypass surgery. The benefits of endarterectomy for asymptomatic patients with critical or severe stenosis are yet to be determined and multicentre trials are in progress to clarify this controversy (Asymptomatic Carotid Surgery Trial, ACST). An endarterectomy itself can cause a stroke in 1–4% of patients. Placement of a saphenous vein or prosthetic patch increases the luminal area and is performed on a selective basis by most surgeons. The use of a Pruitt or Javid bypass shunt during the operation reduces cerebral ischaemia time. Measurement of the carotid 'stump pressure' may help in deciding whether a shunt is necessary. Shunts can, however, cause intimal damage beyond the endarterectomized region. Endarterectomy of the external carotid artery is occasionally performed in patients when a reduced collateral contribution from this artery to cerebral blood flow is considered significant in the production of symptoms.

Intraoperative monitoring

Perioperative duplex scanning, completion arteriography and middle cerebral artery Doppler are the most frequently used methods to assess the immediate success of carotid endarterectomy. These methods may detect intimal flaps, dissection, spasm and residual disease, correction of which could improve the clinical outcome.

Follow-up

The majority of patients receive aspirin (75 mg once per day) after carotid endarterectomy. The benefits of this drug in reducing recurrent symptoms and in preventing restenosis is, however, marginal. Any effect on mortality is due to a reduction in cardiac-related deaths.

Restenosis

The introduction of non-invasive methods of detection, like occuloplethysmography and duplex, has increased the incidence of this condition from 1–4% to 6–37%. Restenosis within two years is usually due to myointimal hyperplasia and thereafter due to recurrent atheroma. Revision surgery is indicated for patients who present with symptoms but the literature is divided as to whether a repeat operation is of benefit in symptomless patients. This has led several centres to discontinue routine postoperative surveillance by duplex. Symptomless patients with recurrent stenosis are marginally more likely to develop symptoms than those with a symptomless primary stenosis, however, revision surgery is technically more difficult with an increase in morbidity and stroke rates.

Carotid angioplasty

The Carotid and Vertebral Artery Transluminal Angioplasty Study (CAVATAS) has increased awareness in using angioplasty as a less invasive alternative to surgery in treating carotid stenosis. Distal and intracranial stenoses can easily be reached. Plaque remodelling and stabilization is the proposed mechanism by which this technique works. Initial results are promising but the considerable amount of particulate microembolization that is detected by transcranial Doppler during this procedure has led many vascular surgeons not to recommend this approach.

Further reading

Bernstein EF, Callow AD, Nicolaides AN, Shifrin EG. *Cerebral Revascularisation*. London: Med-Orion, 1993.
Burnard KG, Lattimer CR. Intraoperative duplex scanning and completion DSA in the assessment of carotid endarterectomy. In: Greenhalgh RM (ed.) *Vascular Imaging for Surgeons*. London: W.B. Saunders, 1995; 129–39.

Related topics of interest

CHEST TRAUMA

Chest injuries may be blunt or penetrating, blast injuries frequently involving a combination of these. Fewer than 15% of chest injuries require surgery. Tube thoracostomy, blood or fluid replacement, oxygen therapy and analgesia are the mainstay of treatment in most patients.

Treatment approach

Primary survey, resuscitation, secondary survey and definitive care are undertaken as described in Trauma management – principles (p. 301).

Specific chest injuries

1. Uncomplicated rib fracture. A common injury. Pain impedes respiration facilitating retention of secretions, atelectasis and infection, particularly in those with pre-existing respiratory disease. Injury to the upper ribs (1–3) usually implies a severe injury. Ribs 4–9 sustain the majority of injuries. Localized pain, tenderness and crepitus indicate a fracture. An erect CXR must be performed to identify associated injuries rather than to identify fractures accurately. A short course of non-steroidal analgesics may be given if not contraindicated. Alternatively, local infiltration of the fractures with bupivacaine or thoracic epidural analgesia may be necessary.

2. Simple pneumothorax. Lung laceration caused by blunt or penetrating injury is the most common cause. Air in the pleural space results in lung collapse and a consequent ventilation–perfusion mismatch. Reduced hemithorax movement, dyspnoea, hyperresonance and reduced breath sounds are usually detected. An erect CXR (especially in expiration) will show the collapsed lung, but needle aspiration will establish the diagnosis if the patient is *in extremis*. Pneumothorax associated with other injuries should be treated using an intercostal tube drain inserted to the apex of the pleural cavity. General anaesthesia, ventilation and air transport should not be undertaken until a drain has been inserted.

3. Open pneumothorax. Most penetrating wounds close themselves, but large defects may persist causing a sucking chest wound and impairing ventilation. The defect should be covered by a large occlusive dressing (taped on three sides to create a flutter valve, allowing air to escape during expiration) until surgical closure can be performed.

4. *Tension pneumothorax.* A one-way valve effect occurs allowing air to pass into the pleural space either from the lung or through the chest wall. The lung collapses and the mediastinum is displaced towards the opposite hemithorax further impairing ventilation and impeding venous return. Dyspnoea, cyanosis, tracheal deviation, hyperresonance, absent breath sounds and raised venous pressure are the cardinal signs. Immediate decompression should be performed by inserting a needle into the second intercostal space in the midclavicular line. An intercostal tube drain should be inserted as soon as possible.

5. *Flail segment.* This occurs where multiple rib fractures allow an island of chest wall to move independently of the rest of the chest wall. The free-floating segment moves paradoxically, reducing the efficiency of the chest wall excursion in expanding and deflating the lung. More important, however, is the injury to the underlying lung which is the more potent cause of hypoxia. Dyspnoea, poor chest movement, the identification of a segment moving paradoxically and crepitus of rib or cartilage fractures are the physical signs. A CXR may show multiple fractures. Patients with flail chest often compensate adequately in the first 24–48 hours and then rapidly develop respiratory failure. Treatment includes adequate analgesia, oxygen therapy, intravenous fluids. Intercostal tube drainage may be necessary if there is a co-existent pneumothorax. Ventilation may be necessary if respiratory failure supervenes.

6. *Haemothorax.* Massive haemothorax (blood loss > 1500 ml) occurs following disruption of major intrathoracic vessels, usually by a penetrating wound. Poor respiratory movement, dullness to percussion, absent breath sounds and shock are prominent. An erect CXR is required to detect even the presence of large volumes of blood. Pneumothorax may co-exist. Intravenous lines for transfusion are necessary and a large-bore intercostal drain is placed to drain the dependent areas of the thorax. Continuing blood loss of 200–300 ml/hour necessitates thoracotomy. Wounds medial to the nipple or the scapula indicate possible mediastinal trauma.

7. *Pulmonary contusion.* Localized oedema may result from blunt trauma, but widespread pulmonary oedema may also occur in response to primary lung injury in the presence of

normal cardiac filling pressures (ARDS). The alveolar transudate impedes gas exchange resulting in respiratory failure. Ventilation may become necessary, especially in those with pre-existing pulmonary disease, impaired consciousness, other concomitant injuries and multisystem organ failure.

8. Tracheobronchial tree injuries. Penetrating tracheal injuries are often associated with oesophageal, carotid and jugular injuries and require prompt surgical exploration and repair. A major bronchial injury is unusual and often fatal. Patients present with haemoptysis, surgical emphysema and pneumothorax. A persisting large air leak after intercostal tube drainage suggests bronchial injury. Surgical repair is necessary in most patients.

9. Cardiac tamponade. This usually results from a penetrating injury. Physical signs include hypotension, raised venous pressure, muffled heart sounds and pulsus paradoxus. Pericardiocentesis should be attempted but open pericardiotomy and arrest of haemorrhage may be required.

10. Aortic rupture. Aortic rupture is the commonest cause of death following major trauma and usually occurs at the ligamentum arteriosum or the aortic root. In survivors, a thin layer of adventitia persists and a contained haematoma extends into the mediastinum. A CXR showing a widened mediastinum is often the first indication, and arteriography and CT scanning should be performed to confirm the diagnosis. Immediate surgical repair is necessary.

11. Myocardial contusion. Blunt trauma, especially to the left chest wall, is the usual mechanism. Premature ventricular contractions, ST segment changes, sinus tachycardia and right bundle branch block may be evident on the ECG. Continuous cardiac monitoring is mandatory because sudden dysrhythmias may supervene.

12. Oesophageal injury. Penetrating trauma (usually by instrumentation) is the commonest injury, but forceful ejection of gastric contents into the oesophagus with the glottis closed may lead to oesophageal rupture (Boerhaave syndrome). Mediastinitis and empyema follow and are usually fatal. Left haemothorax/pneumothorax without rib fracture or the presence of mediastinal air suggest and

Gastrografin swallow confirms the diagnosis. Tube drainage and antibiotics with subsequent direct surgical repair of the defect should be undertaken if possible.

13. Diaphragmatic rupture. Blunt trauma, usually to the abdomen, causes large radial tears leading to immediate herniation and respiratory embarrassment. Over 90% are on the left. Penetrating injuries produce small defects that do not usually cause immediate herniation. The diagnosis is frequently missed, but the CXR may reveal viscera in the chest. Surgical repair is necessary.

Further reading

ATLS Core Handbook. American College of Surgeons, Chicago, 1993.
Goldstraw P. The chest wall, lungs, pleura and diaphragm. In: Burnand KG, Young AE (eds) *The New Aird's Companion in Surgical Studies.* Edinburgh: Churchill Livingstone, 1992; 723–60.
Westaby S. Resuscitation in thoracic trauma. *British Journal of Surgery,* 1994; **81**: 929–31.

Related topic of interest

Trauma management – principles (p. 301)

CHOLANGIOCARCINOMA

Cholangiocarcinoma (bile duct carcinoma) is increasing in incidence. It differs from gall bladder carcinoma in two respects. Firstly, the sex incidence is equal compared with a male-to-female ratio with gall bladder carcinoma of 1:4 and secondly, the presence of bile duct stones occurs in almost 100% of cases of gall bladder cancer whereas they are present in less than 40% of patients with cholangiocarcinoma. It is rare for anyone to survive either condition for more than 2 years. The usual life expectancy for cholangiocarcinoma is 3–6 months.

Classification

Classification is into hilar/intrahepatic (50%), middle third (25%) and lower third (25%), the latter including ampullary lesions. Hilar cholangiocarcinomas are often termed Klatskin tumours and are occasionally classified together with primary liver tumours.

Predisposing factors

In contrast to hepatocellular carcinoma, there is no association with hepatitis B infection. The following factors increase the probability of developing a cholangio-carcinoma.

1. Clonorchis sinensis. A liver fluke infestation common in south-east Asia.

2. Sclerosing cholangitis. This is associated with ulcerative colitis.

3. Anabolic sterioids. In some patients these behave like an exogenous carcinogen.

4. Congenital abnormalities. Choledochal cysts and the intrahepatic cysts of Caroli's disease both predispose.

5. Papillomatosis. Controversy arises as to whether the solitary benign polyp or multiple duct polyps are premalignant.

Presentation

This is usually with jaundice (90%), pruritis or epigastric pains. Occasionally, episodes of cholangitis occur and a right hypochondrial mass may be palpable. Weight loss, anaemia and ascites indicate advanced disease.

Spread

Spread is by local encasement of the bile ducts, the portal vein and the hepatic artery, and then by direct liver invasion. Metastatic spread to surrounding portal, pyloric or coeliac nodes is common. Occasionally, the disease is multifocal with secondary deposits occurring within the duct system or throughout the liver substance.

Investigations

The choice of investigation depends upon whether it is to be undertaken to establish a diagnosis or to determine resectability.

1. Ultrasound. An ultrasound is non-invasive, cheap, usually identifies a dilated duct system and may identify a mass.

2. CT scan. A CT scan is often equally unrewarding because cholangiocarcinoma has a similar density to the liver and enhances to the same extent after the administration of intravenous contrast. It may detect multifocal disease, non-specific enlarged lymph nodes or encasement of the portal vein, hepatic artery and bile ducts, and thereby indicate non-resectability. Suspicious lesions should be biopsied under CT or ultrasound guidance. Histologically, the lesions are adenocarcinomas of varying differentiation (well, moderate or poor).

3. PTC/ERCP. The extent of local spread is best identified with percutaneous transhepatic cholangiography (PTC), endoscopic retrograde cholangiopancreatography (ERCP) or both combined. Bile should be analysed by cytology and culture. Klatskin tumours classically visualize as three strands radiating from the confluence, the so-called 'Mercedes sign'. Care must be taken to inject the right and left duct systems separately and to take delayed films if maximum information is to be obtained with PTC. All bile duct instrumentations should only be undertaken after an international normalized ratio (INR), activated partial thromboplastin time (APPT), haemoglobin and platelet estimations, and a sample for cross-match. The procedure must be covered with intravenous antibiotics against biliary pathogens and full surgical facilities should be available should a need arise. Infected bile is associated with a high mortality.

4. Angiography. This will add to the investigations by confirming vascular involvement and planning operative strategy.

Resection

The aim of treatment is to excise the tumour and restore bile flow into the bowel. This approach offers the best palliation and longer survival time and may offer a chance of cure. Surgery also offers a confident histological diagnosis after resection or bypass that other treatment modalities may fail to provide. Resection, though, is often not possible because of the proximity of the tumour to major vessels, and patient factors like the infirmity of old age or serious concurrent medical illness which result in unacceptable mortality rates. If the obstruction is not relieved, death results from liver failure and cholangitis. Hepatic transplantation has been performed in several centres for these tumours but recurrence (accelerated by immunosuppressive agents) and death usually occur within 12 months. Lower third and ampullary lesions have the highest resectability rates of all the cholangiocarcinomas. They should be treated by local excision or a radical pancreaticoduodenectomy (Whipple's operation).

Bypass

If resection is not possible then bypass should be considered. This can be performed surgically by fashioning a Roux-en-Y loop and joining it to a duct proximal to the tumour. The left hepatic duct is preferred because it is long and has a shallow intrahepatic course, and can be dissected free from the liver by lowering the hepatic plate. It is usually approached by following the round ligament down to the liver hilum. It drains hepatic segment III (segment III by-pass).

Stenting

Palliative stenting has an equivalent mortality to surgical bypass. The methods used are improving due to the use of self-expanding stents and the realization that the larger the stent the less likelihood there is of displacement. They can be deployed percutaneously from above (PTC) or endoscopically from below (ERCP), or by a combined technique. If stent placement fails on the first attempt, a period of biliary decompression should relieve any oedema and may make subsequent passage possible. The Lundquist stent is an intero-external stent that allows both internal and external drainage to take place. External drainage is usually required during the first 24 hours to allow blood and debris to clear before internal drainage commences. Should the internal part of the stent later occlude, external drainage may resume. Intero-external stents also allow the placement of irridium-192 wire. There are no reported controlled trials which accurately assess whether chemotherapy, radiotherapy or brachytherapy improves survival or palliation.

Further reading

Blumgart LH, Studley JGN. Surgical treatment of tumours of the liver and hepatic ducts. *Recent Advances in Surgery*, 1988; **13**: 63–82.
Dawson JL, Heaton ND. Carcinoma of the biliary tree and gallbladder. *Surgery,* 1992; 84–7.

Related topics of interest

Gallstones and their complications (p. 139)
Jaundice – investigation (p. 189)
Ulcerative colitis (p. 305)

CHRONIC PANCREATITIS

Chronic pancreatitis may be defined as repeated episodes of inflammatory pancreatitis combined with evidence of structural damage to the pancreas. The damage usually starts in the duct system, and is characterized by ductal stenoses, which are frequently multiple with dilated portions in between.

Aetiology

The vast majority of cases of chronic pancreatitis result from alcohol, though the exact mechanism remains obscure. The anatomical abnormality of pancreas divisum accounts probably for more cases than is generally thought. This is due to the persistence of the embryological ductal drainage of the ventral and dorsal pancreatic portions. The dorsal part comprising the bulk of the pancreas remains drained by what in the normal pancreas becomes the accessory (smaller) duct of Santorini. The ventral pancreatic bud, which rotates to form the lower part of the pancreatic head and uncinate process, freely drains through a wide duct, which should join the main duct of Wirsung allowing free drainage of the major (dorsal) portion of the pancreas. Gallstones passing through the lower portion of the common bile duct can damage the pancreatic duct and result in not only acute pancreatitis, but rarely chronic pancreatitis. Essentially, any cause of acute pancreatitis may result in chronic pancreatitis if there are repeated episodes, or if damage to the pancreatic ductal system results.

Clinical examination

The symptoms are pain, in 95% of patients, which is usually epigastric and possibly radiating to the back, and weight loss, which is usually marked and clinically evident. The pain may be severe and protracted and, occasionally, patients become reliant on opiate analgesics for relief. Less common symptoms include steatorrhoea, jaundice or symptoms of diabetes mellitus. A raised amylase is not a reliable indicator of chronic pancreatitis, as the exocrine pancreas is very often damaged to such an extent that the production of amylase is limited. Even in acute attacks occurring in chronic pancreatitis, the amylase is rarely raised significantly. Eighty per cent of sufferers are male, and most are middle aged. The prevalence of this condition is approximately 3/100 000.

Investigations

Endoscopic retrograde cholangiopancreatography (ERCP) is the only method to establish the diagnosis of chronic pancreatitis with certainty. This endoscopic procedure is performed under sedation as an out-patient. A side-viewing gastroscope is passed into the duodenum, and the ampulla of Vater is cannulated via a side arm through which contrast is injected. X-rays are taken which show both the biliary tree and pancreatic duct. In the realms of chronic pancreatitis, ERCP is a diagnostic tool rather than therapeutic.

Plain abdominal radiographs may demonstrate small flecks of calcification in the head and body of the pancreas. This is highly suggestive of chronic pancreatitis. The calcification may also be seen on CT scanning. Pancreatic cysts are common in chronic pancreatitis, and these may be visualized by ultrasound, CT, and, if they communicate with the ductal system, by ERCP, an important therapeutic consideration.

The function of the exocrine part of the pancreas may be tested by means of pancreatic function tests such as the pancreolauryl test. This comprises an oral dose of a compound that is intestinally absorbed and excreted in the urine only after, and proportional to, the action of pancreatic enzymes.

Conservative treatment

The principles of managing chronic pancreatitis are to treat any identified underlying cause, to control the pain, to supplement pancreatic exocrine function, and to correct any anatomical abnormality that is amenable to surgery. Most cases are managed conservatively. If severe pain is a feature, then potent analgesics are required. The unfortunate complication of most opiate analgesics is that spasm of the sphincter of Oddi at the duodenal end of the pancreatic duct occurs, and this will further aggravate pancreatic duct obstruction. Pethidine causes less spasm than other opiates and is thus the drug of choice, but it is not as effective an analgesic as most other opiates, and patients may resort to using vast amounts. More lasting pain relief may be achieved with a coeliac ganglion block. However, tolerance may arise, and it may need to be repeated. Transthoracic splanchnotomy has also been advocated. Different preparations of oral pancreatic enzyme supplements are available and should be prescribed, although pain is not affected by this treatment.

Surgical treatment

The role of surgery is limited in chronic pancreatitis but is quite well defined. Mostly, the aims of surgery are to reduce pain but should not be attempted until less invasive means of pain control have been tried. If surgery is planned, anatomical abnormalities (cysts, stenoses, dilatated ducts) may be corrected.

1. Relief of obstruction. Any obstruction at the ampulla of Vater, such as a benign or malignant tumour, should be resected. If there is a cyst obstructing the duct, this should be bypassed as a cystjejunostomy or cystgastrostomy. Cystic dilatation of the duct of greater than 1 cm as a result of downstream obstruction may be treated by pancreatico-jejunostomy.

2. Pancreatic resection. If the duct system is too narrow to bypass, and pain persists despite all conservative measures, and if the patient is fit for major surgery, then the last option is to resect the pancreas. In order to preserve as much of the remaining pancreatic function as possible, a pancreatic resection should be limited in benign disease. Thus, if the distal pancreas is diseased and the head is normal, then a distal pancreatectomy is performed. If the head is abnormal, then a pancreaticoduodenectomy (Whipple's procedure) is performed, preserving the distal pancreas and reanastomosing the duct with the jejunum. If there is no discernible normal tissue worth preserving, or if there has been a previous pancreatic resection, then a total pancreatectomy is performed. This is complicated surgery, with up to 5% mortality, and a high incidence of complications such as pancreatic or duodenal fistula. The results are reasonable, however, with up to 75% of patients pain free and 15% improved as a result of surgery. 10% remain unchanged.

3. Pancreatic cysts and pseudocysts. Rarely, pancreatic cysts may become complicated by infection or may compress the extrahepatic biliary tree giving rise to jaundice, or compress the splenic vein causing left-sided or sectoral portal hypertension. Haemorrhage into a large pancreatic cyst is very rare, but is life threatening. All these complications require surgery, which must be immediate to arrest haemorrhage if present. The cyst is decompressed, and this is best done by internal drainage to the stomach or jejunum. Percutaneous drainage of pancreatic cysts sounds an attractive proposition, but may be fraught with problems. Generally, if a cyst is found not to be communicating with the pancreatic duct system on ERCP, then percutaneous drainage may be performed. However, should a cyst be of proportions that require decompression, then an internal drainage may be a better option. If a cyst is seen to be communicating with the duct system, then attempts at percutaneous drainage will result in a distressing pancreatic fistula.

Further reading

Bornman PC, Russell RCG. Endoscopic treatment for chronic pancreatitis. *British Journal of Surgery*, 1992; **79**: 1260–1.

Grace PA, Williamson RCN. Modern management of pancreatic pseudocysts. *British Journal of Surgery*, 1993; **80**: 577–81.

Russell C. Chronic pancreatitis. *Surgery*, 1992; **10**: 247–50.

Related topics of interest

COLORECTAL CARCINOMA

This is the second highest cause of cancer deaths in men (after lung cancer), and the third highest in women (after breast and lung cancer). 20 000 deaths result annually, and the incidence appears to be rising. The peak incidence is at 60 years, but no age group is immune. Five per cent of colorectal carcinoma occurs below the age of 30, and it has occurred in children.

Pathology

Forty-five per cent occurs in the rectum and 25% in the sigmoid colon, 20% occurs in the caecum. Ten per cent occurs throughout the rest of the colon, in order of frequency in the ascending and transverse colon, splenic flexure, descending colon and hepatic flexure. Synchronous carcinomas are present in 2–5% of cases.

Macroscopically the carcinoma is usually either polypoidal or ulcerating. The latter is prevalent in the rectum, whilst larger polypoidal carcinomas are mostly found in the right colon. Ulcerating carcinomas often spread circumferentially to cause an annular stricturing tumour. Other morphological types are also seen, including colloidal and plaque-like carcinomas.

Predisposing conditions include colonic adenomatous polyps, long-standing ulcerative colitis, and a familial tendency towards colorectal carcinoma has been determined. It is probably true that in all colorectal carcinoma, apart from that complicating ulcerative colitis, the carcinoma arises as a result of the polyp–cancer sequence.

Colorectal carcinoma spreads preferentially via the lymphatics and via the portal blood to the liver. Transcoloemic metastasis and ascites may occur in advanced stages.

Presentation

1. Alteration in bowel habit. Rectosigmoid carcinomas usually present with a recent alteration in bowel habit, more frequently tending towards constipation, but sometimes towards loose motions. Carcinomas of the right colon are less likely to present in this way as flow of semi-solid ileal content is less readily impeded than the solid motions of the left side of the colon. However, diarrhoea can occur in right-sided colonic carcinomas.

2. Bowel obstruction. The rectum is a capacious structure and rectal carcinoma rarely obstructs it. Annular carcinomas elsewhere frequently obstruct. If the ileocaecal valve is incompetent, loops of small bowel will distend, and symptoms may develop slowly. If the ileocaecal valve is competent, then a closed loop obstruction results, with gross caecal distension carrying a high risk of perforation and faecal peritonitis. Caecal carcinomas can obstruct the terminal ileum. Obstructed colonic carcinomas carry a worse prognosis than a similar staged non-obstructing carcinoma.

3. Bleeding. Left-sided carcinomas often present with the passage of dark blood per rectum. This symptom must raise suspicion of underlying colonic malignancy in any patient, and should never simply be put down to minor anorectal conditions such as haemorrhoids. Up to 30% of patients presenting with rectal bleeding have a colonic carcinoma or polyp. Because of the distance from the anus, right-sided carcinomas are less likely to present with overt blood loss per rectum. However, occult bleeding occurs, and anaemia is a very common presentation of caecal carcinoma.

4. Fistula. Colovesical fistula may occur presenting with recurrent urinary tract infection. Rectovaginal fistula is a distressing complication of locally advanced rectal carcinoma. A transverse colonic carcinoma may result in a gastrocolic fistula causing faecal vomiting.

5. Perforation. Faecal peritonitis may result from the spontaneous perforation of colonic carcinoma.

Investigation

- Careful rectal examination and rigid sigmoidoscopy is mandatory in those with rectal bleeding. Over 50% of all colorectal carcinoma will be within the range of an examining digit or sigmoidoscope. If a rectal carcinoma is encountered, its location, circumferential spread and distance from the anal verge, mobility and the relationship to the levator ani will determine the choice of operation to be undertaken.
- Barium enema is requested to confirm a lesion seen at sigmoidoscopy, or demonstrate carcinomas out of reach of the sigmoidoscope. It will detect any synchronous carcinoma or coexistent polyps, which occur in up to 30% of cases. Patients with a colonic obstruction may have an unprepared barium enema to confirm the site of obstruction (bowel preparation in colonic obstruction may result in colonic perforation).
- Colonoscopy should also ideally be performed to confirm a histological diagnosis. Synchronous carcinomas will also be identified and polyps may be snared and removed.

- Liver ultrasound will detect metastases although, if present, this should not deter surgery to remove potentially obstructing or bleeding carcinomas.
- Solitary hepatic metastasis or metastases confined to a single lobe may be treated by hepatic resection, and if this is suspected on ultrasound, a CT scan should be performed for confirmation.
- FBC, group and save, U&E and liver function tests are requested. Anaemia is corrected by transfusion.
- Pre-operative carcinoembryonic antigen is requested if estimation of this will form part of the postoperative follow-up.
- Arrangements are made to admit the patient to the ward at least 1 day prior to the proposed date of surgery for a full bowel preparation. This usually amounts to fluids only and two sachets of picolax on the day before surgery. If endorectal surgery is planned, a rectal washout is performed on the morning of surgery.

Dukes' staging

Colorectal carcinoma is staged according to Cuthbert Dukes' classification.

- Dukes A is carcinoma confined to the bowel wall and does not penetrate through it.
- Dukes B is carcinoma penetrating the bowel wall to involve the serosa or extrarectal tissue.
- Dukes C carcinomas have lymph node metastases. (If the highest resected lymph node is clear of metastasis, this is Dukes C_0 and if involved it is Dukes C_1.)
- Hepatic metastases has been termed stage D, although this is not part of Dukes' original staging.

The value of Dukes' staging lies in prognosis. The 5-year-survival in Dukes A carcinoma is 95%, in Dukes B it is 70% and in Dukes C it is 50%.

Treatment

1. Curative resection. In the absence of hepatic involvement, which can be assessed intraoperatively by careful palpation of the liver, the objective of colonic resection for carcinoma is to achieve a cure. This requires the draining lymph nodes to be excised, and necessitates the interruption of the arterial blood supply as proximally as is feasible. The level at which the arterial supply to the colon is taken governs the extent of the colonic resection. It is important, however, to ensure that the bowel ends to be anastomosed and their adjacent mesentery must have a visibly adequate arterial blood flow. If this is not so, then the doubtful segment is resected further until the bowel is indisputedly viable.

- *Right hemicolectomy.* This is performed for carcinomas from the caecum to splenic flexure. Ileo-colic anastamoses have a reduced incidence of breakdown compared to colo-colic anastomoses.
- *Left hemicolectomy.* This is undertaken for carcinomas of the sigmoid and descending colon.
- *Anterior resection of the rectum.* Carcinomas of the rectum may be resected as low as the level of the levator ani. The requisite clearance from tumour is 1–2 cm. Low colorectal anastomoses may be hand-sewn or stapled. Colo-anal anastomoses may be fashioned transanally.
- *Abdomino-perineal excision of the rectum.* If a low anterior resection of the rectum is not technically possible, the rectum and anus are excised, and a permanent left iliac fossa end colostomy is fashioned. The patient will have been counselled by the stoma therapist preoperatively, and the optimal location for the stoma will have been marked.

2. Emergency bowel resections. Obstructing carcinomas from caecum to the splenic flexure are best treated by (extended) right hemicolectomy with primary anastomosis. Resecting all the proximal obstructed colon avoids potential anastomotic dehiscence resulting from proximal faecal loading, and avoids an anastomosis involving obstructed colon. This is a one-stage procedure.

Obstructing carcinomas of the rectosigmoid may be treated by subtotal colectomy and ileorectal anastomosis. Hartmann's procedure, resection of the tumour, oversewing of the distal end or formation of a mucous fistula, and formation of a left iliac fossa end colostomy, is an alternative. Should the primary tumour be difficult to resect, or the patient be too unwell to have a resection, or if the operator is inexperienced, a simple proximal loop colostomy can be fashioned. This is followed by a staged resection of the obstructing carcinoma and eventually by closure of colostomy, as a three-stage procedure.

Perforated carcinomas of the sigmoid may be dealt with by Hartmann's operation.

3. Palliative surgery. Resection of a colonic carcinoma should be undertaken even if liver metastases are detected to avoid continued bleeding and bowel obstruction. The resection can be limited. If a carcinoma is unresectable, a bypass may be fashioned to avoid obstruction.

In unresectable rectal carcinoma, local symptoms may be controlled by endoscopic transanal resection (ETAR) using a technique identical to that used for transurethral resection of the prostate. Expanding metal stents have also been used. Radiotherapy may be of help if pain results from invasion of pelvic structures.

Adjuvant therapy

Pre-operative radiotherapy to a bulky or locally advanced rectal carcinoma often results in a reduction in size, thus facilitating resection. Postoperative chemotherapy regimens using 5-fluorouracil, whether as a sole oral agent or by continuous low-dose intravenous infusion, or delivered to the liver through a cannulated hepatic artery, have proved disappointing to date. However, there may be a role for postoperative combined 5-fluorouracil and radiotherapy in younger patients with residual disease following surgery.

Follow-up

Metachronous carcinomas occur in 2–5% of patients. Regular review in the outpatient clinic is usual to monitor for this or recurrence. A rise in carcinoembryonic antigen above pre-operative levels may indicate disease progression. Digital rectal examination and sigmoidoscopy must be performed to detect anastomotic recurrence. Further episodes of rectal bleeding require barium enema or colonoscopy. Regular colonoscopic follow-up may be necessary for those with multiple carcinomas or polyps but not in those with advanced disease or fully resected solitary carcinomas.

Further reading

Golligher J. *Surgery of the Anus, Rectum and Colon*, 5th Edn. London: Ballière Tindall, 1984.
Mini Symposium – Large Bowel Cancer. *Current Practice in Surgery*, 1993; **5**: 181–201.

Related topics of interest

COMMON PAEDIATRIC CONDITIONS

Inguinal hernia

This is common, particularly amongst boys, and frequently associated with maldescent of the testis. The hernial sac lies within the spermatic cord. They may contain bowel, and they readily strangulate, and should be repaired as soon as they are discovered. A strangulated inguinal hernia is managed conservatively. The child is sedated and put into bed with a head-down tilt. The majority will reduce and surgery can be planned for the next operating list. The child must be re-examined after 4 hours. If reduction has not occurred, the hernia must be explored urgently. A patent processus vaginalis presents as a hydrocoele.

Congenital hypertrophic pyloric stenosis

Pyloric stenosis affects four in one thousand births. This presents with projectile vomiting, and affects boys more often than girls. In one in seven cases, there is a family history of the condition, mostly on the maternal side. It typically presents in the sixth week of life, though with modern methods of diagnosis and a high degree of suspicion, cases are being identified at younger ages. The child should be admitted under a medical paediatric team for investigation. If vomiting has been persistent, the infant may be dehydrated, hypokalaemic or alkalotic. The child is given a 'test feed' whilst simultaneously being palpated in the right upper quadrant. Prior to vomiting, a palpable 'tumour' may be felt (the hypertrophic pylorus). This should be confirmed by ultrasound, which is the optimal method of investigation. A barium meal also demonstrates pyloric stenosis. Pyloric stenosis is treated by Ramsted's pyloromyotomy.

Undescended testes

Undescended testes are present in 40% of full-term male births. The proportion is higher in pre-term births. Most will come to lie in the scrotum, but in 2% the testes remain in the incorrect position. It is more common on the right, and in 20% it is bilateral.

If the testis has not entered the scrotum at one year of age, it is highly unlikely to do so. Undescent of the testis comprises incomplete descent and maldescent. Incompletely descended testes lie at some point between the retroperitoneum and the neck of the scrotum, having stopped at some point along their normal developmental descent into the scrotum. They usually lie in the vicinity of the internal inguinal ring, where they are impalpable. Maldescended testes take up an ectopic position. Ectopic testes are most commonly in the superficial inguinal pouch, immediately lateral to the external inguinal ring, where they may be easily palpated. Other positions include perineal, femoral, or at the base of the penis. Ectopic testes may be pulled into abnormal sites by extrascrotal gubernacula, the so-called gubernacular 'tails of Lockwood'.

Complications of testicular maldescent include tortion of the testis, loss of seminiferous function and infertility, and a risk of developing seminoma of the testis, which may be as much as 40 times the usual risk, and which is not reversed by orchidopexy. Surgery must be performed before the age of two years to preserve function.

Tortion of the testis

This presents with acute scrotal pain but lower abdominal pain may occasionally be present. Predisposing abnormalities include maldescended testes, transverse lying testes, and 'bell-clapper' testes with a long mesorchium. Torted testes are tender, and lie high in the scrotum. The differential diagnosis includes tortion of a pedunculated hydatid of Morgagni, acute epididymitis or orchitis, testicular trauma and idiopathic scrotal oedema. Acute infections will usually be secondary to urinary tract infections and this may be evident on urinalysis with traces of blood and protein, and leucocytes and bacteria on microscopy. Idiopathic scrotal oedema is painless and may be associated with signs of Henoch–Schoenlein purpura, though the appearance of the scrotum may be similar to a testicular torsion.

The only reliable method of ensuring the correct diagnosis is by surgical exploration of the testis. If this rule is followed, then no testicular tortion will be missed. The contralateral testis should also be fixed.

Gastrointestinal obstruction

1. Intussusception. Four out of 1000 children develop intussusception, which carries a 1% mortality. The intussusception is usually ileo-colic, but may be colo-colic or ileo-ileal, in which case it may occur at multiple sites. There is usually a lead point to intussusception in children, which may be a Meckel's diverticulum, a polyp, or a reactive Peyer's patch. Intussusception typically causes screaming episodes interspersed with periods of silence and pallor, and the passage of bloody mucus per rectum, which has been likened to redcurrant jelly. A sausage-shaped mass may be palpable in the abdomen. The diagnosis is confirmed by barium enema. Barium may enter the space between the intussusceptum and the intussuscepiens, giving rise to the 'coiled-spring' appearance of oedematous mucosal folds.

The instillation of barium frequently reduces the intussusception. The reduction should not be deemed to be complete until there is free passage of barium into the terminal ileum. Despite this, there is a 1–3% recurrence rate, which may be dealt with by repeated barium reduction (though this is less likely to succeed the second time) or surgery. Surgery is performed through a transverse incision, and the intussusceptum is gently pushed back through the investing intussuscepiens. Surgery must be undertaken if there are signs of peritonitis, and bowel must be resected if either a manual reduction is impossible, or if it is gangrenous.

2. Congenital causes of bowel obstruction. Malrotated bowel is prone to volvulus (volvulus neonatorum). Ladd's bands are congenital peritoneal adhesions that usually tether the right colon to the liver, and may result in obstruction. A Meckel's diverticulum often has a band at its apex which may tether it to the umbilicus, or to the mesentery of the distal ileum. The former acts as a fulcrum for volvulus of the ilium, and the latter can result in adhesion obstruction or internal herniation. Neonatal duodenal stenosis or atresia, common in Down's children, results in intractable vomiting. This is often identified *in utero* and gastrojejunostomy planned for the first few days of life. Strangulated inguinal hernia must never be overlooked as a cause of intestinal obstruction at any age.

Acute abdomen

The acute abdomen in children may not be due to a surgical condition. However, surgical problems can prove life-threatening if left to develop. Bowel ischaemia and perforation may occur over a very short period of time in children. It is important to review the child frequently and to have a low threshold for surgical exploration.

1. Acute appendicitis. Only 7% of all acute appendicitis occurs in the under-6-years age group, but this is responsible for up to one-third of deaths from appendicitis. The child is usually still, may have vomited and will not be hungry; facial flushing is prominent, there is a low grade pyrexia (high fever if seen late), a tachycardia, and there is firm evidence of right-sided abdominal peritonism. A leucocytosis is common, but not requisite for the diagnosis. A child suspected of having acute appendicitis must undergo appendicectomy as soon after diagnosis as possible. If acute appendicitis is not apparent, a Meckel's diverticulum is sought.

2. Constipation. This may cause peritonism and can cause a leucocytosis, and often occurs without a history of prior episodes, unless the patient has megacolon or Hirschprung's disease. The diagnosis may be very difficult to establish without a plain abdominal X-ray, which shows faecal loading throughout the colon. Underlying causes such as fissure-in-ano should be excluded. Faecal impaction is diagnosed by rectal examination, and requires manual evacuation of faeces under general anaesthesia.

3. Mesenteric adenitis. A generalized viral infection may result in mild enteritis with reactive enlarged mesenteric lymph nodes. This causes a diffuse, poorly localized, often peri-umbilical pain, which is not associated with vomiting. There is a history of a recent coryzal infection, and the child may have a high pyrexia and palpable cervical adenopathy. The abdomen may be tender but there will not be signs of peritonism. If there is doubt about the diagnosis, the child is admitted. Paracetamol will relieve the pyrexia and the pain.

4. Gastro-enteritis. Colicky abdominal pain with vomiting and diarrhoea, often a pyrexia and abdominal tenderness but no signs of peritonism should suggest a diagnosis of gastroenteritis. There may be others in the family with the same problem. Most causes are viral, but some prove to be bacterial, including *Salmonella* and *Campylobacter.* All are self-limiting, and the child may be admitted for assessment of hydration and correction with i.v. fluids if necessary.

5. Other causes. These include lower and upper urinary tract infections, renal and ureteric calculi, hydronephrosis, gallstones, pancreatitis, pneumonia, hepatitis, Henoch–Schoenlein purpura, diabetes, sickle-cell crisis, porphyria, and lead poisoning.

Further reading

Davenport M. Surgically correctable causes of vomiting in infancy. *British Medical Journal,* 1996; **312**: 236–9.
Davenport M. Acute abdominal pain in children. *British Medical Journal,* 1996; **312**: 498–501.
Drake DP. Neonatal surgery. In: Burnand KG, Young AE (eds) T*he New Aird's Companion in Surgical Studies.* Edinburgh: Churchill Livingstone, 1992; 1373.

Related topics of interest

CRITICAL LEG ISCHAEMIA

The term 'critical leg ischaemia' implies the presence of limb-threatening impairment of arterial flow, but attempts to define chronic critical leg ischaemia objectively have met with difficulty.

Acute ischaemia

The clinical features are pain, pallor, pulselessness, paraesthesia, paralysis and coldness. The causes are listed below.

1. Acute on chronic ischaemia. Rupture or ulceration of an atheromatous plaque may lead to thrombosis and occlusion.

2. Emboli. These may arise from the heart (mural thrombus on an area of recent infarction; left atrial thrombus in atrial fibrillation; thrombus on diseased or artificial valve), atherosclerotic plaques or aneurysms.

3. Aneurysm thrombosis. This is more likely to affect aneurysms of smaller vessels (e.g. popliteal aneurysm thrombosis).

4. External compression. Tourniquets, inadvertant application of compression bandages.

5. Ligation

6. Traumatic arterial disruption. This may occur following closed injuries (e.g. supracondylar fracture of the humerus) or penetrating injuries (e.g. stab wound, gunshot injury, diagnostic catheter study).

Chronic ischaemia

The most widely accepted definition is that stated in the European consensus document: "Chronic critical leg ischaemia, both in diabetic and non-diabetic patients, is defined by either of the two following criteria:

1. Persistently recurring rest pain requiring regular adequate analgesia for ≥ 2 weeks, with an ankle systolic pressure ≤ 50 mmHg and/or a toe systolic pressure of ≤ 30 mmHg.

2. Ulceration or gangrene of the foot or toes, with an ankle systolic pressure ≤ 50 mmHg and/or a toe systolic pressure of ≤ 30 mmHg."

Approximately 15–20% of non-diabetic patients with intermittent claudication progress to critical leg ischaemia.

Diabetic claudicants are far more likely to progress to critical ischaemia. Approximately 60% of patients presenting with chronic critical leg ischaemia undergo early vascular reconstruction or angioplasty and 20% undergo early primary amputation. One year after initial presentation 25% of patients have undergone major amputation, 55% still have both legs and 20% have died.

Pathophysiology

The changes that occur in the microcirculation during ischaemia are not well understood. When they become irreversible infarction and gangrene occur. Platelets, white cells and their products, endothelial cells, and the components of the coagulation and fibrinolytic systems are all implicated in the microcirculatory changes taking place in the face of severe ischaemia.

Assessment

Having assessed the leg clinically for pulses, ulceration, temperature capillary refilling, movement and sensory loss, the ankle–brachial Doppler pressure indices should be recorded. Either conventional or intra-arterial digital subtraction arteriograms should be obtained to define the arterial anatomy. Even where embolus is the likely cause, an arteriogram should be undertaken to define co-existent atheroma. Evidence of coronary or cerebrovascular disease should be sought.

Treatment

Limb salvage is sought to avoid the mutilation, morbidity, mortality and expense associated with amputation.

1. General measures. Effective pain relief is essential. Positioning of the leg in a dependent position maximizes arterial inflow, but should be avoided if there is oedema. Co-existent infection should be treated with parenteral antibiotics or surgical drainage if indicated. Necrotic areas should be kept dry.

2. Medical conditions. It is important to treat any co-existing or causative medical conditions such as cardiac failure, which may impair perfusion pressure, diabetes mellitus or renal failure. Atrial fibrillation should be treated. Beta-blockers should be replaced by calcium channel blockers.

3. Thrombolysis/angioplasty. Intra-arterial catheter infusion of streptokinase, urokinase or tissue plasminogen activator is frequently successful in clearing arterial segments and is particularly useful in distal occlusions (e.g. following embolization from popliteal aneurysms). A stenosis or occlusion may then become apparent that can be dilated or recanalized using angioplasty. Thrombolysis can occasionally give rise to catastrophic limb ischaemia, probably through destabilization of thrombus and consequent embolization. Thrombolysis should be abandoned if this occurs and surgical reconstruction attempted. Frequent monitoring in a high dependency unit is mandatory during thrombolysis.

4. Surgical reconstruction. The patient's general health, mobility and social circumstances should be considered when planning reconstruction. Embolectomy may be performed via a groin approach under general or local anaesthesia, depending on the age and condition of the patient. An approach via the popliteal artery may be necessary less frequently. Intraoperative thrombolysis by injection down an irrigating embolectomy catheter is sometimes a useful adjunct if the embolectomy has failed to clear the distal circulation. Bypass of an occluded segment (aortofemoral, femoropopliteal, femorodistal) is frequently necessary. Arteriographic demonstration of a patent distal vessel is necessary, and an autogenous vein should be used for distal bypasses wherever feasible. Where multiple stenoses/occlusions are present, the proximal segments should be cleared or bypassed first. Femorodistal bypass procedures are time-consuming and demand considerable dedication in achieving patency. Various techniques (Miller cuff, Taylor patch, St Mary's boot) have been devised to enlarge the distal anastomosis and improve patency rates where prosthetic grafts are used. High reocclusion rates frequently mean that secondary procedures are frequently required. Unfortunately, graft patency does not always ensure limb salvage.

5. Primary amputation. In some patients, amputation is inevitable and should not be delayed by misplaced attempts at revascularization. An epidural prior to amputation relieves pain and may lessen postoperative phantom limb pain.

6. Pharmacological agents. A trial of pharmacological agents may be justified where a patient's ischaemia is not deteriorating rapidly. Prostanoids (PGI_2, PGE_1, iloprost) inhibit platelet activation, aggregation, adhesion and release actions, stabilize leucocytes and endothelial cells, and cause vasodilatation. They have been used in end-stage critical ischaemia and there is some evidence of ulcer healing, relief of rest pain and improved limb salvage. These agents should be considered for patients in whom surgery or interventional radiology are inappropriate or in whom several weeks' delay for a course of treatment is unlikely to be detrimental.

Trials have recently shown that long-term administration of low-dose aspirin reduces the frequency of fatal cardiovascular events in patients with peripheral vascular disease.

7. Phenol sympathectomy. Destruction of the lumbar sympathetic nerves supplying the lower limb arteries causes vasodilation and improvement of the cutaneous circulation. Ischaemic ulcers are encouraged to heal and pain is lessened. Diabetic patients are usually refractory to sympathectomy because their neuropathy often results in an autosympathectomy.

Further reading

Dormandy J. Critical leg ischaemia. In: Clement DL, Shepherd JT (eds) *Vascular Diseases in the Limbs.* St Louis, MO: Mosby Year Book, 1993; 91–102.
Berridge DC. Advances in thrombolytic therapy. *British Journal of Surgery*, 1994; **81**: 1249–50.

Related topics of interest

Amputations (p. 24)
Intermittent claudication (p. 180)
Vascular imaging and investigation (p. 332)

CROHN'S DISEASE

This is a chronic granulomatous inflammatory condition that can involve any part of the gastrointestinal tract. It may occur at any age, and the sex distribution is equal. The most common site affected is the terminal ileum. This is involved in 70% of patients, giving rise to the soubriquet of 'terminal ileitis' or 'regional ileitis'. The colon may also be involved, and Crohn's colitis is the only manifestation of disease in 20% of cases. Multiple sites are common: Crohn's disease occurs in a discontinuous pattern within the bowel such that affected areas may be separated by quite normal bowel. These affected areas are termed skip-lesions.

Pathology

Macroscopically the bowel wall becomes grossly thickened, and enveloped in mesenteric fat (fat wrapping). The histological hallmark is a non-caseating granuloma. This may not be found in up to 40% of specimens, however. There is transmural chronic inflammation of the affected bowel with local lymphadenopathy.

Various theories exist regarding the aetiology of the disease, including genetic or autoimmune disease, viral and mycobacterial infections.

Presentation

Crohn's disease presents in a varied fashion. In children, failure to thrive and loss of weight may be the only features. In adults, the most common presentation is diarrhoea, which occurs in 80% of cases. Perianal lesions are present in 70%, and this may be the presenting feature of the disease. Abdominal pain is present in 60% of cases. Other features include abdominal distension, rectal bleeding, pyrexia, abdominal mass, or abdominal wall fistula.

Clinical manifestations and complications of chronic inflammatory bowel disease

There are many extra-intestinal manifestations of Crohn's disease, many of which also occur in ulcerative colitis.

- Oral and rectal aphthous ulceration.
- Clubbing of the nails.
- Pyoderma gangrenosum.
- Erythema nodosum.
- Large joint mono-arthritis and sacroileitis.
- Uveitis and episcleritis.
- Renal oxalate stones.

Hepatobiliary complications of both Crohn's disease and ulcerative colitis include:

- Cholelithiasis.
- Fatty change of the liver.
- Pericholangitis.

- Cirrhosis.
- Chronic active hepatitis.
- Cholangiocarcinoma.
- Sclerosing cholangitis.
- Amyloid deposition may occur in Crohn's disease.

Investigations

A barium enema or small bowel enema may reveal characteristic features of Crohn's: rose thorn ulceration, deep fissures, skip lesions, fistulae, thickened bowel, string sign of Kantor (terminal ileal stricture) or a featureless (drain pipe) colon. The ESR and C-reactive protein are invariably raised in acute episodes, and the LFTs are often elevated. Anaemia is common.

Complications

1. Acute inflammation. This can result in peritonitis and any of its sequelae, particularly intra-abdominal abscess formation. Rarely, involved bowel may perforate. Crohn's colitis, as with any form of colitis, can become fulminant and develop into a toxic megacolon.

2. Bleeding. This may be a feature of a Crohn's colitis, but rarely occurs if small bowel is involved alone, and it rarely requires emergency surgery.

3. Recurrence. Up to 30% of patients having a bowel resection for Crohn's disease will require further procedures for recurrent disease. It has a predilection for recurring at anastomoses from previous resections.

4. Bowel obstruction. This results from a stricture, which is common in Crohn's, particularly in the small intestine. These are best treated by either a conservative bowel resection, or stricturoplasty if the strictures are multiple or there have been previous resections. It has been shown that bowel healing is not affected by the presence of Crohn's disease. Therefore wide resections of affected bowel are both unnecessary and counterproductive in the long term.

5. Perianal disease. Anal conditions such as perianal tags, perianal abscess, chronic fissures and fistula-in-ano are common. Acute perianal conditions need to be treated as they arise. Histologically the affected tissue may show changes of Crohn's disease. Fistulae may be very numerous and wide ranging, with openings throughout the perineum ('watering can perineum'). The chronically inflamed and infected perianal skin that results has been shown to be histologically indistinguishable from hidradenitis suppuritiva. The end result of multiple procedures on the anus in the presence of Crohn's disease is a distorted, scarred and chronically inflamed anus that may be the source of great distress to the patient.

6. *Malignancy.* There is a risk of developing carcinoma in colon or small bowel affected with Crohn's disease. The prognosis is poor as the diagnosis is usually made late because the symptoms are put down to existant inflammation. The risk of malignancy in Crohn's disease is less than the risk of developing colonic carcinoma in ulcerative colitis.

7. *Abdominal mass.* Persistent inflammation in affected bowel may result in a phlegmanous mass. This usually occurs in the right iliac fossa, representing terminal ileal disease, but may occur at any site. An inflammatory mass may resolve with continued anticolitic drugs and metronidazole, but persistence despite these measures is an indication for bowel resection.

8. *Fistula.* Crohn's disease has a tendency to form fistulae. Entero-enteric, entero-colic, and entero-cutaneous fistulae are the most commonly encountered. These frequently follow surgery, however carefully undertaken.

Medical treatment

- 5-Aminosalicylic acid-containing preparations may be of benefit. Colitis responds better than small bowel disease.
- Steroids are used in acute episodes, though there is little to suggest that maintenance treatment with steroids prevents recurrence.
- Immunosuppression with azathioprine may be successful in severe disease, particularly in combination with steroids.

Surgical treatment

1. *Small bowel.* The principle of surgery in small bowel Crohn's disease is to conserve as much bowel as possible. Stricturoplasty is preferred to resection, and if resection is necessary, then limited resection is performed. If a fistula becomes unmanageable, the affected segment may need to be removed. Intra-abdominal abscess must be drained.

2. *Colonic.* Should symptoms persist in Crohn's colitis despite maximal medical therapy, the colon may be

defunctioned by the formation of a split (loop) ileostomy. This has been shown to improve colonic inflammation. A subtotal colectomy with a permanent right iliac fossa end ileostomy may however become necessary. Crohn's disease is an absolute contraindication for the formation of an ileoanal pouch.

Further reading

Alexander-Williams J. Small bowel Crohn's disease - surgical strategy. *Current Practice in Surgery*, 1991; **3**: 118–24.
Golligher J. *Surgery of the Anus, Rectum and Colon*, 5th Edn. London: Ballière Tindall, 1984.
Schofield PF. Inflammatory disease of the large bowel. *Surgery*, 1990; **85**: 2020–6.

Related topics of interest

Enterocutaneous fistula (p. 128)
Intestinal obstruction (p. 183)
Nutrition in the surgical patient (p. 213)
Ulcerative colitis (p. 305)

CUSHING'S DISEASE

Cushing's disease was first described in 1932 by Harvey Cushing. Women predominate with the condition (4:1) with a peak incidence in the fifth decade. The primary lesion is a basophil adenoma of the pituitary gland wich secretes excess levels of ACTH. This acts upon the zona fasciculata of the adrenal cortex to stimulate an over-production of cortisol which is responsible for the features of the disease.

Cushing's syndrome

Excess levels of circulating cortisol can be produced in a number of other ways but their effects on metabolism are similar, all resulting in Cushing's syndrome. This syndrome comprises of truncal obesity, buffalo hump, plethoric moon face, proximal muscle wasting, skin atrophy, poor wound healing, osteoporosis, hirsuitism, acne, excessive bruising, impotence, amenorrhoea and growth retardation in children. Diabetes, hypertension and psychiatric disturbances can also be precipitated. Fatal complications include cerebral thrombosis and myocardial infarction. Cushingoid striae are purple. They can thus be distinguished from the white striae of simple obesity.

Aetiology

Cushing's disease is diagnosed by excluding the other causes of glucocorticoid (mainly cortisol) excess.

1. Ectopic ACTH. This can be secreted by an oat cell carcinoma of the lung or a bronchial carcinoid (ectopic ACTH syndrome).

2. Exogenous ACTH. This can be administered therapeutically in excess.

3. Adrenal cortisol. Both benign and malignant tumours of the adrenal gland can secrete a variety of inappropriate glucocorticoids and corticosteroids. The condition of nodular adrenal hyperplasia (NAH) occurs at around 18 years of age. It is characterized by the presence of multiple adrenal nodules up to 3 mm in diameter. In this condition, an excess of cortisol is produced with ACTH suppression.

4. Exogenous cortisol. The commonest cause of Cushing's syndrome is the therapeutic administration of corticosteroids for conditions like rheumatoid arthritis, autoimmune diseases and chronic inflammatory disorders.

Investigations

The aim of the investigations is firstly to establish the presence of hypercortisolism, secondly to determine its origin and finally to image the suspected organ involved.

1. Diagnosis. Hypercortisolism is determined by an elevated plasma cortisol and loss of the diurnal variation. The level at 6:00 a.m. is normally higher than the 6:00 p.m. dip (a level less than 5 µg/dl is normal). The 24 hour urinary free cortisol should normally be less than 320 µg per day. All patients with non-pituitary Cushing's syndrome should exhibit resistance to suppression with a low-dose dexamethasone suppression test (0.5 mg is given every 6 hours for 2 days) by maintaining their hypercortisol state.

2. Origin. The high-dose dexamethasone suppression test (2 mg is given every 6 hours for 2 days) can further localize the problem. Pituitary Cushing's syndrome hypercortisolism is suppressed with this level of dexamethasone but hormone production continues with the hypercortisolism of adrenal or ectopic origin. ACTH levels can be measured by a radioimmunoassay. This should distinguish an ectopic ACTH source from hypercortisolism of adrenal origin, because in the latter condition ACTH levels are low. A chest radiograph should not be forgotten.

3. Adrenal imaging. A $[^{131}I]$6-β-iodomethyl-19-norcholesterol (NP-59) scintigram images the adrenal glands. Bilateral increased uptake is indicative of excess ACTH stimulation, whereas asymmetrical uptake is more indicative of nodular adrenal hyperplasia. Lateralized uptake is pathognomic of an adrenal adenoma. Adrenal carcinoma often shows poor uptake and the cortisol it produces suppresses the contralateral gland resulting in bilateral non-visualization. Furthermore, compared to that of benign disease, the hormone profiles of adrenal malignancy demonstrate increased levels of a large variety of steroid metabolic by-products. CT and MRI may be used in a complementary fashion to image the adrenal glands. With these investigations a 'histological' diagnosis can be inferred in the majority of patients.

4. Pituitary imaging. Only half of the patients with pituitary microadenomas are visualized on a CT scan which makes the confirmation of Cushing's disease difficult. If a chest radiograph or whole body CT fails to show evidence of an ectopic ACTH source in lung, pancreas or mediastinum, bilateral selective petrosal venous sampling for ACTH can confirm excess pituitary ACTH production. This is a difficult, but invaluable, technique only carried out at specialist centres.

Treatment

The treatment of Cushing's disease in patients where a pituitary microadenoma has been identified is carried out with a trans-spenoidal microsurgical dissection and excison of the adenoma. Ninety per cent of patients are cured in this way. In patients demonstrating supra sellar tumour extension, direct excision together with hypophysectomy is associated with recurrence of Cushing's disease of over 50%. In these patients, bilateral adrenalectomy is indicated with autotransplantation of 8 g of sliced adrenal into the rectus abdominis muscle. This prevents dependence on glucocorticoid and mineralocorticoid replacement, preserves reproductive function and prevents Nelson's syndrome. The major disadvantage to autotransplantation is that exogenous steroids may not be required and any residual pituitary lesion will be freed from steroid inhibition and encouraged to expand. External pituitary irradiation or interstitial radiotherapy can be administered as adjuvant therapy and primary therapy. The latter is especially indicated in children. Complete adrenal blockade can be achieved with Metyrapone which acts by inhibiting the conversion of 11-deoxycortisol to cortisol. It can be used as a poor alternative to surgery in Cushing's syndrome and has prophylactic value prior to surgery. Replacement steroid therapy is required following adrenalectomy, and prophylactic antibiotics are helpful to prevent the wound infections cushingoid patients are prone to developing. Wound sutures should be left undisturbed for several more days than for normal patients.

Nelson's syndrome

In 1960, Nelson described a syndrome of hyper-pigmentation, pituitary enlargement and ACTH elevation in patients following bilateral adrenalectomy for pituitary-dependent Cushing's disease. The hyper-pigmentation is due to the increased levels of ACTH and melanocyte-stimulating hormone (MSH). Treatment involves prophylactic pituitary irradiation at the time of adrenalectomy. If the syndrome becomes established (this occurs in 30% of patients), hypophysectomy or pituitary irradiation is indicated.

Further reading

Farndon JR, Dunn JM. Adrenal tumours. *Recent Advances in Surgery*, 1992; **15**: 55–68.

Lucarotti M, Farndon JR. Cushing's syndrome. *Current Practice in Surgery*, 1993; **5**: 172–7.

Related topics of interest

Adrenal tumours (p. 16)

Renal tumours (p. 258)

DAY CASE SURGERY

The concept of complete hospital care for the surgical patient during the course of an 8 h period arose primarily out of the lack of adequate inpatient resources as well as from the rapid developments of surgical technique and anaesthesia. Although the publication of the *Guidelines for Day Case Surgery* in 1985 by the Royal College of Surgeons recommended 35% of patients eligible for day case surgery, under 20% are actually treated in this way. In contrast to the UK, North America carries out over 60% of their surgery on a day case basis.

Benefits

The benefits of day case surgery are plentiful, as follows.

1. Early ambulation. This is preventative of the complications of venous thromboembolism.

2. Reduced waiting list. Seventy-five per cent of patients on the waiting list for greater than 3 months are suitable for treatment as a day case. Offering them such a service decreases the waiting lists by approximately 20% and reduces the cancellation rate because the competition with emergency admissions for beds is eliminated. There is also less time spent in hospital which is a positive benefit for many patients who fear hospitals, especially children.

3. Job satisfaction. This increases for the nursing staff as they can rotate within the unit between theatre, anaesthesia, recovery and ward care as well as be guaranteed time off at Christmas, Easter and weekends.

4. Efficient management. Protocols are easier to establish and their implementation can be supervised because many patients require similar procedures which all require similar after care.

5. Reduced complications. If day case surgery is to be successful the complication rates must be reduced to an absolute minimum. Surgeons and anaesthetists recognize this need and should ensure the procedures are carried out by fully trained and experienced staff. This would be beneficial to patients.

Unit management

The management and running of a day surgery unit should be consultant based. This requires an additional commitment to the already busy consultant program and, consequently, this has not found universal favour. Whilst the principle of day surgery has many benefits, especially for the patient, it is an exception rather than the rule, that such a unit is correctly and optimally managed. Over 50% of centres have their beds separated from the operating theatres. Either day beds are borrowed from the main ward, or main theatre facilities are used for the day patients. There is considerable variation in consultant practice in the same hospital and between practices in neighbouring districts as to the type of surgery that should take place in a day surgery unit. Some use the unit exclusively for minor local anaesthetic operations and outpatient procedures like colposcopy, whilst others use the facilities extensively for operations like breast lumpectomy and varicose vein surgery. Such inconsistencies between the classification of a day surgical operation has created audit problems and invalidated many of the statistical comparisons that are made to indicate performance and efficiency.

Patient selection

The ideal day surgery patient should have a confined day surgical problem, good social circumstances for rehabilitation and domestic support, and be reasonably fit and healthy. Unfortunately, these criteria are not always met. It is suggested that the patient book in to the day surgery unit at the time of outpatient consultation where a nurse, with the aid of a standard pro forma, will assess general fitness and the social support required. This will also confirm the appointment date for operation, reduce patient anxiety on the day of surgery and dramatically decrease the patient cancellation rate. An anaesthetic pre-surgical check clinic has similarly been suggested to avoid these problems.

Complications

All patients should be forewarned of any general complications if the risk is greater than 5%. The signs of postoperative haematoma, haemorrhage and dehiscence should be looked for before discharge. A supply of adequate prophylactic analgesia is given with general postoperative advice, an information leaflet and a phone number to call in case of emergency. In comparison to main ward patients, there is a small increase in the readmission rate due to early postoperative complications.

Patient satisfaction

Day patients themselves often have increased anxiety and frequently admit that they would have preferred to stay in overnight; however, if recently discharged ward patients are asked the same question many would also have elected to remain a further night. Increased patient anxiety at being discharged too soon and being totally responsible for their own management has led to a slight increase in the use of the GP and the community nurse.

Cost

The cost of a day surgery unit must be balanced with its benefits to the working community and to improved patient care. Money is only saved in nursing salaries and hotel services if one ward patient bed is closed or substituted for every day surgical bed that is opened. This is not often the case and the resulting cost is usually in addition to the services that are already provided. Costs are further increased if consultant numbers increase to manage the service. More skilled nurses would be required to manage the greater proportion of severely dependent inpatients if comparatively more straight-forward and self-caring patients were removed from the main wards. A well-run unit is also likely to attract boundary patients to the hospital who would otherwise go elsewhere for their treatment. This is not without even further cost.

Further reading

Ralphs DNL. Day surgery revisited. *Current Surgical Practice*, 1993; **6**: 32–42.

Related topic of interest

Audit (p. 46)

DEEP VEIN THROMBOSIS/PULMONARY EMBOLISM

The significance of deep vein thrombosis (DVT) lies in its potential to cause pulmonary embolism (PE) and post-thrombotic calf pump failure. Virtually all venous thrombi arise in the deep veins of the legs or pelvis. The incidence of DVT in the general population is approximately 0.5%. Where no preventative measures are employed, the incidence of DVT in general surgical patients over 40 years undergoing major surgery is 30%, and 60–80% in patients undergoing hip or knee replacement, or surgery for hip fracture. In patients recovering from myocardial infarction or cerebrovascular accident, the incidence is 20–60%.

Aetiology

1. *Virchow's triad*
- *Hypercoagulability*: antithrombin III, lupus anti-coagulant, heparin cofactor, protein C, protein S, alpha II macroglobulin, alpha I antitrypsin, fibrinolytic impaiment, oral contraceptive. Smoking increases plasma fibrinogen.
- *Stasis*: surgery, bed rest.
- *Vein wall damage*: surgical injury, trauma, radiotherapy.

2. *Risk factors*. Smoking, age, sex, race, operation, anaesthetic, pregnancy, trauma, immobilization, bed rest, malignancy, previous thrombosis, varicose veins, obesity, cardiac failure, myocardial infarction, contraceptive pill, congenital venous abnormalities.

Pathology

Thrombosis is frequently initiated in the vein valve sinuses of the soleal plexuses. Platelets adhere to the venous endothelium initially and fibrin and red cells are deposited between the layers of platelets giving rise to a laminated thrombus. This propagates to extend up the vein, being free or loosely attached to the wall initially. Thrombus then becomes firmly adherent to the endothelium, organizes, retracts and recanalizes, to varying degrees, destroying the endothelium and valves as it resolves.

Clinical features

Limb swelling, pain, tenderness, erythema and dilated superficial veins are the classic signs but are frequently absent, even in a major thrombosis. A swollen white leg (phlegmasia alba dolens) or blue leg (phlegmasia cerulea dolens) may follow an extensive ileofemoral thrombosis. Clinical diagnosis is incorrect in 50% of patients when compared with venography. The differential diagnosis includes ruptured Baker's cyst, cellulitis, lymphoedema, torn calf muscles and calf haematoma.

Ascending venography remains the gold standard, although colour duplex ultrasound is non-invasive and is being used increasingly. It is, however, time-consuming and relatively insensitive in the detection of below knee thromboses. Plethysmography is used to detect reduced venous capacitance after a thrombosis, but has low accuracy in non-occlusive thrombi.

Prophylaxis

1. General measures. Early mobilization, hydration, cessation of smoking.

See sheet

2. Mechanical methods. Graduated compression stockings, perioperative pneumatic compression and electrical calf stimulation all reduce the incidence of perioperative DVT.

3. Pharmacological. Warfarin – postoperative bleeding can be troublesome. Low-dose heparin (5000 IU b.d.) is effective in preventing DVT and pulmonary embolism (PE), but at the risk of increased bleeding complications. Low molecular weight heparins have the advantage of once daily administration and are at least as effective as unfractionated heparin. A reduction in bleeding complications is most marked in patients undergoing hip or knee surgery. Dextran 70 has not been demonstrated to reduce the incidence of DVT, although it appears to reduce the incidence of PE. Problems with fluid overload and hypersensitivity have occurred.

Combinations of prophylactic techniques appear additive in their reduction of DVT risk, but even with careful prophylaxis, 5–20% of patients undergoing general surgical operations sustain DVT and up to 0.2% have a fatal PE.

Treatment

Because clinical diagnosis is unreliable, objective venographic or duplex evidence of DVT should be obtained, wherever possible, before starting treatment. Both legs should be studied. A confirmed thrombosis should be treated with a bolus of 70 IU/kg heparin followed by an infusion of 20–30 IU/kg/hour to maintain the activated partial thromboplastin time (APTT) at 1.5–2.5 times the control. Intermittent i.v. or s.c. bolus injections are also effective. Warfarin should be started once the patient is stable and an international normalized ratio (INR) of 2.5–3.0 obtained. Warfarin should be continued for 3–6 months. Warfarin is not always given to patients who have suffered a minor calf thrombosis, since these rarely cause major PE. Most extensive DVTs start as calf thromboses, however, and the long-term effects on critical areas of the calf pump mechanism remain uncertain.

Thrombolysis may be used to resolve extensive, fresh thrombus. Surgical thrombectomy has no place in the treatment of distal thrombosis, but may prevent limb loss in the acutely ischaemic limb caused by extensive thrombosis.

Caval interruption by ligation, plication, clip, Mobin-Udin umbrella or Greenfield filter may be required when there is fresh, non-adherent thrombus floating in the iliofemoral segment, especially where there are contraindications to anticoagulation or there has been an initial minor PE. The percutaneously inserted Greenfield filter is the device of choice.

Pulmonary embolism

DVT is the source of 98% of PE, generally arising from the iliofemoral veins. Approximately 2–5% of DVTs give rise to significant PE. Death occurs immediately or within the first hour in 10% of patients sustaining PE. A firm diagnosis of PE is made in a minority of the remaining 90%. Up to 70% of patients presenting with the features of PE have normal pulmonary angiograms.

Clinical features	Dyspnoea, haemoptysis, pleuritic chest pain and sudden death, caused by interruption of venous return to the left heart, are the cardinal features. A pleural rub may be detected.
Investigations	The chest radiograph may show oligaemia, consolidation and hilar enlargement. The electrocardiograph may show the S1 Q3 T3 pattern of right heart strain and the arterial blood gas analysis may show hypoxia and hypocarbia. Ventillation–perfusion isotope scintigraphy shows varying probability of PE, but the definitive investigation is the pulmonary angiogram.
Treatment	Minor PE requires heparin anticoagulation once the source of the embolus has been confirmed. Acute massive PE requires emergency surgical embolectomy where there is marked pulmonary outflow obstruction. Fibrinolytic treatment may suffice where the haemodynamic effects are less severe. Once the PE has been confirmed, the legs should be studied with venography or duplex ultrasound to determine the extent of the DVT in case thrombectomy or venous interruption is required. Recurrent PE in the face of adequate anticoagulation is a strong indication for filter insertion.

Further reading

Browse NL, Burnand KG, Lea Thomas M. *Diseases of the Veins: Pathology, Diagnosis and Treatment*. London: Edward Arnold, 1988.

Burnand KG, Scurr JH. The veins. In: Burnand KG, Young AE (eds) *The New Aird's Companion in Surgical Studies*. Edinburgh: Churchill Livingston, 1992; 385–413.

Related topics of interest

Calf pump failure and venous ulceration (p. 67)
Postoperative care and complications (p. 247)
Pre-operative assessment (p. 255)
Vascular imaging and investigation (p. 332)

DIVERTICULAR DISEASE

Diverticular disease is an acquired condition of the colon. Mucosal pouches herniate outward through the submucosa and muscularis externa (congenital diverticula occur in the jejunum and duodenum although these comprise all layers of the bowel wall). Colonic diverticula arise between the antimesenteric taenia and the omental and free taenia, at the site of entry of blood vessels. The appendix and rectum have a continuous longitudinal muscle layer rather than taenia, and thus do not have diverticula.

This is a common condition which affects upwards of 30% of individuals aged more than 60 years. The condition is rare in those aged less than 30. It is more common in females than males. The association of diverticulosis, cholelithiasis and hiatus hernia is known as Saint's triad. The presence of colonic diverticula is 'diverticulosis' or 'diverticular disease'.

Diverticulosis is a disorder of modern civilization, probably reflecting dietary fibre content. Diverticular disease does not occur in rural African populations where the diet is rich in fibre and colonic transit time is greatly reduced compared with Westernized populations. Colonic diverticula often contain inspissated faecal matter.

Sixty per cent have involvement of the sigmoid colon. This is the part most commonly affected in isolation, and which results in most of the complications of diverticular disease. However, any part of the colon may be affected; 7% of cases have total colonic involvement. Diverticula may be giant, in which case the wall is particularly attenuated and prone to rupture. These often occur singly and are found in the sigmoid and the caecum equally.

Pathology	Diverticula probably form because of disordered colonic peristalsis. Peristalsis occurs in neighbouring segments of the colon causing high intraluminal pressure in between. This may cause the herniation of mucosa out through the bowel wall at weaker locations, often the site of entry of blood vessels. The dysmotility may result from constipation. A constant finding is hypertrophy of the circular and longitudinal muscle resulting in a contracted, tortuous often gnarled colon with a narrowed lumen.
Complications and immediate management	*1. Pain.* Ninety per cent of patients with diverticulosis are symptomless. It may be associated with lower abdominal colic.
	2. Acute diverticulitis. A diverticulum may become inflamed when an inspissated faecolith obstructs the neck of the diverticulum. Acute diverticulitis, causes lower abdominal colic followed by constant left iliac fossa pain. Rebound tenderness and guarding result (this has been called 'left-sided appendicitis'). Most of the inflammatory and infective complications of diverticular disease affect the sigmoid colon, although the caecum is occasionally affected.

3. Diverticular abscess. Acute diverticulitis may result in purulent peritonitis or a localized diverticular abscess. There is severe pain, a high swinging pyrexia and a prominent leucocytosis. If an abscess becomes established, then diagnosis by ultrasound or CT scan may enable percutaneous drainage. Paracolic or subphrenic abscess may occur.

4. Diverticular mass. The local response to acute diverticulitis may be phlegmonous rather than purulent, resulting in a palpable and tender diverticular mass.

5. Diverticular stricture. Repeated episodes of inflammation in the sigmoid colon will eventually result in fibrosis, and thickening of the bowel wall. A stricture may result, often presenting with acute colonic obstruction.

6. Faecal peritonitis. Diverticula may perforate causing faecal peritonitis, which is a life-threatening complication, carrying a mortality of 50%. The patient may be endotoxic, requiring resuscitation with i.v. fluids and high doses of antibiotics.

7. Haemorrhage. This results from the neck of a diverticulum being sandwiched between a faecolith and colonic blood vessel. The vessels can erode, and bleeding is typically very brisk with the passage of bright red blood from the sigmoid (common), or dark red blood from the caecum (unusual).

8. Fistula. Inflamed segments of sigmoid colon may adhere to adjacent viscera via a diverticular abscess, which points and ruptures into it, establishing a fistula. The most common is a colovesical fistula. These result in recurrent lower urinary tract infections. Pneumaturia and faecaluria may occur. Colovaginal fistula is very debilitating and necessitates urgent correction. A paracolic abscess may rupture laterally through the parietes presenting as a left groin abscess (if on the right, consider an underlying appendicitis). If this discharges, a colocutaneous fistula arises. Coloenteric fistulae may cause diarrhoea.

Investigation

Diverticula can be seen on flexible sigmoidoscopy and colonoscopy. These examinations should not be carried out if acutely inflamed distal colon is suspected as perforation of the bowel may result. Diverticular disease is best diagnosed by barium enema 6 weeks following the resolution of symptoms.

Treatment

Acute diverticulitis or a diverticular mass requires a broad-spectrum cephalosporin combined with metronidazole. Should symptoms or a mass persist it is worth continuing metronidazole for some weeks. During the acute phase the patient is allowed a soft diet. A high-fibre diet is started when the inflammation has settled. If simple dietary measures do not prevent constipation, additional fibre supplements may be prescribed. Antispasmodics may relieve cramping pains, but may slow colonic transit time, and should be avoided.

Surgery

Diverticulitis is a common cause of an acute abdomen. If there is peritonitis, a laparotomy must be performed. The usual operation is a Hartmann's procedure, involving excision of the affected colon (usually the sigmoid), and fashioning of a left iliac fossa end colostomy. The distal end is either oversewn and fixed to the side of the pelvis, or brought to the abdominal skin as a mucous fistula, considerably facilitating the reversal of the end colostomy at a later date. This operation is applied to most acute conditions of the left colon presenting with either peritonitis or obstruction. It has been shown that excision of diseased sigmoid carries a better prognosis, compared with drainage and proximal loop colostomy, and left colonic anastomoses have high leak rates if performed in obstructed bowel or if there is peritonitis. However, many gastrointestinal surgeons regard Hartmann's procedure as obsolete. Sigmoid resection with a primary colonic anastomosis can be safely performed following pre-operative (on table) colonic lavage.

Elective resection may be performed for chronic symptoms, usually pain, resulting from diverticulosis. A sigmoid colectomy with primary anastomosis is usually sufficient.

Further reading

Golligher J. Diverticulosis and diverticulitis of the colon. In: *Surgery of the Anus, Rectum and Colon*, 5th Edn. London: Ballière Tindall, 1984.

Morgan PG, Hyland JMP. Management of diverticular disease. *Current Practice in Surgery*, 1994; **6**: 102–7.

Related topics of interest

ENDOSCOPY

Endoscopy is the visualization of the luminal surface of hollow viscera. A large number of organs can be inspected. The need for exploratory operations has thus diminished and diagnostic potential is greatly enhanced. Similar techniques have been applied to the visualization of coelomic cavities and even fascial compartments, and these will be mentioned.

Gastroscopy

Gastroscopy (oesophagogastroduodenoscopy) allows visualization of the oesophagus, stomach and duodenum under light sedation. The patient is placed in the left lateral position, head on a pillow, and the neck slightly flexed. The throat is sprayed with lignocaine, and either diazemuls or midazolam is used for sedation. The gastroscope is manoeuvred into the pharynx, and the patient is asked to swallow, while the endoscope is gently inserted into the oesophagus. The endoscope has channels that allow for biopsies, suction, flushing. Air is blown through the endoscope to distend the gastrointestinal lumen in order to pass the endoscope under a clear field of view.

Gastroscopy is used for diagnostic purposes, for example, to localize the source of upper gastrointestinal bleeding or in the investigation of dyspepsia. It may also be therapeutic. Bleeding gastric or duodenal ulcers may be injected with a solution of adrenaline which may reduce the incidence of rebleeding. Oesophageal strictures may be dilated after introduction of a guidewire past the stricture. Similarly, pyloric stenosis may be dilated. Malignant strictures of the oesophagus may be palliatively treated by laser via the endoscope.

Colonoscopy

This allows the full length of the colon to be examined under sedation. The bowel must be prepared prior to colonoscopy. It may be used for a great number of purposes: to confirm and assess the extent of colitis; to biopsy lesions identified on barium enema; to snare polyps and retrieve them for histology; regularly to follow-up colitics to check for malignant or dysplastic changes; to differentiate acute colonic pseudo-obstruction from organic causes of obstruction and to deflate the colon; to identify angiodysplasias in the colonic mucosa (a source of bleeding) and to treat them.

Proctosigmoidoscopy

In the general surgical outpatient department, proctoscopy and rigid sigmoidoscopy are invaluable. Proctoscopy examines the anus and the distal folds of rectal mucosa, and sigmoidoscopy is used to visualize the rectum. In the presence of an acute anal condition such as thrombosed haemorrhoids, fissure-in-ano or anorectal abscess, proctoscopy and sigmoidoscopy should not be performed. The anal canal will almost certainly be in spasm, and the procedure will be exceptionally painful, if not impossible.

On proctoscopy, first degree (bleeding) haemorrhoids can be injected with 3% phenol to good effect, and second degree (prolapsing) haemorrhoids can be banded. Sigmoidoscopy will identify proctitis and biopsies can be taken. Polyps and rectal carcinomas may be seen and biopsied. Flexible sigmoidoscopy enables a view through to the sigmoid colon, and this can be performed in the outpatient setting.

Endoscopic retrograde cholangiopancreatography (ERCP)

ERCP is performed using a side-viewing gastroduodenoscope. The ampulla of Vater is identified and cannulated. Contrast is injected and radiographs outlining both the biliary tree and pancreatic duct are obtained. Biliary strictures and bile duct calculi can be identified. Chronic pancreatitis results in characteristic pancreatic duct strictures with intervening dilated segments. Brushings and biopsies of neoplastic obstructions of the common bile duct or ampulla may be obtained for diagnostic purposes. ERCP also has important therapeutic roles. The sphincter of Oddi can be incised (sphincterotomy) to extract biliary calculi thus relieving obstructive jaundice. Stents can be inserted to bypass structures or obstructing calculi. The combination of ERCP followed by laparoscopic cholecystectomy has almost replaced the operation of open cholecystectomy, intraoperative cholangiography and exploration of the common bile duct. ERCP may be complicated by acute pancreatitis or (rarely) haemorrhage following a sphincterotomy.

Intraoperative endoscopy

1. Enteroscopy. This is intraoperative visualization of the interior of the small bowel and this has been of use in the surgery of Crohn's disease to identify co-existing skip lesions and to dilatate stenoses.

2. Choledochoscopy. The extrahepatic biliary tree and its larger intrahepatic branches are visualized. The choledochoscope is inserted through a longitudinal choledochotomy during exploration of the common bile duct. Choledochoscopy can determine whether an obstruction is calculous or neoplastic.

3. Colonoscopy. This may be of use in the identification of sites of colonic bleeding during surgery when no source can easily be identified.

Chest

Brochoscopy is performed under local anaesthesia. Thoracoscopy requires a general anaesthetic. It provides a view of the pleural cavity enabling biopsy of pleural masses, aspiration of effusions, and insufflation pleurodesis. Mediastinoscopy requires general anaesthesia, and enables a view of the superior and anterior mediastinal structures through a small suprasternal incision. Masses, particularly enlarged lymph nodes, can be biopsied.

Urinary tract

Cystoscopy with a rigid cystoscope is performed under general or spinal anaesthesia, and enables transurethral resection of the prostate, bladder neck or bladder tumours, extraction of calculi, or insertion of ureteric stents. The bladder is best viewed using a 60° angled cystoscope and the bladder base and ureteric orifices using a 30° cystoscope. The ureters may be entered with a ureteroscope enabling laser or contact lithotripsy of ureteric calculi. The urethra is viewed using a 0° urethroscope prior to cystoscopy, and strictures may be incised with a urethrotome. Nephroscopy is performed under general anaesthesia after percutaneous nephrostomy followed by dilatation of the tract. Renal calculi may be extracted.

Laparoscopy

The peritoneal cavity is insufflated with carbon dioxide using a Veres needle inserted immediately below the umbilicus. A 10 mm diameter port is inserted and the peritoneal cavity is visualized directly. This may be used for diagnostic purposes but, increasingly, laparoscopy is used to achieve an operative procedure, such as cholecystectomy, gastric fundoplication, biopsy of intraperitoneal or hepatic lesions, rectopexy, herniorrhapy, tubal ligation, or colonic mobilization prior to colectomy. Surgery is performed following insertion of 10 mm or 5 mm operating ports, through which a variety of laparoscopic equipment can be inserted.

The complications of laparoscopic procedures include haemorrhage from the anterior abdominal wall port sites or retroperitoneal vessels, port site incisional hernia, and it may predispose to lower limb venous thromboembolism because of raised intra-abdominal pressure.

Other

There are many applications of 'endoscopy'.

- Angioscopy using fine flexible angioscopes has been applied to peripheral arteries and veins. Arterial occlusions can be located and recanalized. Carotid arteries may be angioscoped following endarterectomy to check for suture line thrombus or intimal flaps. Veins have been screened *in situ* by angioscopy prior to use as arterial bypass grafts.
- Angioscopy has been used to identify incompetent deep vein valves to allow accurate positioning of plicating sutures to restore valvular competence.
- Cruroscopy allows inspection and interruption of incompetent perforating veins passing through the deep fascia of the lower leg.
- The interior of the cerebral ventricles may be visualized during a craniotomy by ventriculoscopy.

Related topics of interest

ENTEROCUTANEOUS FISTULA

An enterocutaneous fistula is an abnormal connection between the gastrointestinal tract and the skin. In an end fistula the gastrointestinal tract is discontinuous (e.g. as in an end duodenal fistula), while in a lateral fistula, the connection is between the side of an intact viscus and intestinal continuity is maintained. A simple fistula has a single tract from involved bowel to the abdominal wall, whereas a complex fistula will have multiple tracts and often is associated with an abscess cavity.

Aetiology

There are five main causes of an enterocutaneous fistula and these are important when establishing a plan of treatment.

1. Anastomotic leakage. This is principally due to poor surgical technique or judgement (e.g. inadequate blood supply to bowel ends, tension on suture line, construction of an anastomosis in a high risk situation (intraperitoneal sepsis, distal obstruction)). Thus intestinal continuity should not be immediately restored after bowel resection in high risk patients as a stoma is easier to manage than a fistula.

Fistulae may occur following sepsis without prior surgery. Following acute diverticulitis on the left, and acute appendicitis on the right, localized infection may track through the parietes and present at the groin as an abscess. If this points and bursts, a fistula results.

2. Inflammatory bowel disease. This is mainly due to Crohn's disease, especially as the incidence appears to be rising in developed countries, but other inflammatory causes include intestinal tuberculosis and diverticular disease.

3. Malignancy. This causes fistulae by direct invasion of the abdominal wall or after spontaneous perforation and abscess formation with discharge through the abdominal wall, thus leading to the formation of a complex fistula. Radical surgical resection can be therapeutic, though this may be inappropriate in patients with disseminated malignancy.

4. Radiotherapy. Especially pelvic irradiation may lead to damage of small or larger bowel.

5. Trauma. Penetrating wounds to the abdomen can cause fistulas, particularly when the trauma results in multiple intestinal perforations with subsequent sepsis and abscess formation.

Management

1. General principles. Fistulas should be closed while maintaining the patient in good physical and mental health. This requires a team approach with the participation of both clinical and support staff (including nutritional and stoma nurses, pharmacist, physiotherapist). Initial resuscitation needs to be followed by longer-term nutritional support and then detailed assessment of the fistula with appropriate imaging to delineate it. A treatment plan including surgical or non-operative options can then be formulated, however, special attention needs to be directed to the following areas:

- *Fluid and electrolyte loss.* A high output fistula (>500 ml/day) can lead to large fluid and electrolyte losses with eventual circulatory collapse. Appropriate resuscitation needs to be guided by accurate measurement of all fluid losses. Serum levels of electrolytes need to be tested frequently until fluid balance is achieved. Thereafter twice-weekly estimations of haematological and biochemical indices should be sufficient.
- *Skin protection.* Proteolytic enzymes, especially in the upper gastrointestinal tract, can rapidly cause skin excoriation and damage. Adequate skin protection is essential to keep the intestinal contents away from the surrounding skin. Reducing the volume of a high output fistula not only helps skin management but also reduces fluid and electrolyte losses. This can be achieved by restricting oral intake, however, a number of pharmacological agents (H2 antagonists, omeprazole and somatostatin analogues) have been used with varying degrees of success.
- *Nutritional support.* Correction of nutritional deficiencies and long-term parenteral nutrition are often necessary for patients with high output fistulae. Oral intake should be stopped, which reduces fistula output and intestinal secretions. Intravenous feeding should be commenced in any patient with an enterocutaneous fistula other than a simple low output terminal ileal or colonic fistula. This rests the bowel and restores nutritional status, providing optimal conditions for spontaneous fistula closure. Enteral feeding should be considered for patients with gastric, duodenal or high small bowel fistulae, however, fluid and electrolyte losses will still need to be replaced intravenously and the ensuing diarrhoea can be troublesome.
- *Control of sepsis.* An abscess cavity may complicate an enterocutaneous fistula and should be suspected in the

presence of persisting pain, pyrexia, tachycardia, leucocytosis and a falling serum albumin. Confirmation and delineation of an abscess cavity is best achieved by intubation and instillation of dilute barium sulphate. Ultrasound and CT scanning are also useful and may allow needle drainage. Abscess cavities need to be drained either radiologically or surgically to control and eliminate sepsis with the aim of converting a complex cavity into a simple fistula tract which can close spontaneously. Antibiotics should not be used unless there is septicaemia (confirmed by blood cultures) or surrounding cellulitis.

• *Haemorrhage*. This can be life-threatening from eroded vessels within the fistula tract or abscess cavity. Erosion of arteries occurs as a result of sepsis or the action of digestive enzymes (especially in the stomach). Treatment may require urgent resection of the fistula but arterial embolization should also be considered.

2. Conservative or operative management. Accurate prediction of the likelihood of spontaneous closure is generally possible after detailed investigation of the patient and the anatomy and cause of the fistula. Closure will not occur if there is: total discontinuity of bowel ends, distal obstruction, a chronic abscess cavity or mucocutaneous epithelial continuity and is less likely if the involved bowel is diseased (e.g. Crohn's or malignancy), the patient is malnourished or the fistulae are internal. Approximately 60% should close within 1 month of conservative treatment after control of sepsis. If after 6–8 weeks closure has not occurred, the underlying cause should be determined and surgical closure undertaken.

Related topics of interest

Crohn's disease (p. 106)
Nutrition in the surgical patient (p. 213)

FEMORAL HERNIA

Epidemiology and aetiology

Herniation through the femoral canal is commoner in women than in men (F : M = 2.5 : 1). In women, indirect inguinal hernias and femoral hernias are equally common. Femoral hernias account for 11% of all groin hernias, but account for between 35% and 50% of all strangulated groin hernias. Approximately 50% of femoral hernias present with strangulation. The cumulative probabilities of strangulation at 1 month and 21 months after diagnosis are 22% and 45% respectively. Bowel resection is twice as likely during operations for strangulated femoral hernia as for strangulated inguinal hernia and the mortality for such surgery lies between 3% and 15%.

Femoral hernias are almost exclusively acquired and usually occur from middle age onwards. They are commonest in multiparous women and may follow a period of weight loss. Ten per cent of femoral hernias follow a previous operation for inguinal hernia. Femoral hernias are usually irreducible and frequently exhibit no cough impulse. Omentum is the usual content of a femoral hernia, but if bowel is contained it is frequently in the form of a Richter's hernia, this phenomenon occurring most frequently on the right.

Femoral hernias share the same basic pathology with all other lower abdominal hernias. A defect in the transversalis fascia occurs, allowing a peritoneal protrusion to appear.

Differential diagnosis

- Inguinal hernia.
- Enlarged lymph node.
- Saphena varix.
- Psoas bursa or abscess.
- Obturator hernia.
- Lipoma.
- Femoral aneurysm.
- Sarcoma.
- Ectopic testis.

Management

Because of the high risk of strangulation, femoral hernia should always be repaired promptly after diagnosis. The principles of repair include isolation and removal of the peritoneal sac, repair of the transversalis fascia, and reinforcement of this repair. Three approaches are described below.

1. *Abdominal, preperitoneal (Henry, McEvedy).* A vertical midline or Pfannenstiel incision is used to repair bilateral hernias, or an oblique incision over the lateral border of rectus abdominis (linea semilunaris) for unilateral hernias (McEvedy). The hernias are reduced and the femoral canal closed without breaching the peritoneum, unless there is a suspicion of strangulated bowel. This is a good approach for a strangulated hernia.

2. *Inguinal or high (Lothiessen).* The posterior wall of the inguinal canal is opened to give access to the femoral canal from above. Femoral and inguinal hernias may be repaired simultaneously by this method which is therefore useful if the exact nature of the hernia is unclear. The inguinal canal must be repaired carefully to avoid a subsequent inguinal hernia.

3. *Crural or low (Lockwood).* An incision is made directly over the hernia, just below and parallel to the medial half of the inguinal ligament. The sac is identified, opened and ligated. The femoral canal is closed using either non-absorbable sutures or a plug, taking care not to damage or narrow the femoral vein. An upturned flap of pectineal fascia may be used to reinforce the repair. This approach should be reserved for elective operations, but if compromised bowel is discovered, a separate incision should be performed.

The chance of recurrence following the extraperitoneal high approach or the crural low approach is 5–10%. A higher recurrence rate accompanies the inguinal approach, although this can be substantially reduced if the inguinal canal is carefully repaired using the Shouldice or Lichtenstein technique.

Further reading

Clinical Guidelines on the Management of Groin Hernias in Adults. Royal College of Surgeons of England, 1993.
Devlin B. The abdominal wall and hernias. In: Burnard KG, Young AE (eds) *The New Aird's Companion in Surgical Studies.* Edinburgh: Churchill Livingstone, 1992; 845–75.

Related topics of interest

FISTULA-IN-ANO

More reputations have been damaged by the unsuccessful treatment of fistula-in-ano than by excision of the rectum. The notoriety of anal fistula led Salmon (who operated on Dickens for the condition) to found St Mark's Hospital in 1835 for the treatment of fistula and other diseases of the rectum.

Epidemiology

Men predominate (5:1) with a maximal incidence between the third and fifth decades.

Pathogenesis

The cryptoglandular hypothesis of Eisenhammer for the pathogenesis of anal fistula postulates that infection starts in an anal gland lying within the intersphincteric space, at the line of the anal valves (dentate line). As the abscess expands, pus may tract longitudinally, up or down, in the intersphincteric, submucous or extrasphincteric planes to present as a perianal, ischiorectal or supralevator abscess. Circumferential tracking can similarly occur along these planes and form a horseshoe abscess. The fistula is 'complete' when the abscess spontaneously discharges or the surgeon provides this communication. Secondary tracts complicate the situation and represent upward extension into the supralevator space or lateral extension into the ischiorectal fossa.

Classification

The most widely used system to classify fistulae is by Parks who divided them into four groups.

1. Intersphincteric. These fistulae occur between the internal and external sphincter. Downward extension presents as a perianal abscess, but they can also extend upwards to drain into the rectum without a perineal opening. This can be detected clinically by the presence of supralevator induration. In rare circumstances a pelvic abscess, for example from the appendix or a sigmoid diverticulum, can extend downwards in the intersphincteric plane to produce a perianal abscess.

2. Trans-sphincteric. These fistulae occur when the tract penetrates through the external sphincter and consequently presents as an ischiorectal abscess.

3. Suprasphincteric. These fistulae tract upwards to loop over the puborectalis. They penetrate through levator ani to reach the perineal skin via the ischiorectal fossa. Presentation is usually with an ischiorectal abscess.

4. Extrasphincteric. These fistulae are rare. They occur when a pelvic abscess drains into the ischiorectal fossa.

Evaluation

Accurate operative evaluation of the anatomy of an anal fistula is essential if the two major problems of recurrence and incontinence are to be avoided. The principle of surgery is to lay open the primary tract and to drain any secondary tracts. Preoperative examination allows assessment of sphincter tone (internal sphincter) and squeeze (external sphincter), and will aid in the determination of the level of the internal opening in relation to the puborectalis. In difficult cases, a full electrophysiological assessment of the anorectum is required together with anal ultrasound. Sigmoidoscopy is essential to exclude underlying pathology like Crohn's proctitis. If any doubt arises a rectal biopsy should be taken.

Surgery

The initial aim is to locate the internal and external openings, the primary tract and secondary tracts, and seek the presence or absence of an underlying disease process. Digital examination with a well-lubricated finger and an Eisenhammer retractor can identify the hallmark of fibrosis: induration. Massage of this area may be all that is necessary to identify the internal opening with a bead of emerging pus. The careful use of the four standard Lockhart–Mummery probes together with a lachrymal probe are usually essential for identification. Injection of 1 mm of hydrogen peroxide into the tract may result in the emergence of bubbles from the internal opening. Further tricks used include methylene blue injection, but this has a habit of staining everything blue and not just the granulation tissue. Finally, traction on the external opening may cause the internal opening to dimple. Granulation tissue that will not curette away is a helpful guide to the presence of secondary tracts. All suspicious fistulae should be examined histologically for evidence of Crohn's disease.

Goodsall's rule

Goodsall's rule states that fistulae with an external opening around the posterior half circumference of the anus have their internal opening in the midline posteriorly. Those with an external opening around the anterior half circumference have their internal opening directly opposite, the tract coursing radially. Exceptions to this rule occasionally occur which is why it is no substitute for an accurate operative evaluation.

The seton

Ninety per cent of fistulae are easy to treat and are readily managed by fistulotomy or excision (fistulectomy).

Complicated or high fistulae are usually managed by setons (seta = bristle in Latin). These are ligatures, usually made of nylon, placed through tracts and around important sphincters. They may be applied loosely, when used as a drain, or tightly to stimulate fibrosis. This fibrosis prevents separation of the anal sphincter muscle when gradual fistulotomy, by fortnightly seton tightening, is performed. Although puborectalis is the most significant muscle in controlling continence, all the sphincters play a role and should be preserved as much as possible.

Anorectal abscess

More than 50% of patients with acute first time anorectal abscesses can be treated primarily by de-roofing. Those that reoccur demonstrate anaerobes in their initial abscess culture. There is a good argument for performing a subsequent examination for the detection of fistulae in all patients whenever anaerobes are demonstrated. This strategy should prevent recurrent abscess presentations. If an internal opening is found, it should be documented or marked with a seton until the acute situation is over. Overzealous or inexperienced attempts at probing may spread the sepsis and result in false passages. Digital examination can identify supralevator induration, indicating the presence of a secondary tract, which can often be drained by opening the intersphincteric plane and using a seton. All diabetics and the immunosuppressed require antibiotics because anorectal sepsis in these patients can become rife, leading, in some cases, to sacrococcygeal osteitis or even retroperitoneal extension.

Infancy

Anal fistulae in infancy occur usually in males under 1 year of age. They are due to a congenital abnormality of the anal glands. The majority are intersphincteric and managed along adult lines.

Further reading

Seow-Choen F, Nicholls RJ. Anal fistulae (Review). *British Journal of Surgery*, 1992; **79**: 197–205.

Related topics of interest

AIDS (p. 20)
Anorectal investigation (p. 35)
Crohn's disease (p. 106)

FLUID REPLACEMENT

The Confidential Enquiry into Perioperative Deaths (CEPOD) has recognized that inadequate rehydration and oliguria prior to surgery carries with it a high mortality. Total body water is distributed into the intracellular compartment (two-thirds) and the extracellular compartment (one-third). A quarter of the extracellular fluid exists as plasma. These ratios are maintained together with electrolyte balance and acid–base balance by various homostatic mechanisms. The approximate water compartments for a 70-kg man are tabulated below.

Compartment	Volume (1)
Total body water	42
Intracellular fluid	28 (2/3)
Extracellular fluid (ECF)	14 (1/3)
Plasma volume	3.5 (1/4 of ECF)

Renin–angiotensin–aldosterone

This mechanism is activated by sympathetic stimulation, falls in blood pressure and alterations in Na^+ flux across the renal tubules. Renin is secreted by the juxta-glomerular apparatus, and activates circulating angiotensinogen to form angiotensin I. This is then converted to angiotensin II by converting enzyme, found in high concentrations in the lungs. Angiotensin II is itself a powerful vasoconstrictor and stimulates the release of aldosterone from the zona glomerulosa of the renal cortex. Aldosterone acts mainly on the distal convoluted tubule to encourage the preferential resorption of sodium at the expense of potassium and hydrogen ions. This system is the most powerful single mechanism for the control of plasma volume, electrolyte and acid–base balance.

Antidiuretic hormone (arginine vasopressin)

This hormone is released from the posterior pituitary in response to anxiety, operative trauma, falls in blood pressure and changes in plasma osmolality. It acts upon the collecting ducts to reduce the excretion of water.

Atrial naturetic peptides

These have been identified in cardiac tissue and are released in response to increases in plasma volume. They act on the kidney to provide an increased diuresis independent of the renin–angiotensin–aldosterone mechanism.

Sodium

Sodium is considered the skeleton upon which the extracellular fluid hangs. The normal plasma concentration is maintained between 135 and 145 mmol/l. The normal daily requirement is 100 mmol. Excess loss of sodium and therefore water occurs in vomiting, diarrhoea, high output fistulae, profuse sweating, Addison's disease and third space sequestration like intestinal obstruction or peritonitis. Assuming that the total body water is three-fifths of the body weight the saline deficit can be estimated:

Saline deficit (mmol) = 3/5 Body weight (kg) × (140 − Plasma Na conc.)

Potassium

Potassium is 97% intracellular. Normal plasma values are between 3.5 and 4.5 mmol/l. The normal daily requirements vary from 60 to 90 mmol.

1. Hypokalaemia. Deficiency from gastrointestinal fluid loss or a metabolic alkalosis (pyloric stenosis) results in weakness, confusion and ileus, or even cardiac arrest in systole. Diagnostic ECG changes include a prolonged PR interval, depressed ST segments and inverted T waves.

2. Hyperkalaemia. This is often secondary to renal failure and can be treated with 10% dextrose (1 l) with 10 units of added Actrapid as a single infusion. Ionic exchange resins can be administered rectally. Severe cases require dialysis. Characteristic ECG changes include peaked T waves, absent P waves and a widened QRS complex. Eventually, cardiac arrest occurs in diastole.

Metabolic response to trauma

The duration and extent of the metabolic response to trauma (release of cortisol, ADH, aldosterone) depends upon the severity of the insult. Burns and crush injuries are particularly strong stimuli whereas day case procedures hardly elicit any response. Awareness of this has important implications in postoperative fluid balance.

Postoperative management

During the first postoperative day it is essential to establish a urinary output of greater than 30 ml/hour. This should be effected primarily by ensuring the patient is adequately hydrated without precipitating cardiac failure. A 200 ml crystalloid fluid challenge is a useful way of establishing this. If a hydrated patient continues to produce only small volumes of urine, frusemide should be administered to challenge the metabolic response to trauma and provide a diuresis. Occasionally, some hypertensives or patients in poor cardiovascular health fail to establish a good urinary output despite adequate filling and frusemide. Restoration of blood pressure to 'normal' levels (i.e. in a hypertensive patient) or the commencement of a renal (low-dose) dopamine infusion can often encourage the kidneys to perform again. Maintenance of an adequate diuresis is a requisite for renal health and the prevention of renal failure. Intensive monitoring of the CVP and the pulmonary artery wedge pressure should be performed if problems in maintaining normal blood pressure (in the presence of presumed adequate filling) still arise. The response of the CVP to a fluid challenge is a more useful indicator than the absolute value alone. A rising potassium, urea or creatinine indicates renal failure. Potassium supplements should not be given in the first postoperative day because tissue damage and blood transfusions provide a rich source of plasma potassium.

Fluid and electrolyte maintenance

The normal fluid requirement is 3 l/day. Pyrexia, nasogastric aspirate, ileus, peritonitis, fistula, diarrhoea and unhumidified ventilation increase these requirements, and adjustments should be made in the replacement regime. Up to 1 l of fluid can be lost each hour during a laparotomy. Serial haematocrit, electrolyte, urea and creatinine estimations give an indication as to the state of hydration. A typical short-term fluid maintenance regime involves 1 l of normal saline followed by 2 l of 5% dextrose with 60–80 mmol of KCl added in divided doses. This will provide 150 mmol of sodium. Alternatively, 3 l of dextrose saline can be administered, but this only provides 90 mmol of sodium. Patients on long-term dextrose saline infusions may consequently become sodium deficient. Gastrointestinal losses should be replaced with saline, volume for volume, with added potassium supplements.

Pyloric stenosis

The repetitive vomiting of pyloric stenosis results in a metabolic alkalosis. It also provides a situation where acid is lost from the stomach and a paradoxical acid urine may be excreted. This happens because the distal convoluted tubule preferentially conserves potassium rather than hydrogen ions when sodium is resorbed.

Further reading

Smith JAR. Fluid balance and electrolyte disturbance. *Recent Advances in Surgery*, 1992; **15**: 209–23.

Related topics of interest

GALLSTONES AND THEIR COMPLICATIONS

Gallstones are common, affecting about 20% of the population. Although the typical patient is said to be 'fat, fertile, fair, female and over forty', men and women are probably equally affected, and gallstones may even occur in childhood. They frequently co-exist with diverticular disease and hiatus hernia (Saint's triad). Most gallstones are symptomless, but a wide variety of clinical entities may result. Surgery for removal of the gallbladder, cholecystectomy, is the most common elective operation performed.

Formation and composition

Eighty per cent of gallstones have alternate laminae of cholesterol and calcium salts (mixed). Such stones are invariably multiple, numbering from a few to many hundreds, and are faceted. Twelve per cent of stones are small, multiple and dark, containing bilirubin salts (pigment stones). They may be separate or concreted together (mulberry stones). These may complicate haemolytic anaemias. Eight per cent of gallstones are composed primarily of cholesterol. These stones are usually single (solitaires) and tend to be soft and large.

The formation of gallstones revolves around three factors:

- Bile is rendered 'lithogenic' by an increase in cholesterol relative to bile salts which render it soluble. A reduction in bile salts, as may follow ileal resection or Crohn's disease of the terminal ileum, may effectively precipitate cholesterol in the bile.
- A nidus may be necessary for the stones to form, and this may be provided by bacteria or foreign bodies.
- Some degree of stasis is also required.

Diagnosis

1. Clinical. Gallstones may cause flatulence, dyspeptic symptoms, nausea, and postprandial discomfort. This overlaps with other foregut pathologies, particularly peptic ulceration and hiatus hernia, and a clinical diagnosis may be difficult. Murphy's sign, the arrest of inspiration (due to pain) while pressure is being applied to the right hypochondrium, is indicative of cholecystitis.

2. Ultrasound scan. Ultrasound scanning is a rapid non-invasive test demonstrating stones in the gallbladder with acoustic shadows behind them. The gallbladder wall may be thickened in acute cholecystitis. The gallbladder is usually small and shrunken. The scan will also identify bile duct dilatation if there are stones within the extrahepatic bile ducts, though stones in the distal common bile duct are rarely visualized due to overlying intra-duodenal gas.

3. Plain radiology. Plain abdominal X-rays will detect only 10% of gallstones. Rarely, a thin rim of calcification is seen within the wall of the gallbladder (porcelain gallbladder). Limey bile may be visible rarely.

4. Oral cholangiography. This concentrates an oral bolus of contrast in the gallbladder. Radiolucent stones become obvious filling defects on X-rays.

Complications: stones within the gallbladder

1. Biliary colic. Intermittent epigastric pain may radiate to the right and may be induced by fatty food. The patient may need to be admitted and opiate analgesia may be required. The pain usually subsides within 24 hours. The pain is not caused by gallbladder contraction as in cholelithiasis the gallbladder is non-contractile.

2. Acute cholecystitis. Stasis in a hollow viscus allows infection to supervene. In the gallbladder this results in severe pain in the right upper quadrant which is constant. The patient has a pyrexia and a tachycardia, and a leucocytosis will be present. The signs include rebound tenderness or guarding. This requires antibiotics covering Gram-negative organisms. Approximately 10% of patients with acute cholecystitis may be transiently jaundiced. This may arise from compression of the common bile duct from oedematous tissue in the region of the neck of the gallbladder where a calculus has impacted.

3. Empyema of the gallbladder. Very severe acute cholecystitis with a high swinging pyrexia suggests an empyema of the gallbladder. This may result from infection within a mucocoele or from a severe cholecystitis. An air-fluid level is seen on a plain abdominal X-ray.

4. Acute acalculous cholecystitis. Rarely, the gallbladder may become inflamed in the absence of gallstones. This may occur in those who are already severely debilitated, particularly patients in intensive care. This commonly results in a necrotic gallbladder.

5. Emphysematous cholecystitis. Severe infections with anaerobic gas-forming organisms may occur in diabetics.

Gas is seen in the wall of the gallbladder on a plain radiograph. This may occur in the absence of stones.

6. Mirizzi syndrome. A gallstone impacted in Hartmann's pouch, usually a single large solitaire, may result in obstructive jaundice by impinging on the common bile duct. This is Mirizzi type 1 syndrome, and should be diagnosed pre-operatively, as there is a risk of damage to the common bile duct. Pressure on the common bile duct from the large calculus may result in necrosis of the intervening tissue, with a resultant cholecystocholedochal (or cholecysto-hepatodochal) fistula. This is Mirizzi type 2 syndrome. ERCP should demonstrate these conditions.

7. Mucocoele. Impaction of a calculus in the neck of the gallbladder resulting in stasis and continued formation of mucus results in a mucocoele.

8. Carcinoma. There is a small risk of malignancy in the gallbladder mucosa in association with gallstones. It is five times more common in females than males. Up to 0.5% will have carcinoma-*in-situ* if closely examined histologically. Rarely, advanced gallbladder carcinoma presents as a hard right upper quadrant mass and jaundice through lymph node involvement at the porta hepatis. This is usually unresectable, and the prognosis is poor.

Complications: stones outside the gallbladder

1. Pancreatitis. Acute and chronic pancreatitis may result from the passage of gallstones through the common bile duct. Approximately 50% of pancreatitis is gallstone-related.

2. Biliary stricture. Chronic calculous inflammation may result in a benign bile duct stricture. This may cause obstructive jaundice and predispose to ascending cholangitis, with further inflammation and further tendency for stricture formation. This requires careful evaluation by ERCP before cholecystectomy and a biliary drainage procedure.

3. Obstructive jaundice. This results from impaction of a calculus in the distal common bile duct. Multiple calculi may be present. ERCP will identify the problem, and a sphincterotomy can be performed through which stones can be retrieved. Any residual stones fall through the sphincterotomy. If ERCP is unsuccessful or unavailable, surgery to remove stones from the bile ducts is required. This procedure entails cholecystectomy with exploration of the common bile duct.

4. Ascending cholangitis. This is a severe infection, usually complicating benign obstruction of the biliary tree. The infecting organisms are usually Gram-negative bacilli. Endotoxic shock may result. A diagnosis may be made clinically in the presence of Charcot's triad: fever with rigors, jaundice, and an enlarged tender liver. It requires prompt diagnosis, i.v. fluids, antibiotics directed toward coliforms, and urgent relief from the obstruction. ERCP and sphincterotomy with stone extraction or temporary stenting is urgently undertaken. Open surgery is hazardous in the acute cholangitis.

5. Gallstone ileus. A large solitaire may erode into the duodenum and impact at the narrowest point of the small bowel, typically two feet proximal to the ileocaecal valve or at an existent pathological stricture. This presents as a small bowel obstruction. A plain abdominal X-ray may show obstructed small bowel, a large calcified gallstone in the right iliac fossa, and air outlining the biliary tree, although the whole triad is rarely seen.

Management of gallstones

1. Gallbladder calculi. Elective cholecystectomy is required if symptomatic. Surgery should be urgent in severe acute cholecystitis, empyema, or emphysematous or necrotizing cholecystitis.

2. Common bile duct calculi. Following acute pancreatitis or obstructive jaundice, or if the LFTs are abnormal or the common bile duct is dilated on ultrasound, the bile ducts should be screened prior to cholecystectomy by ERCP. This is essential in established jaundice or ascending cholangitis. Alternatively, intra-operative cholangiography is performed.

Surgery

1. Cholecystectomy. Right subcostal (Kocher's) or transverse incisions are ideal for open surgery. Tiny incisions may be used (mini-cholecystectomy), but laparoscopic cholecystectomy is the preferred technique.

2. Intra-operative cholangiography. Cholangiography may be performed during open or laparoscopic surgery. The X-rays are scrutinized for filling defects (calculi), biliary dilatation and flow of contrast into the duodenum. If common bile duct calculi are suspected, the duct is explored.

3. Exploration of the common bile duct. The duodenum is mobilized (Kocher's manoeuvre). The opened common bile duct is irrigated to flush out loose calculi. Choledochoscopy locates impacted calculi which are extracted with Desjardin's forceps or a Fogarty catheter. Transduodenal sphincteroplasty plus stone extraction is rarely required. The common bile duct is closed over an external biliary drain (T-tube), through which a cholangiogram is performed at 10 days. The T-tube is removed if there are no stones and there is free flow into the duodenum.

Treatment of retained common bile duct calculi

T-tubes may be repeatedly flushed with saline if cholangiography confirms small retained calculi. Alternatively, methyl terbutyl ether instilled through a T-tube will dissolve residual stones. Larger calculi may be extracted using forceps introduced along a dilated T-tube tract (Burhenne technique). Extracorporeal lithotripsy has been used successfully. The results of these techniques may be improved by endoscopic sphincterotomy.

Postcholecystectomy syndrome and recurrent symptoms

Early recurrence of the often vague epigastric or dyspeptic symptoms for which the patient was relieved of their gallbladder is frequently referred to as the post-cholecystectomy syndrome. In some of these patients, the true cause of their symptoms may be discovered, but often the problem persists, and proves very difficult to treat.

Medical treatment

Gallstones may dissolve with oral ursodeoxycholate and chenodeoxycholate (bile acids). Treatment takes many months to complete, and has been shown to dissolve only small uncalcified stones successfully. A functioning gallbladder is necessary for bile acids to work. There is a high recurrence rate, as the root cause of the problem, the gallbladder, remains *in situ*. Their use is thus limited.

Further reading

Cheslyn-Curtis S, Russell RCG. New trends in gallstone management. *British Journal of Surgery*, 1991; **78**: 143–9.

O'Leary DP, Johnson AG. Future directions for conservative treatment of gallbladder calculi. *British Journal of Surgery*, 1993; **80**: 143–7.

Perissat J, Huibregtse K, Keane FBV *et al.* Management of bile duct stones in the era of laparoscopic cholecystectomy. *British Journal of Surgery*, 1994; **81**: 799–810.

Related topics of interest

GASTRIC CANCER

Nearly all gastric cancers detected in the UK are advanced adenocarcinomas with an overall 5-year survival rate of 5–10%. In comparison, in Japan, where the disease is commonest, over 30% of all gastric cancers are detected early and the overall 5-year survival rates exceed 50%. Japanese experience in mass screening, appreciation of the radical R2 gastrectomy and different disease behaviour patterns all contribute to improved survival.

Demography

Gastric cancer is twice as common in males, peaks in incidence between 55 and 65 years, is associated with blood group A and occurs more frequently amongst the lower social classes. A fourfold increase is noted amongst patients with a family history, which suggests powerful genetic factors, but Japanese migrants to Hawaii develop significantly lower incidences within their second generation suggesting an environmental influence, for example, diet.

Types

Gastric cancer can be divided into intestinal and diffuse types. The intestinal type matches geographical areas of increased incidence and is usually accompanied by an area of chronic gastritis. The diffuse type bears no such relationship.

Risk factors

Chronic gastritis, gastric ulcers and gastric polyps are lesions often considered precancerous. The gastric remnant following a partial gastrectomy for benign disease has an increased risk of developing a gastric carcinoma. Autoimmune gastritis (pernicious anaemia) is subject to dysplastic change which may then become neoplastic. Populations where gastric cancer is common have a high incidence of chronic gastritis, mucosal atrophy and subsequent intestinal metaplasia. Over 90% of carcinomas are found in areas of gastritis and 10% of patients with chronic gastritis develop a carcinoma. Gastric adenomatous polyps are considered premalignant. They are composed of dysplastic glands and the larger the polyp the higher the incidence of malignancy. There is no convincing evidence that chronic gastric ulcers undergo malignant change.

Presentation

Clinical presentation depends upon lesion site and disease advancement. The commoner antral lesions may cause outlet obstruction with vomiting and a succussion splash or fistulate into the colon. Cardial lesions may cause dysphagia or regurgitation. Fundal lesions are often silent, with anorexia and increasing satiety after meal times. Irrespective of site, many first present with indigestion pains and dyspepsia. Carcinomas may perforate, ulcerate causing anaemia and lead to ill health with weakness and weight loss. A knobbly liver or the carcinoma itself may be palpable. A left supraclavicular node mass (Virchow's node) (Troisier's sign) or ascites indicates advanced disease. Jaundice may be caused by nodal compression at the porta hepatis, direct ductal involvement or by progressive liver replacement.

Diagnosis

The mainstay of diagnosis for early lesions is to perform an upper GI endoscopy on all patients with a recent onset of dyspepsia or indigestion-like pains. All suspicious lesions and unusual areas of gastritis should be biopsied or undergo brush cytology. Linitis plastica (leather bottle stomach) is suggested if the stomach fails to distend on insufflation. Repeat biopsies at the same site (trench biopsy) may be required to reach the areas of submucosal infiltration that are typical for these carcinomas. Double contrast barium radiology is complimentary to diagnosis. A filling defect, mucosal irregularity or stricture may be visualized. Ultrasound, CT scan and laparoscopy may be useful in assessing disease advancement and preventing an unnecessary laparotomy.

The R2 gastrectomy

All the lymph node groups which drain the stomach are classified according to their site (supra/infra pyloric, right/left cardiac, greater/lesser curve and those groups along and at the origins of the arterial supply to the stomach). The primary tumour is documented in the upper, middle or lower third of the stomach. N1 nodes are situated within 3 cm of the primary. N2 nodes are all those mentioned above greater than 3 cm from the primary. N2 nodes could all become N1 nodes if the tumour was sited in a different region. An R2 resection involves removing all the N1 and N2 nodes with a 5 cm clearance of the tumour. The operative mortality for an R2 gastrectomy should not exceed 5%.

Anastomosis

Gastrointestinal continuity is restored after a radical lower partial gastrectomy with a Polya or a Roux-en-Y anastomosis. A Billroth 1 gastrectomy is ill advised because the anastomosis will be sited on the original tumour bed. Continuity after total gastrectomy is usually with a Roux-en-Y or an omega jejunal loop with a side-to-side enteroenterostomy. These anastomoses are protected with a naso-jejunal tube until radiological evidence of anastomotic integrity. Oral feeding can then be reinstituted.

Post-gastrectomy symptoms	Gastrectomy is associated with post-gastrectomy symptoms in 20% of cases. These include biliary reflux, diarrhoea, osmotic (early) and hypoglycaemic (late) dumping, anaemia and malnutrition. A Roux-en-Y construction with an anastomosis at least 50 cm distal to the upper resection limit can lessen biliary reflux. Vitamin B12 injections and oral ferrous sulphate are often-needed supplements.
Prognosis	Disease stage is the best prognostic indicator. Well-differentiated lesions carry a better prognosis than the poorly differentiated or signet cell types. Vascular invasion is associated with future liver metastasis. Serosal invasion, perforation and poor differentiation are associated with peritoneal dissemination. Lymph node metastases are associated with both. Upper gastric lesions are often advanced with a poor prognosis. There is no convincing evidence that chemotherapy or radiotherapy prolongs survival.
Lymphoma	Gastric lymphoma is the commonest extranodal primary site for non-Hodgkin's lymphoma. Therapy involves resection and adjuvant chemotherapy and/or radiotherapy. Careful observation is required if chemotherapy or radiotherapy is initiated when resection has not been possible, because gastrointestinal lymphomas have a tendency to perforate.
Carcinoid tumour	Carcinoid tumours usually form a polypoidal mass. The carcinoid syndrome of flushing, diarrhoea and bronchospasm occurs when liver metastases secrete excessive amounts of 5-HT (serotonin). Resection offers 5-year survival rates of over 75%.
Leiomyosarcoma	Gastric leiomyosarcomas most often present with bleeding. They can occur *de novo* or arise within a leiomyoma. Resection offers 5-year survival rates approaching 50%.

Further reading

Sugimachi K. Treatment of gastric cancer. *Current Opinion in General Surgery*, 1993; 216–18.

Wastell C, Fielding JWL. The stomach and duodenum. In: Burnand KG, Young AE (eds) *The New Aird's Companion in Surgical Studies*, Edinburgh: Churchill Livingstone, 1992; 980–8.

Related topics of interest

GASTROINTESTINAL POLYPS

Polyps are swellings arising from the gastrointestinal epithelium. Occasionally, through the action of normal peristalsis, they may develop a stalk, which can become very long indeed. Polyps that have a stalk are called pedunculated, and those arising directly from the bowel wall on a broad base are termed sessile. Polyps may be single or multiple and can occur at any age. The majority of gastrointestinal polyps occur in the colon, however, the stomach and small intestine are other sites.

Pathology

Polyps may be classified as malignant or benign, however, this can be confusing as many benign polyps have malignant potential. The best classification has four major groups: adenomatous (or neoplastic), hamartomatous, inflammatory and miscellaneous.

1. Adenomatous. Adenomatous polyps are benign neoplasms arising from the gastrointestinal epithelium. They are almost always found in the colon, but may occur in the stomach, duodenum or small bowel. There are different types based on morphology. All adenomatous polyps comprise glandular tissue, but this may be arranged differently giving rise to a pathological classification. Eighty per cent of adenomatous polyps are found in the rectosigmoid. They are an important cause of rectal bleeding, although they may be discovered incidentally. Large rectal polyps may present as a prolapsing mass at the anus. Any polyp may act as the lead point of an intussusception.

(a) *Tubular adenoma.* These are polyps that are macroscopically solid and consist of many curled acini. They comprise about 65% of all colonic polyps and may occur anywhere in the gastrointestinal tract, but are most common in the colon. They often develop a stalk, and thus become pedunculated.

(b) *Villous adenoma.* These are usually sessile, and appear fronded, soft and velvety macroscopically. Microscopically they consist of multiple villi. These are more common in females, and comprise about 15% of all polyps. They are most frequently found in the rectum or the caecum, are usually solitary, and may be large at presentation, possibly involving the full circumference of the colon. Large rectal villous adenomas produce inordinately large amounts of mucus. Copious amounts of mucus and slime are passed per rectum, best described as a clear and somewhat lumpy jelly. This is a potassium-rich alkaline mucus. If this is lost in excess over a long period, patients will become hypokalaemic and may even develop a metabolic acidosis.

(c) *Tubulovillous adenoma.* If there are tubular and villous histological features, the polyp is a tubulovillous adenoma. These are more common in males than females, and account for about 20% of gastrointestinal polyps. In 20% of cases these are multiple.

2. *Hamartomatous*

(a) *True hamartoma.* These occur sporadically or as part of the Peutz–Jehger's syndrome. They vary greatly in size, and have well-defined fibrous and smooth muscle layers interspersed with epithelial structures histologically. They may carry a small increased risk of malignancy.

(b) *Juvenile polyps.* These are large, fleshy, hamartomatous polyps that usually occur in childhood. They are more common in boys, and there may be a family history.They cause rectal bleeding and may intussuscept. They have a typical histological appearance of a well-defined fibrous stroma interspersed by large cystic epithelial lined spaces. They are usually solitary, but may be multiple in juvenile polyposis coli. Juvenile polyposis is associated with an increased risk of malignancy, although solitary juvenile polyps are not.

3. *Inflammatory.*
These arise in inflamed colonic mucosa, typically in ulcerative colitis. They represent islands of regenerating epithelium, are usually multiple, and are often called pseudopolyps.

4. *Miscellaneous*

(a) *Metaplastic polyps.* These are usually small and are of no clinical significance. They are commonly encountered in the colon, and are differentiated from neoplastic polyps by their fronded or serrated microscopic appearance. They are usually sessile, but may, rarely, be pedunculated. They are common in the rectum and at stomas.

(b) *Lymphoid.* These are sessile accumulations of benign lymphoid cells, and have little clinical significance.

(c) *Other benign tumours.* Any submucosal tumour may become pedunculated and appear polypoid. In the colon, this is usually a submucosal lipoma or leiomyoma. They may be the cause of intussusception.

The polyp cancer sequence

All adenomatous polyps carry the potential to become malignant. Features most likely to be associated with malignancy in a polyp are size (greater than 2 cm diameter), number, the presence of cytological atypia in the epithelium, polyp morphology and villous adenomas. The epithelium of an excised or biopsied polyp must be scrutinized carefully for the presence of signs of developing malignancy. Hyperplasia, atypia or mitotic figures all suggest epithelial dysplasia, and if this is ignored, then invasion and frank malignancy will result. If a pedunculated polyp is excised, the stalk must be examined for invasion in view of the above. Excluding the colonic carcinomas developing in ulcerative colitis, probably all carcinomas arise as a consequence of the polyp–cancer sequence. Villous adenomas have a higher risk than tubular adenomas of developing malignant change.

Polyposis syndromes

1. Familial adenomatous polyposis. This comprises multiple colonic adenomatous polyps, otherwise known as polyposis coli. This is inherited as an autosomal dominant gene. The sheer quantity of colonic polyps combined with their early onset, give rise to the very high risk of gastrointestinal carcinoma, usually occurring by the age of 30. The treatment for this condition is total colectomy with formation of an ileo-anal pouch, or subtotal colectomy and ileorectal anastomosis with frequent endoscopic screening of the rectal mucosa. Polyps may also occur at other sites in the gastrointestinal tract, particularly in the duodenum. The family must also be screened for the disorder.

2. Gardner's syndrome. This represents multiple colonic adenomatous polyps associated with multiple extracolonic tumours, often hamartomatous. These include dental and epidermoid cysts, bone exostoses, and abdominal wall desmoid tumours. There is debate as to whether this is an individual clinical entity or if there is overlap with familial adenomatous polyposis.

3. Peutz–Jeghers syndrome. This is the association of multiple, variably sized small bowel hamartomatous polyps with perioral pigmentation. The polyps may cause multiple episodes of entero-enteric intussusception. The polyps may, rarely, occur in the colon or stomach.

Treatment

Polyps should be removed by diathermy snare polypectomy during colonoscopy. These must be retrieved for histological examination. Should a polyp be found to harbour non-invasive carcinoma or dysplasia, or if there are multiple polyps or recurrent polyps, then colonoscopic follow-up is mandatory. If a pedunculated polyp is frankly malignant, but with no evidence of invasion into the stalk, then the patient may be similarly followed-up. However, if there is evidence of an incomplete excision, then the patient should undergo colonic resection.

Pedunculated rectal polyps may be snared through an operating sigmoidoscope under general anaesthesia. Alternatively, if they are sessile, they may be excised locally after infiltration of saline to separate the lesion from the muscularis. The mucosal defect is often left open.

Large benign polyps may be removed colonoscopically or using the operating sigmoidoscope in a piecemeal fashion, but if this is not possible, a laparotomy, colotomy and open polypectomy or a limited colectomy may be better. If a polyp is seen to be histologically malignant after initial biopsy, then there is no option other than a colectomy.

Further reading

Campbell WJ, Spencer RAJ, Parks TG. Familial adenomatous polyposis. *British Journal of Surgery*, 1994; **81**: 1722–33.

Desai DC, Neale KF, Talbot IC *et al.* Juvenile polyposis. *British Journal of Surgery*, 1995; **82**: 14–7.

Talbot IC. Colonic polyps. *Surgery*, 1992; **10**: 182–6.

Related topics of interest

Colorectal carcinoma (p. 93)
Lower gastrointestinal haemorrhage (p. 192)

GASTRO-OESOPHAGEAL REFLUX

Gastro-oesophageal reflux is a normal physiological process but if it becomes prolonged symptoms like heartburn can arise. Excessive reflux, hiatus hernia and oesophagitis are distinct disease entities. Most patients with hiatus hernia do not have reflux symptoms. Severe heartburn can occur in the absence of oesophagitis, and be treated successfully with an anti-reflux operation. Reflux prevention depends upon the lower oesophageal sphincter, acid clearance, gastric content and function, and local anatomy.

Lower oesophageal sphincter
The lower oesophageal sphincter is 1–4 cm long and cannot be identified anatomically. It has a resting pressure of 20–40 mmHg, relaxes with coffee, fatty foods, chocolate, secretin, glucagon and cholecystokinin, and contracts after the administration of cholinergic and α-adrenergic drugs. Reflux is encouraged with a hypotensive sphincter, increases in abdominal pressure, such as obesity, and episodes of inappropriate sphincter relaxation from vagal overactivity.

Acid clearance
The acid clearance mechanism is effected by the primary peristaltic wave of saliva rich in bicarbonate. A reflex secondary peristaltic wave occurs in response to lower oesophageal distension. Smoking acidifies saliva, and reduced peristalsis is characteristic of achalasia and scleroderma.

Gastric content
Duodeno-gastric reflux, gastric outlet obstruction, gastric distension and the acid nature of the gastric content all promote gastro-oesophageal reflux. The hyperacidity of duodenal ulcer disease and the Zollinger–Ellison syndrome both encourage oesophagitis.

Anatomy
Anatomical factors are least important. The length of the intra-abdominal oesophagus may be preventative; however, in sliding hiatus hernias reflux still occurs with an intra-abdominal oesophagus. The right crus of the diaphragm may indent the lower oesophagus at endoscopy and the acute angle (angle of His) of the gastro-oesophageal junction was believed to act as a valve. Of greater significance is the redundancy of the mucosal rosette which occludes the lumen of a contracted oesophagus.

Presentation
Heartburn and regurgitation are the commonest symptoms. They are relieved by milk and antacids and are precipitated by heavy meals and stooping. Dysphagia can be due to stricture, oedema from oesophagitis or a motility disorder. Globus (feeling of a lump in the throat) is caused by reflux

cricopharyngeal spasm in response to acid stimulation of the lower oesophagus. Chest pain mimicking angina can also occur. Rarer symptoms include odynophagia (painful swallowing), aspiration pneumonitis, bronchospasm and upper gastrointestinal haemorrhage with anaemia.

Investigations

1. Endoscopy. Endoscopy is the investigation of choice allowing direct mucosal visualization and tissue sampling. Oesophagitis is graded by endoscopic appearance.

Grade	Description
I	Erythema
II	Non-confluent linear ulceration
III	Confluent circumferential ulceration
IV	Complications: Barrett's, stricture, shortening

The pinchcock action of the right crus, seen when the patient is asked to sniff, identifies the diaphragm, the landmark for diagnosis of a hiatus hernia. A Barrett's oesophagus is identified when the squamocolumnar junction is at least 3 cm higher than the gastro-oesophageal junction. Islands of the deeper pink columnar mucosa at the distal oesophagus are characteristic of this condition.

Oesophageal pH

Twenty-four hour ambulatory oesophageal pH recordings are essential for accurate diagnosis of reflux, especially in patients with symptoms and the absence of oesophagitis on endoscopy. A pH electrode is placed 5 cm above the gastro-oesophageal junction and the patient is asked to record the onset, severity, character and duration of any painful episodes during everyday activity. Combined refluxers (supine and upright) or reflux lasting more than 5% of the time indicates a positive test.

Other

Other investigations include barium swallow (stricture visualization), manometry for associated motility disorders, oesophageal scintigraphy and the Bernstein acid perfusion test. Symptom reproduction following lower oesophageal perfusion with 0.1 M HCl indicates a positive test.

Treatment

1. General. General treatment includes weight reduction, bed tilting for nocturnal symptoms, the avoidance of fatty foods, chocolate, coffee, large meals and smoking, and antacid therapy. In established oesophagitis, a H2-receptor antagonist is given until endoscopic evidence of healing. The dose can then be reduced. Metoclopromide, Domperidone or the pro-kinetic drug Cisapride are all useful to enhance oesophageal clearance. Omeprazole is a proton pump antagonist which is used in resistant cases and is indicated for the treatment of benign strictures.

2. Dilatation. Oesophageal strictures are dilated periodically either by dilators passed over a guide wire (Eder-Puestow olives, Celestin dilators) or by hydrostatic balloon inflation. The frequency of dilation usually decreases with time. An anti-reflux operation is indicated in young people with resistant strictures.

3. Surgery. Anti-reflux operations include fundoplication procedures or the placement of an Angelchick prosthesis. They probably act by protecting the cardia from the distracting force exerted by a distended stomach. The Nissen fundoplication involves mobilization of the distal oesophagus and wrapping the mobilized fundus around it through 360°. The high incidence of gas bloat and dysphagia can be diminished by making the wrap short and loose. A short oesophagus can be lengthed by a Collis gastroplasty before a fundoplication around the neo-oesophagus. The Angelchick prosthesis is a C-shaped silicone ring which is tied around the gastro-oesophageal junction. It is less effective than the Nissen and 10% need to be removed due to displacement, infection or intolerable dysphagia.

Barrett's oesophagus

The acquired condition of Barrett's oesophagus has a 44-fold increased risk of development of an aggressive adenocarcinoma. It is treated traditionally by endoscopic surveillance and biopsy. Severe dysplasia, *in situ* disease or carcinoma is an indication for oesophagectomy. Anti-reflux procedures sometimes induce regression.

Further reading

Mughal M, Bancewicz J. Gastro-oesophageal reflux – pathophysiology and treatment. *Recent Advances in Surgery*, 1991; **14**: 17–35.

Related topic of interest

Oesophageal dysmotility (p. 220)

GOITRE

The term goitre is used to describe any form of enlargement of the thyroid gland. Morphologically, three varieties of goitre are recognized:

- Diffuse goitre.
- Multinodular goitre.
- Solitary nodule (50% are actually dominant nodules in a multinodular goitre).

Pathologically, thyroid abnormalities causing goitre are as follows:

- Simple goitre.
- Multinodular colloid goitre.
- Graves' disease.
- Thyroid 'cyst'.
- Thyroiditis.
- Thyroid adenoma.
- Malignant thyroid neoplasms.

Simple goitre

May be diffuse or nodular. Results from increased thyroid-stimulating hormone (TSH) drive in the face of relative T_4 and T_3 deficiency. Physiological goitres occur to meet increased demand for thyroxine (puberty, pregnancy, lactation).

Iodine-deficiency goitres occur endemically in regions (usually mountainous – Alps, Andes) of iodine deficiency or are sporadic. They can also be caused by antithyroid drugs (iodides, propylthiouracil, carbimazole, thiocyanate, lithium) and foodstuffs (halogens, cassava, soya beans). Dyshormogenesis (absence of an enzyme involved in thyroxine synthesis) is familial and rare. Iodine transport, oxidation, coupling or thyroglobulin synthesis may be affected. Radiation to the head and neck may cause nodular goitre and thyroid cancer.

Multinodular colloid goitre

Usually euthyroid. Symptoms include visible swelling, discomfort, cough, dyspnoea, dysphagia, hoarseness and anxiety about malignancy. Troublesome hyperthyroidism sometimes occurs (Plummer's syndrome).

Graves' disease

This is an autoimmune disorder caused by polyclonal immunoglobulins stimulating the thyroid cell membrane TSH receptors. Female:male = 10:1. The peak incidence occurs at 20–40 years. The goitre is usually diffuse, often with a bruit. Exophthalmos, pretibial myxoedema and thyroid acropachy are other classic signs. Patients are hyperthyroid and describe weight loss, fatigue, heat intolerance, palpitations, tremor, diarrhoea and menstrual disorders. Treatment is by antithyroid drugs, radioiodine or thyroidectomy. Mild disease may resolve spontaneously but the majority will require treatment.

Thyroid 'cyst'

True cysts (a space containing fluid lined by epithelium) are rare. Nodules containing colloid degeneration, necrosis or haemorrhage are however quite common. Aspiration of clear fluid with negative cytology does not exclude malignancy notably papillary carcinoma. If aspiration does not provide complete and lasting resolution, surgical excision is required.

Thyroiditis

The aetiology of these conditions is largely unknown. Some varieties have an autoimmune basis in which reduced suppressor T-cell function probably allows sensitization to thyroid antigens of helper T cells which stimulate B cells to produce autoantibodies. These are common conditions, usually affecting women.

1. Acute suppurative thyroiditis. Now rare. Results from the spread of haematogenous infection (*Staphylococcus aureus*, β-haemolytic *streptococcus*, *Streptococcus pneumoniae*) usually to a goitrous gland. The signs are of acute infection and treatment is by antibiotics or, occasionally, surgical drainage.

2. Sub-acute thyroiditis
- de Quervain's thyroiditis. Self-limiting and probably caused by viral infection. The gland enlarges diffusely and flu-like symptoms are prominent. Mild hyperthyroidism occurs initially, followed by slight hypothyroidism. Isotope scanning reveals low uptake. Treatment is symptomatic.
- Postpartum thyroiditis. Affects 5% of women. An autoimmune condition causing thyroid dysfunction within a year of delivery. There is a modest, firm goitre and hyperthyroidism or hypothyroidism may occur. Antithyroid drugs, radioiodine and surgery are contraindicated and the condition resolves spontaneously.
- Silent thyroiditis. A painless, diffuse goitre with mild hyperthyroidism, but none of the features of Graves' disease. It occurs at any age and affects males more frequently than do other varieties. Usually self-limiting, but may recur.

3. Chronic thyroiditis

- Riedel's thyroiditis. Dense fibrosis of the gland occurs which is of normal or reduced size. The thyroid remains non-tender but becomes very hard ('woody'). Patients are usually middle-aged and euthyroid. Malignancy must be excluded.
- Hashimoto's thyroiditis is characterized by a large, rubbery goitre with hyperthyroidism progressing to hypothyroidism as the immune process destroys the gland. Antithyroid drugs or thyroxine may be necessary, but steroids are unhelpful. Surgery may be required if the gland is unresponsive to thyroxine and if malignancy is suspected.
- Atrophic thyroiditis. The end result of autoimmune thyroiditis, leaving a fibrotic, shrunken gland, usually with hypothyroidism. Thyroxine is the only treatment required.

Thyroid adenoma

See Thyroid neoplasms (p. 297).

Malignant thyroid neoplasms

See Thyroid neoplasms (p. 297).

Investigation of goitre

Morphological and functional aspects are important. Ultrasound scanning demonstrates single or multiple solid or 'cystic' lesions but is of little practical value. Standard CXR views will indicate retrosternal extension and tracheal deviation. CT scanning is more informative and will often show tumour transgression of the thyroid capsule or retrosternal extension. Scintiscanning using iodine-123 or technetium-99m is rarely justified. FNAC is very accurate (in experienced hands) in the diagnosis of goitres and is easily performed in the clinic. The technique will not distinguish between follicular adenoma and follicular carcinoma.

Thyroid function is assessed by TSH, T_3 and T_4. Total T_4 may be misleading because hyperthyroidism may be caused by raised T_3; thyroid-binding globulin (TBG) may be increased during pregnancy or oestrogen therapy, e.g. oral contraceptives (low T_4); TBG may fall during liver disease or nephrotic syndrome (high T_4). For these reasons TSH is the most helpful single investigation and 'free' T_3 and T_4 measurements should be reviewed for the situation described above. Thyroid autoantibody titres should be measured if thyroiditis is suspected.

Treatment for goitre

Endemic goitre can be treated with thyroxine, but older patients with established goitre rarely benefit from thyroxine. Thyroxine is commonly given to suppress multinodular goitre and may be effective in the early stages, but frequently does not reduce the size of an established, nodular goitre. It is usually effective in suppressing dyshormogenetic goitres.

Propylthiouracil and carbimazole are used to treat hyperthyroidism. These drugs are usually given for 14–24 months and more than 50% of patients relapse after cessation of treatment. Agranulocytosis may occur on treatment and regular FBC is necessary. Beta-blockers are used to control tachycardia, sweating and tremor.

Radioiodine as ^{131}I can be offered to patients beyond reproductive age. The choice between radioiodine and surgery should rest with the patient when the pros and cons of each treatment have been explained.

Surgery is appropriate in the following circumstances:
- Discomfort.
- Unacceptable appearance of goitre.
- Dyspnoea, dysphagia or retrosternal extension.
- Failure of thyroxine to suppress goitre.
- Possible malignancy – solitary cold nodule.
- Thyrotoxicosis.

Further reading

Weetman AP. Thyroiditis. *Current Practice in Surgery,* 1992; **4**: 118–22.
Young AE. The thyroid gland. In: Burnand, KG, Young AE (eds) *The New Aird's Companion in Surgical Studies.* Edinburgh: Churchill Livingstone, 1992; 633–60.

Related topics of interest

HAEMORRHOIDS

Although haemorrhoids (Greek: haima = blood, rhoos = flowing) are almost never life-threatening, they cause immense unhappiness. At least 50% of people over fifty will suffer from them.

Aetiology

Haemorrhoids are associated with high anal pressures, sphincter overactivity and the low-fibre diet in Western countries. They probably result from chronic downward displacement of the anal cushions during straining and defecation, with distension of the internal and external (depending on the relation to the dentate line) haemorrhoidal venous plexuses. Bouts of constipation may precede the complication of acute thrombosed haemorrhoids which appears more likely to occur in young adults with high anal pressures (the tight executive anus). Piles (Latin: pila = ball) consist of a vascular moiety and a fleshy connective tissue moiety. Portal hypertension can cause anal varices which must not be confused with haemorrhoids.

Presentation

Presentation is with bleeding, prolapse, pruritis or pain.

1. Bleeding. This is usually a fresh smear on the toilet paper or occasionally a spectacular spatter into the pan.

2. Prolapse. This often occurs on defecation requiring manual reduction (third-degree piles). If interference of venous drainage occurs, acute thrombosis and strangulation with progression to gangrene ensues. Second-degree piles reduce spontaneously after defecation and first-degree piles bleed without any prolapse.

3. Pruritis. This results from excessive mucous discharge secreted from the congested mucosa.

4. Pain. This is usually experienced as a severe throb which can distinguish piles from the sting of an anal fissure. Strangulated piles are extremely painful.

Examination

A general abdominal examination may indicate constipation. Anal inspection often reveals skin tags or obvious prolapse (third-degree piles) when dark red fleshy masses are seen covered by variable pale areas of squamous metaplasia. This must be distinguished from rectal prolapse where the mucosa is paler, bowel mucosa is palpable and anal tone is diminished.

| **Proctoscopy** | Proctoscopy demonstrates haemorrhoidal tissue, usually in the 3, 7, and 11 o'clock positions, which flop into the lumen of the scope as the scope is withdrawn. Identification of the dentate line is necessary to determine if the piles are mainly internal or external. A sigmoidoscopy is essential to exclude other pathology which may present with haemorrhoidal symptoms, especially if there has been a change in bowel habit. |

Outpatient therapy

1. General advice. Symptomless piles should not be treated other than with the general advice of increasing dietry bran, ensuring the stool remains soft and discouraging straining.

2. Rubber band ligation. The mainstays of surgical outpatient therapy are rubber band ligation (RBL) and injection sclerotherapy, the former being the most favoured. In a large controlled trial, RBL achieved 89% success compared with 70% for sclerotherapy. The technique was first described by Barron and involves grasping the pile to be banded with forceps, sliding the band applicator over the forceps and releasing the band. Even though the band is placed well above the dentate line, RBL is more uncomfortable than sclerotherapy with a report of severe pain in 7.5% of patients. A suction bander has recently been introduced and can be operated with just one hand, leaving the other free to hold the proctoscope. RBL is not universally accepted since there has been a report of a death from secondary haemorrhage.

3. Injection sclerotherapy. This involves placement of 3–5 ml of sclerosant (usually 5% phenol in arachis oil) submucosally above each pile at the level of the anorectal ring. This should cause the pile to thrombose, and eventually retract by fibrosis. Patients are warned that they may experience rectal bleeding and tenesmus over the next 24 hours.

4. Miscellaneous. Other methods of outpatient treatment include cryotherapy, infrared photocoagulation and bipolar diathermy.

Haemorrhoidectomy

The standard method for surgical treatment in the USA is by day case ambulatory haemorrhoidectomy. At St Mark's Hospital the time-tested method for intero–extero piles is by the Milligan–Morgan haemorrhoidectomy. This involves dissection, transfixion and excision of up to three piles, preserving the intervening skin as three bridges and leaving the wounds open. These bridges should not be left too narrow so that the complication of anal stenosis can be avoided. A paraffin-gauze wick is used as an anal drain to avoid a concealed haemorrhage. The operation can also be performed by diathermy. This is carried out after adrenaline infiltration, is said to produce less bleeding and pain, and requires no pedicle transfixion. Closed haemorrhoidectomy techniques are popular in the USA and are performed in the jack-knife position. They involve closure of the haemorrhoidal excision beds by suturing together the skin bridges. Simple transfixion and ligation has earned a place in developing countries.

Circumferential haemorrhoids

These can be treated by the Whitehead operation. This involves excision of a circumference of haemorrhoidal tissue and resuture of the rectal mucosa to the dentate line. The complication of stricture and anal ectropion is common in untrained hands if the excision extends below the dentate line.

Strangulation

Acute strangulated piles or a thrombosed saccule of the external haemorrhoidal plexus (perianal haematoma) are both painful self-limiting conditions usually treated with topical cloth-covered ice, laxatives and strong analgesia. Manual reduction by constant firm pressure is occasionally beneficial in limiting the oedema, but recurrence is common. Emergency limited haemorrhoidectomy by just removing one pedicle can often achieve a permanent cure.

Complications

Specific postoperative problems are bleeding, pain and urinary retention (10%). Bleeding is often secondary when infected slough separates off a patent vessel. Pain can be reduced by concomitant lateral sphincterotomy, stool softeners or the omission of anal packs.

Further reading

Barron J. *American Journal of Surgery*, 1963; **105**: 563–70.
McDonald P. Haemorrhoids and anal fissures. *Recent Advances in Surgery*, 1992; **15**: 107–18.
Milligan ETC, *et al. Lancet*, 1937; **2**: 1119–24.

Related topics of interest

Anal fissure (p. 28)   Crohn's disease (p. 106)
Anorectal investigation (p. 35)

HEAD INJURY

Pathology of head injury

The Monroe–Kelly doctrine confirms that the skull cannot easily accommodate an increase in volume of its contents without a significant rise in intracranial pressure (ICP). Cerebral perfusion pressure (CPP) equals the systemic arterial pressure (SAP) minus the ICP. This relationship is fundamental and explains the pathophysiology of brain injury.

Brain injury causes swelling. This volume increase causes a rise in ICP and thus a fall in CPP, resulting in brain ischaemia. Deterioration in cerebral function causes respiratory failure resulting in reduced PaO_2 and a rise in $PaCO_2$, which both cause cerebral vasoconstriction, further aggravating ischaemia. This leads to infarction which causes more brain swelling. If this vicious cycle is not interrupted, the inevitable outcome is death, as total brain failure occurs when ICP = SAP, and the CPP is zero.

A rise in the ICP results in displacement of parts of the brain. In earlier phases this is seen as midline shift. Later stages result in herniation of the cingulate lobe under the adjacent falx (subfacial herniation), the uncus through the tentorial hiatus to compress the oculomotor nerve and midbrain, and the cerebellar tonsil through the foramen magnum compressing the medulla oblongata. These are terminal events.

Mechanism of brain injury

Trauma may either injure the brain, or the extracerebral vessels. Rupture of extracerebral vessels results in intracranial bleeding, indirectly causing further brain injury. Trauma severe enough to cause brain injury usually also results in skull fracture. However, skull fracture is not requisite for either direct brain injury or intracranial bleeding.

Brain injury may occur at the site of the trauma ('coup' injury). Acceleration of the brain away from the source of injury with an abrupt stop at the opposite side also results in injury. ('contre-coup' injury).

1. Intracranial bleeding. Extracerebral bleeding occurs in the extradural or subdural spaces. Intracerebral bleeding results from coup or contre-coup injury. All result in haematomas that raise the ICP.

(a)   *Cerebral contusion.* Injuries range from mild contusion to large intracerebral haematoma. Mild contusions resolve. Large haematomas are acute space-occupying lesions, and need to be evacuated.

(b) *Extradural haematoma*. The thin pteryon anterior to the ear fractures easily, and rupture of the underlying middle meningeal artery may result. A compact haematoma lying between the periosteal layer of the dura mater and the inner table of the skull results. The classical sequence of events is loss of consciousness as a result of the blow, followed by some recovery (the so-called 'lucid-phase'), before consciousness is lost again. CT scan shows characteristic convex haematoma. Treatment is by craniotomy, evacuation of the haematoma, and clipping of the bleeding artery. Small extradural haematomas may result from blood oozing from skull fractures.

(c) *Acute subdural haematoma*. This is far more common than extradural haematoma. It results from bleeding communicating veins in the less restricted subdural space, and thus develops rapidly. Prompt evacuation is required.

(d) *Chronic subdural haematoma*. The elderly are prone to develop subdural haematomas. Cerebral atrophy places the communicating veins under tension, and these rupture easily. Because of cerebral atrophy, there is a greater space for blood to accumulate. The haematoma may remain undiscovered for a long time. As the contents alters, it becomes osmotically active, slowly expanding, and presenting as a chronic confusional state.

2. Direct parenchymal injury. The brain has a layered structure. A force applied to the parenchyma causes shearing stresses and the layers may move over each other. This direct parenchymal disruption is impossible to visualize by any means, and may occur without any appreciable intracranial bleeding. The prognosis is poor.

Evolution of clinical signs

With cortical disruption, convulsions may occur, the level of consciousness reduces, and there may be Cheyne–Stokes respiration. As corticospinal tracts are disrupted, contralateral weakness occurs. With involvement of the midbrain, hyperventilation may occur. The ipsilateral pupil becomes fixed and dilated. With involvement of the upper pontine respiratory centre, the respiratory pattern develops with episodes of hyperventilation separated by periods of apnoea. If the lower pons is involved, there may be prolonged inspirations and expirations. Blood pressure elevation and bradycardia signify involvement of the medullary cardiovascular regulatory centre.

Evaluation of clinical signs

Conscious level may be rapidly evaluated using the Glasgow Coma Scale (GCS). The highest score possible is 15, and the lowest is three. This serves to assess neurological state in standard terms, and second, to monitor the progress of a patient following a head injury and to identify quickly any deterioration in condition.

External examination may reveal signs of a brain skull fracture: blood or CSF issuing from the ear, Battle's sign (bruising around the mastoid area), bilateral periorbital haematomata ('panda eyes') or haemotympanum.

The Glasgow Coma Scale

Motor response	Obeying commands	6
	Localizing to pain	5
	Withdrawal to pain	4
	Flexion to pain	3
	Extension to pain	2
	No movement	1
Eye opening	Spontaneous eye opening	4
	Eyes open to request	3
	Eyes open to pain	2
	No eye opening	1
Verbal response	Orientated	5
	Confused	4
	Inappropriate speech	3
	Incomprehensible sounds	2
	No verbal response	1

Management of head injury in casualty

Indications for skull X-ray include loss of consciousness, convulsions, amnesia, severe trauma, global or focal neurological signs, GCS less than 15, and the presence of large scalp haematoma or tenderness. Evidence of facial injuries requires facial X-rays and nasal views. If the skull is fractured, if there is any neurological abnormality or if there is any difficulty in assessing neurological state (e.g. due to intoxication) the patient must be admitted and hourly neurological observations undertaken. There should be low thresholds for admission for children and the elderly. CT scan must be considered if there is a skull fracture or if there is any neurological abnormality. Patients with depressed skull fractures must be referred to a neurosurgical unit, as these need to be elevated.

Management of severe head injuries

1. Initial

- The patient's neck must be stabilized until either a CT scan or X-rays have shown no fracture of the cervical spine.
- Early assessment must be made of the GCS, arterial blood gases, pupillary response, respiratory pattern, and cardiovascular state. If there is evidence of respiratory dysfunction, or if the blood gases show respiratory failure, the patient must be ventilated immediately.
- The brain swelling is treated by infusing 1 g/kg mannitol intravenously, and a urinary catheter is inserted.
- In the presence of gross neurological changes, a CT scan of the head and neck is performed to exclude a surgically correctable focal lesion.

2. Surgical

- The presence of an intra- or extracerebral haematoma necessitates referral to a neurosurgical unit for evacuation.
- Depressed skull fractures must be referred for debridement and elevation. There is a high risk of epilepsy if bone fragments are in contact with the brain.
- Multiple burr holes in the parietal, frontal and occipital bones may achieve decompression in diffuse cerebral oedema.
- If there is any doubt about the potential for surgery in a patient with a severe head injury, the case and CT scans must be discussed early with neurosurgeons.

3. Supportive

- Continued management should be undertaken in an intensive care unit.
- The ICP may be monitored by the insertion of an ICP bolt through which the ICP can be transduced.
- Bolus doses of intravenous mannitol are given, titrated against the ICP, and continued for 4 days.
- Ventilation is continued, and if there is evidence that this is likely to be required for more than 1 week, a tracheostomy (open or percutaneous) is performed.
- Two litres of fluid are given intravenously per day and U&E are monitored daily.

- If prolonged unconsciousness is likely, a nasogastric tube is passed for enteral feeding.
- Care is taken to avoid pressure sores, and physiotherapy is given to chest and limbs.
- Continuous cerebral monitoring by EEG may be useful.
- Phenytoin is given intravenously if there have been seizures, a penetrating head injury, a depressed skull fracture, or if the patient requires longer than 48 hours of ventilation.

Further reading

Jennett B, Teasdale G. *Management of Head Injuries*. Philadelphia: Davis, 1981.
Molloy C. Head injuries Part 1: management of the unconscious patient. *Surgery*, 1993; **11**: 545–9.

Related topics of interest

HYPERPARATHYROIDISM

Parathyroid surgeons often work in close liaison with a renal unit because patients on dialysis provide a large proportion of the workload. The routine use of biochemical screening identifies a symptomless hypercalcaemic population. The upper parathyroids develop from the fourth pharyngeal pouch and the lower ones, together with the thymus, develop from the third pharyngeal pouch.

Parathormone

Parathormone is secreted in response to a lowering of the serum ionized calcium. Parathormone acts by mobilizing calcium from bone and by encouraging calcium resorption and phosphate excretion at the renal tubule. It also hydroxylates the 1α-part of the inactive vitamin D3 to form the active 1,25-dihydroxycholecalciferol; this also takes place at the renal tubule. Activated vitamin D acts by increasing calcium absorption from the gut.

Classification

1. *Primary hyperparathyroidism.* This is characterized by a persistently elevated calcium and a low serum phosphate. It is due to a parathyroid adenoma (90%), parathyroid gland hyperplasia (9%) or a carcinoma (1%).

2. *Secondary hyperparathyroidism.* This develops in response to a chronic calcium-losing state like renal failure or the gastrointestinal malabsorption syndromes. Here, calcium levels may be normal but parathyroid hormone levels are usually elevated. Four hyperplastic glands are usually identified at operation.

3. *Tertiary hyperparathyroidism.* This condition occurs if the parathyroid glands secrete parathormone autonomously after correction of the chronic calcium-losing state. It may develop after a renal transplant.

Differential diagnosis

Distinction must be made between other causes of hypercalcaemia like skeletal carcinomatosis, myeloma, milk-alkali syndrome, vitamin D intoxication, sarcoidosis, tuberculosis or Paget's disease. Protein electrophoresis, bone scan, skeletal survey, parathyroid hormone assays, urinary calcium excretion, the Kveim and Tuberculin tests, if indicated, should exclude the other causes.

Presentation

The highest incidence of hyperparathyroidism occurs in postmenopausal women. Clinical presentation can be summarized with the well-known tetrad of 'stones', 'bones', 'moans' and 'abdominal groans'. The rare manifestation of osteitis fibrosa cystica (von Recklinghausen's disease of bone) has been replaced with the commoner musculoskeletal discomfort of arthralgia and myopathy. Abdominal discomfort could be due to peptic ulceration or pancreatitis, both conditions being precipitated by hypercalcaemia. Mental confusion and mood changes are also often a feature. The renal problems include nephrocalcinosis, calculi and frank renal failure. Hypertension has a strong association with hypercalcaemia. Corneal band keratopathy is diagnostic of hyperparathyroidism but is very rare.

Investigations

Calcium, phosphate and parathormone assays are established in all patients. Radiological appearances may demonstrate subperiosteal bone resorption at the radial side of the middle and terminal phalanges of the hands with erosions of the terminal phalangeal tufts. A 'pepperpot' skull is less common and cystic bone lesions are rare (osteitis fibrosa cystica or the brown tumour/osteoclastoma). A radioisotope thallium/technetium subtraction scan helps to establish the diagnosis and aids in the pre-operative localization of the glands or adenoma. Gland localization by infusion of methylene blue (5 mg/kg in 500 ml of 5% dextrose), 1 h before operation and extending into the time of surgery, allows rapid parathyroid identification. CT scanning or selective venous sampling with a parathormone assay may be required to localize a gland following a failed neck exploration.

Consent

Pre-operatively, patients are warned of the possibility of a failed neck exploration, recurrent laryngeal nerve injury and postoperative hypocalcaemia.

Surgery

The aim of surgery is to remove the abnormal glands and leave the patient normocalcaemic. The normal gland is split-pea sized and tongue shaped and is best recognized in a bloodless field. Thorough familiarity with the normal anatomical positions and variations is mandatory. The upper glands are usually found superior to where the recurrent laryngeal nerve crosses the inferior thyroid artery. The lower ones are more variably situated in posterior relation to the inferior pole of the thyroid gland. The anterior mediastinum, the thymus (10%), within the carotid sheath, or intracapsular within the thyroid itself, can be occasional locations for the lower glands. Five per cent of patients have supernumary glands.

Management

If all four glands are hyperplastic, three-and-a-half glands are removed, marking the remaining gland with a black silk suture should re-exploration be required later. If the remaining gland is inadvertantly devascularized, it can be portioned into about 12 pieces and autotransplanted into the sternomastoid or the flexor compartment of the forearm. Occasionally, thymectomy with amputation of the upper and lower thyroid poles is required if not all the parathyroids are identified. Symptomless hypercalcaemic patients should be treated with a three-and-a-half gland excision, if their serum calcium is greater than 3.0 nmol/l, to prevent the renal, vascular and bone complications. Postmenopausal women with HRT are particularly at risk from femoral neck fractures.

Parathyroid carcinoma

Parathyroid carcinoma is recognized by gland firmness, grey colour and attachment to neighbouring structures or markedly elevated calcium levels. Recurrent laryngeal nerve palsy is a late manifestation. If suspected, a frozen section helps to confirm the diagnosis and an *en bloc* removal with ipsilateral hemithyroidectomy is performed.

Hypocalcaemia

Postoperative management includes regular serum calcium measurements and an intravenous calcium infusion if hypocalcaemia is profound. Prolonged hypocalcaemia is treated with vitamin D supplements and 1α-hydroxy-cholecalciferol. Pre-operative loading with 1α-hydroxy-cholecalciferol in patients with bone disease helps to manage postoperative hypocalcaemia and thereby mitigate the dangers of prolonged hypocalcaemia such as cataract formation.

Familial hypocalciuric hypercalcaemia

In rare cases, the autosomal condition of familial hypo-calciuric hypercalcaemia is responsible for a failed neck dissection. This should be diagnosed pre-operatively by a low 24 hour urinary calcium and a family history, with possibly a failed neck exploration in a parent/sibling.

Multiple endocrine neoplasia

The familial MEN syndromes often present with parathyroid hyperplasia. In MEN type I, pancreatic islet cell and pituitary tumours occur in addition. In MEN type II, medullary thyroid carcinomas and phaeochromocytoma are included. Screening for these familial conditions by hormonal and biochemical analysis is mandatory once an index case has been identified.

Further reading

Collins REC. Parathyroid disease. *Surgery*, 1988; 1486–9.
Gunn A. Parathyroidectomy. *Current Practice in Surgery*, 1990; **2**: 161–7.

Related topics of interest

HYPERTHYROIDISM – TREATMENT

Causes of hyperthyroidism

- Diffuse toxic goitre (Graves' disease).
- Toxic multinodular goitre.
- Toxic solitary nodule.
- Thyroiditis.
- Metastatic thyroid carcinoma.
- Factitious thyroxine ingestion.
- Pituitary tumours secreting TSH.
- Choriocarcinoma / hydatidiform mole.
- Neonatal thyrotoxicosis.

Treatment

Normal thyroid function should be restored as quickly and safely as possible.

1. Antithyroid drugs. Thionamides (propyluracil, carbimazole) prevent the binding of iodine with tyrosine residues and the coupling of iodotyrosines to form iodothyronine. Carbimazole also suppresses thyroid-stimulating antibody production. These drugs act quickly and are usually given for 6 months initially. Relapse occurs within 1 year of stopping treatment in 65% of patients. A small dose of thyroxine given with the drug will prevent iatrogenic hypothyroidism. These drugs are particularly suitable for rendering patients euthyroid prior to surgery. Adverse effects include nausea, pruritis, rashes, arthritis, agranulocytosis and aplastic anaemia.

Iodide (Lugol's iodine) inhibits T_4 and T_3 release and may be given for 10 days pre-operatively in patients who are unable to take thionamides or are poorly controlled. The vascularity of the thyroid may be reduced marginally.

Beta-blockers (propranolol) control the manifestations of thyrotoxicosis and can be used in combination with thionamides to prepare patients for surgery. If used, propranolol should be continued for 1 week postoperatively as thyroxine has a long half-life.

2. Radioiodine. ^{131}I effectively destroys thyroid tissue and is cheap, easy to use and safe. It should not be used in children or pregnant women, and is best avoided in patients in their reproductive years, although there is no evidence that radio-iodine causes leukaemia, thyroid cancer, foetal or genetic damage. Radioiodine takes 2 months to control hyper-thyroidism and antithyroid drugs are required to cover this period. More than one dose may be required if the initial response is inadequate. Hypothyroidism occurs at 3% per year after treatment and prolonged follow-up is therefore required, and treatment with thyroxine may be necessary.

3. Surgery. Pre-operative control of hyperthyroidism is essential, using carbimazole in most patients, with the addition of beta-blockers in the severely thyrotoxic patient. The vocal cords should be checked for a pre-existing paresis, particularly if there has been previous thyroid surgery.

Where surgery is indicated (see below), bilateral subtotal thyroidectomy is performed for diffuse conditions such as Graves' disease and multinodular goitre, leaving 3–4 g (the area of a thumbnail) of thyroid on each side. This reduces the likelihood of postoperative hypothyroidism, and parathyroid or recurrent laryngeal nerve damage. Patients with a toxic solitary nodule should be treated by unilateral subtotal lobectomy.

Possible postoperative complications are:

- Bleeding causing airway obstruction. Equipment to open the wound must be available.
- Recurrent laryngeal nerve damage.
- Parathyroid damage causing hypocalcaemia. Serum calcium should be monitored.
- Hypothyroidism. May affect up to 40%. Give thyroxine replacement.
- Recurrent hyperthyroidism. Antithyroid drugs or radio-iodine should be used.

Treatment strategies

1. Graves' disease (diffuse toxic goitre). Patients over 45 years are best treated with radioiodine. Antithyroid drugs should be given for several weeks until the isotope has been effective. Younger patients should be treated with anti-thyroid drugs (carbimazole) initially. Propranolol should be added in severe cases or where tachycardia and tremor are prominent. Treatment should be stopped after 6 months and patients reviewed regularly. Relapse will affect 65% and these patients should then undergo subtotal thyroidectomy. Patients with large, toxic goitres may benefit from early surgery.

2. Toxic multinodular goitre. Surgery is the treatment of choice as radioiodine and antithyroid drugs do not substantially reduce the size of the gland or resolve the local symptoms.

3. Toxic adenoma. Subtotal lobectomy is the treatment of choice.

4. Recurrent hyperthyroidism after surgery. Repeat surgery is hazardous and, in young patients, antithyroid drugs are used. Radioiodine is preferable for patients over 45 years.

5. Children. Antithyroid drugs should be given for 2 years and repeated in the 50% who relapse. If surgery is required, a radical resection is necessary, as the gland has a great tendency to grow back. Parathyroids and recurrent laryngeal nerves must be preserved. Prolonged follow-up is necessary, to detect abnormal thyroid function. Radioiodine is contraindicated.

6. Thyrotoxicosis occurring in pregnancy. Antithyroid drugs should be given, but hypothyroidism must be avoided. Foetal hypothyroidism may be induced. Free, unbound hormones must be measured during pregnancy, since TBG levels are abnormal. Surgery during the second trimester may be preferable in patients who are difficult to control. Radioiodine is contraindicated.

7. Thyroid crisis. Rare. A life-threatening condition occurring in patients inadequately controlled before surgery or hyperthyroid patients enduring stress (infection, other surgery). Dyspnoea, tachycardia, hyperpyrexia, restlessness, confusion, delerium, vomiting and diarrhoea occur. Carbimazole, Lugol's iodine and propranolol should be given. Cooling, rehydration and oxygen therapy should be carried out, and other respiratory, cardiovascular and psychiatric measures employed as necessary.

Further reading

Vora J, Hall R. Non-surgical treatment of thyrotoxicosis. *Currect Practice in Surgery*, 1990; **2**: 8–15.
Young AE. The surgical management of thyrotoxicosis. *Current Practice in Surgery*, 1990; **2**: 3–7.

Related topics of interest

INCISIONAL AND OTHER ABDOMINAL HERNIAS

Incisional hernia

Incisional hernias occur when a weak surgical or traumatic wound allows the protrusion of a peritoneal sac. A swelling appears which gradually enlarges. The hernia may affect the whole wound or just one small portion, frequently the lower end. The contents may become irreducible and episodic sub-acute intestinal obstruction, incarceration and strangulation may follow. The overlying skin may become thin, atrophic and ulcerated.

Incisional hernia affects 6% of abdominal wounds at 5 years and 12% at 10 years. The incidence in males and females is approximately equal. Predisposing factors include:

- Postoperative haematoma.
- Wound infection.
- Poor technique.
- The presence of drains and stomas in wounds.
- Age.
- Obesity.
- Diabetes, jaundice, renal failure, immunosuppression.
- Malignant disease.

Incisions particularly liable to hernia formation are lower midline, lateral muscle splitting incisions and subcostal incisions.

Incisional hernias may be left untreated where symptoms and deformity are minor, they may be controlled by the use of a corset or surgical belt, or they may be repaired surgically. Prior to surgical repair, patients with large hernias may undergo induction of pneumoperitoneum to enlarge the peritoneal cavity, facilitating hernial reduction at operation without impairing respiratory function. Surgical repair may be performed using:

- Layer-to-layer repair where the defect is of moderate size with no tissue loss.
- The Keel repair (Maingot). The old scar is excised but the underlying peritoneum is left intact and reduced by invagination into the abdomen where it is sutured. Successive layers of the abdominal wall are further invaginated and sutured using non-absorbable material.
- Synthetic mesh. This technique should be used if the defect to be closed is large and there is tissue loss. It is

now commonly used for all incisional hernias and many surgeons regard it as the operation of choice.

Para-umbilical and umbilical hernia

In adults, the hernial defect occurs through the linea alba, resulting from stretching of the abdominal wall by obesity. They rarely occur before the age of 40. Males and females are affected equally. Untreated, they may reach very large dimensions with ulceration of the overlying skin. Abdominal pain and a lump are the commonest symptoms. Intestinal obstruction and strangulation are common complications. Surgical repair should be undertaken, although patients are frequently obese and in poor health.

Epigastric hernia

Epigastric hernias occur in the midline, through a small defect in the linea alba, usually halfway between the xiphoid process and the umbilicus. They usually comprise a pea-sized protrusion of fat which may draw a small peritoneal sac into the defect. They are frequently acutely painful, particularly during exercise.

Repair involves closure of the linea alba defect after reduction of the fat and/or sac.

Spigelian hernia

Spigelian hernias account for less than 1% of abdominal hernias. They occur in the linea semilunaris on the lateral border of the rectus abdominis. The sac usually lies intraparietally between internal and external oblique just medial to the iliac crest at the level of the arcuate line. Patients present with a painful, reducible lump. The diagnosis can be confirmed by ultrasound scanning. Repair is by excision of the sac and closure of the defect.

Obturator hernia

These are rare and the male-to-female ratio is 6:1. They are commoner in middle and old age and the incidence on the right side is twice that on the left. The peritoneal sac passes through the obturator canal into the thigh, lying deep to pectineus, and emerging in the femoral triangle between the pectineus and adductor longus as it enlarges. Strangulation is frequently the initial presentation, and the diagnosis is usually made at laparotomy. The hernia may compress the geniculate branch of the obturator nerve causing pain in the medial aspect of the knee (Howship-Romberg sign). There is usually tenderness medial to the femoral vessels. Vaginal examination allows palpation of the hernia.

Repair is performed via an abdominal incision. The obturator membrane is stretched or divided from within and the sac reduced. Closure of the canal is not usually required.

| **Lumbar hernia** | A lumbar hernia may be primary (occurring usually through the inferior lumbar triangle of Petit, or less frequently through the superior lumbar triangle), or secondary following a renal operation, perinephric abscess or local muscular paralysis following poliomyelitis or spina bifida. |

A primary hernia is easily repaired by direct suture of the defect or by using an extraperitoneal prosthetic mesh. Secondary incisional hernias usually require prosthetic mesh.

| **Gluteal and sciatic hernia** | Both are very rare. A gluteal hernia passes through the greater sciatic notch, above or below the piriformis. A sciatic hernia passes through the lesser sciatic notch. Intestinal obstruction is the usual presentation and the diagnosis is rarely made before laparotomy. Pain may be referred through the sciatic nerve. Repair is performed via an abdominal incision, reducing the hernia from within and closing the defect with sutures or prosthetic mesh. |

| **Perineal hernia** | An anterolateral perineal hernia occurs in multiparous women, spontaneously or after childbirth or trauma. The hernia protrudes into the posterior vaginal wall or labium majus. A posterolateral perineal hernia passes through the levator ani into the ischiorectal fossa. The commonest perineal hernia occurs postoperatively following vaginal hysterectomy or abdominoperineal excision of the rectum. The other varieties are all rare. |

Further reading

Devlin B. The abdominal wall and hernias. In: Burnand KG, Young AE (eds) *The New Aird's Companion in Surgical Studies*. Edinburgh: Churchill Livingstone, 1992.

Related topics of interest

INGUINAL HERNIA

Epidemiology and aetiology

A hernia is a protrusion of an organ through an abnormal defect in its surrounding structures. In the abdomen this invariably means the protrusion of a viscus through a muscle or fascial defect. Abdominal hernias comprise a defect, sac (peritoneum) and sac contents.

Inguinal hernias are the commonest type of groin hernia and are present in 2% of live born babies (4% of male babies), the incidence rising with prematurity and low birth weight. The development of inguinal hernia is commonest in the first 3 months of life and is caused by failure of the processus vaginalis to close. The neck of the hernia is at the internal inguinal ring, lateral to the inferior epigastric vessels, and such hernias are indirect by definition. All indirect hernias pass along the same tissue plane as the processus vaginalis. Direct inguinal hernias (defect and neck of the hernial sac medial to the inferior epigastric vessels) virtually never occur in infants. The ratio of males to females affected is 9:1. At all ages, inguinal hernias are commoner on the right than the left. Approximately 60% of children with an inguinal hernia present with incarceration but this rarely progresses to strangulation, 95% resolving with sedation and elevation in gallows traction.

The incidence of inguinal hernia in adults is difficult to calculate, but approximately 5–10% of males are affected. In adult males and females, inguinal hernias occur in a ratio of 10:1 and, in males, 60% are indirect, 35% direct and 5% combined. Young men tend to develop indirect hernias, whilst older men tend to develop the direct variety. In women, indirect inguinal hernias are as common as femoral hernias, but direct hernias are rare. Indirect inguinal hernias are much commoner in Africans than in Europeans. Inguinal hernia patients account for 6% of all general surgical admissions and currently occupy 5% of all general surgical beds. Approximately 80,000 inguinal hernia repairs are performed annually in England and Wales, 10% of these for recurrence.

Clinical features and differential diagnosis

Pain, a dragging sensation and swelling in the groin are the commonest symptoms. The onset of severe pain suggests strangulation. Examination of the patient lying supine may reveal a swelling in the inguinal canal or, if the hernia has reduced, a defect at the internal ring. A cough impulse may be felt at the external ring. Invagination of the scrotal skin into the inguinal canal is painful and should be avoided. Control of the hernia by pressure applied directly over the internal ring suggests indirect herniation, although it is often difficult to differentiate. The patient should also be examined standing when the hernia is more likely to be apparent. The opposite groin should always be checked for undetected hernias and, in men, the testes should be examined for hydrocoele or epididymal cyst.

Other conditions that may mimic inguinal hernia include:

- Femoral hernia.
- Saphena varix.
- Hydrocoele of the cord or of the canal of Nuck.
- Lipoma of the cord.
- Ectopic testis.
- Inguinal lymph nodes.
- Psoas abscess.
- Ilofemoral aneurysm.

Complications
- Incarceration (irreducibility).
- Intestinal obstruction.
- Maydl's hernia.
- Richter's hernia.
- Strangulation.
- Reduction *en masse*.
- Testicular oedema, ischaemia or infarction.
- Littre's hernia.
- Sliding hernia.
- Herniation of ovaries/fallopian tube.

The annual probability of strangulation in an inguinal hernia is 0.3–3.0% with the risk weighted towards the first 3 months after the hernia is first noticed. Indirect hernias are 10 times more likely to undergo strangulation than direct hernias. The mortality of strangulated inguinal hernia in adults is 7–14%.

Management
A working party of the Royal College of Surgeons of England (Clinical Guidelines on the Management of Groin Hernias in Adults) issued the following guidelines in 1993:

(i) Indirect and symptomatic direct inguinal hernias should be repaired to relieve symptoms and to eliminate the small long-term risk of strangulation.

(ii) Easily reducible direct inguinal hernias which are not at significant risk of strangulation need not necessarily be repaired, especially in the elderly. Such patients should be reviewed within 1 year.

(iii) Recurrent hernias should be managed as in (i) and (ii).

(iv) Irreducible inguinal hernias and those presenting with a history of less than 4 weeks should be repaired promptly to avoid strangulation.

(v) The risk of strangulation in all other inguinal hernias does not warrant waiting list priority, but other considerations such as employment status may do so.

The results of inguinal hernia surgery depend largely on the technical skills of the surgeon. Many different operative techniques have been described. Recurrence rates for primary hernias are approximately 10% and for recurrent hernias, 20%. Specialist centres report rates of 1.5 and 5%, respectively. A technique based on the Shouldice repair is recommended, the principal features of which are:

- Division of the cremaster muscle.
- Primary incision and repair of the transversalis fascia with medial closure of the internal inguinal ring.
- Inspection of all potential hernial orifices.
- Apposition and suturing without tension.
- The use of monofilament sutures for the repair.

The use of prosthetic mesh is currently under examination for the repair of primary hernias. Trials indicate that the Lichtenstein mesh technique provides low recurrence rates, even when employed by junior surgeons. It can be performed under local anaesthetic as a day case procedure.

Laparoscopic repair of inguinal hernias is currently under investigation. The technique is not currently recommended outside the constraints of a clinical trial. Early recurrence rates were high.

Simultaneous repair of bilateral inguinal hernias may be performed with no increase in wound infection or respiratory problems, but there may be scrotal oedema, urinary retention and possibly an increased recurrence rate.

Simple recurrent hernias may be repaired by the standard technique or by use of a prosthetic plug. Multiple or complex recurrent defects are best repaired using a prosthetic mesh.

The use of local anaesthesia for the repair of inguinal hernias is safer in high-risk patients and allows prolonged analgesia with consequent early mobilization and reduced risk of urinary retention. DVT and PE rates are reduced and recurrence rates are not affected.

In appropriate patients, day case hernia repair is desirable and the majority of uncomplicated inguinal hernias should now be treated this way.

Further reading

Clinical Guidelines on the Management of Groin Hernias in Adults. Royal College of Surgeons of England, 1993.
Devlin HB. *Management of Abdominal Hernias.* London: Butterworth, 1988.

Related topics of interest

Common paediatric conditions (p. 98)
Femoral hernia (p. 131)
Incisional and other abdominal hernias (p. 173)

INTERMITTENT CLAUDICATION

This term is derived from the Latin 'claudicatio' ('I limp') and refers to pain arising due to inadequate arterial blood flow in exercising muscle, which is relieved by rest. Intermittent claudication occurs most commonly in the legs, but can also occur in the arms.

Pathology

Atherosclerosis is the cause in the great majority of patients and the common sites affected include the origin of the common iliac arteries, the superficial femoral arteries, particularly at the adductor hiatus, and the popliteal artery. The principal risk factors are cigarette smoking, diabetes, hypertension, hypercholesterolaemia and family history. Other causes (trauma, popliteal entrapment syndrome, compartment syndrome) should be considered, particularly in younger patients.

Pathophysiology

Patients with intermittent claudication have near normal limb blood flow at rest, but cannot increase blood flow adequately during exercise. According to Poiseuille's Law, flow is proportional to the fourth power of the radius of the tube and, thus, increasing degrees of stenosis lead to an exponential decline in flow. Multiple stenoses are effectively resistances in series and have an additive effect.

Natural history

Claudication affects 1.5% of patients under the age of 60 years and 50% of those over 70 years. Claudication remains static in many patients, approximately 20% deteriorating over a 5-year period. Arterial reconstruction is required in 5–10 % over a similar period and a similar proportion will progress to amputation (this rises to 30% in patients over 75 years). The overall mortality of these patients is higher than that of an age-matched normal population, 5- and 10-year survival being 75% and 40%, respectively. The excess mortality is mainly attributable to myocardial infarction and stroke.

Clinical features

Patients complain of pain in single or multiple muscle groups which occurs on walking and resolves at rest. Pain occurs at a predictable walking distance which decreases on an incline or in cold weather. Pain usually begins in the calf if there is superficial femoral/popliteal artery involvement, but extends to the thighs and buttocks if there is iliac artery involvement. Examination may reveal absent or weak pulses and possibly a bruit over the stenotic segment. There may be accompanying manifestations of hypertension, diabetes, hyperlipidaemia, and cardiac and neurovascular disease. The differential diagnosis includes degenerative hip disease, lumbosacral arthritis and lumbar spinal stenosis.

Investigation

Ankle–brachial Doppler index is the simplest non-invasive measurement and ratios of 0.4–0.8 are typical in claudicants. The measurement of Doppler indices before and after exercising on a treadmill together with symptomatic correlation is also helpful and will reveal more subtle changes than resting examination alone. Although techniques of colour duplex sonography are currently being investigated, the arteriogram remains the mainstay of investigation in patients with intermittent claudication where the severity is such that treatment is indicated. Digital subtraction arteriography is gradually replacing conventional arteriography and may be performed using a venous or, more usually, an arterial contrast injection. Assessment of co-existing cardiac and coronary disease is necessary in some patients and diabetes, hypertension, hyperlipidaemia and bronchial carcinoma should be sought.

Treatment

Many patients whose mild claudication remains stable require only an explanation of the problem and reassurance. All patients should be strongly advised to stop smoking and encouraged to exercise. Co-existing conditions (diabetes, hypertension, anaemia) should be treated. Obese patients should be advised to lose weight. Beta-blockers should be avoided where possible, particularly in conjunction with calcium antagonists. Oxypentiphylline is reputed to enhance red cell deformability and reduce platelet aggregation, but trials have failed to demonstrate more than mild subjective improvement in some patients. There has been no significant improvement in Doppler indices. All patients should be treated with low-dose aspirin (unless contraindicated) to reduce their excess propensity to cardiac and cerebrovascular events.

Where the above measures are inadequate, arteriography should be performed. Percutaneous transluminal angioplasty is suitable for stenoses less than 5 cm in length occurring in large arteries (iliac, femoral). Expandable stents enhance patency, especially following restenosis. Laser-assisted angioplasty and atherectomy have proved disappointing and cannot be recommended for routine use.

Where angioplasty is inappropriate, endarterectomy or, more commonly, bypass grafting of the diseased segment may be undertaken. Endarterectomy is most suitable for short stenoses or occlusions, but bypass grafting has become more widely used over the past 20 years as prosthetic graft materials have developed. Aortofemoral grafting can be performed with 2–3% mortality, low morbidity and 5-year patency rates greater than 90%. Femoropoliteal bypass carries a low mortality (1%) and 5-year patency rates of 75%, where vein is used for the conduit, or 55%, where polytetrafluoroethylene (PTFE) is used. Several series report similar patency rates for vein and PTFE in the above knee position. Femorotibial bypass is rarely indicated for claudication alone. Extra-anatomic grafting (femoro-femoral, axillofemoral, axillobifemoral) may be used where there is a good donor vessel and contraindications to an anatomic bypass.

Lumbar sympathectomy does not improve muscle blood flow and is of no benefit in most patients with intermittent claudication.

Further reading

Jamieson CW, Yao JST (eds). *Rob and Smith's Operative Surgery – Vascular Surgery.* London: Chapman and Hall Medical, 1994.

Jarrett F. Claudication. *Current Practice in Surgery*, 1992; **4**: 70 –5.

Related topics of interest

INTESTINAL OBSTRUCTION

Intestinal obstruction is a surgical emergency. Delay in operative intervention may lead to an unnecessary bowel resection, an increased risk of perforation and an overall worsening of patient morbidity and mortality. Appreciation of fluid balance, acid–base–electrolyte disturbance and the importance of pre-operative resuscitation is essential. Small bowel obstruction accounts for about 85% of cases and the other 15%, large bowel obstruction.

Small bowel obstruction

Classification

Mechanical small bowel obstruction can be conveniently classified by percentage aetiology or by the site of the pathological process.

Aetiology	Incidence (%)
Adhesions	70
Hernia	20
Malignancy, other	10

Site	Pathology
Luminal	Meconium, bezoars, gallstones, worms, foreign bodies, faeces
Mural	Atresia,inflammatory bowel disease (IBD), tumours, intussusception, ischaemia, tuberculosis
Extrinsic	Adhesions, hernia, volvulus, congenital bands, malignancy, inflammatory mass

In Third World countries, hernias form the majority of cases and when adhesion obstruction does occur it is usually the aftermath of pelvic sepsis rather than a prior laparotomy. Disseminated peritoneal malignancy (gastric, ovarian, breast, colon) commonly obstructs by mesenteric vascular encroachment or extrinsic compression from subserosal deposits. Any inflammatory mass (diverticular, appendiceal) may involve the small bowel, causing a localized ileus. The narrowest part of the small bowel is the terminal ileum which is the preferred site of obstruction of most of the luminal causes.

Presentation

Clinical presentation is with pain, vomiting, distension and absolute constipation.

1. Pain. The pain is characteristically intermittent and visceral, lasting for about 10–100 sec, increasing in frequency and poorly localized around the umbilicus. Continuous somatic pain that is localized or an area of peritonism suggests strangulation and requires immediate operative intervention. Pyrexia, tachycardia and foetor also infer complicated obstruction.

2. Vomiting. Vomiting becomes more profuse the higher the level of obstruction. Initially, the vomitus contains recognizable food and later it becomes faeculent, often exhibiting the ground coffee appearance of altered blood. The 24 hour secretory function of the proximal gut is illustrated below. It gives an indication of the amount of fluid that can be sequestered in the intestines or lost in the vomitus.

Secretion	Amount (l)
Saliva	1.5
Gastric juice	3.0
Bile	0.5
Pancreatic juice	1.0
Intestinal juice	3.0
Total	9.0

3. Distension. Abdominal distension is more an indication of the site than the extent of obstruction. Central distension suggests small bowel obstruction and flank distension suggests large bowel obstruction. Swallowed air, gas from bacterial fermentation and nitrogen diffusion from the congested mucosa are all responsible for the increased intestinal gas.

4. Constipation. Absolute constipation, the passage of neither flatus nor faeces, indicates complete obstruction. The reliability of this symptom becomes more consistent the lower the level of obstruction. Patients with partial obstruction may develop diarrhoea because fluid faeces is all that can pass through a stenosed segment.

| Examination | Examination should be directed towards all the hernial orifices and the presence of abdominal scars should be noted. High pitched bowel sounds are indicative of obstruction although they may later disappear. The abdomen is characteristically silent in paralytic ileus (neurogenic small bowel obstruction) when all that can be heard are transmitted respiratory and cardiac sounds. This occurs in peritonitis, after a laparotomy, following trauma or in the presence of a retroperitoneal haemorrhage or hypokalaemia. A succussion splash is often present. Visible peristalsis may be an unreliable sign as it is sometimes seen in thin patients who are not obstructed. |

| Investigation | A supine abdominal radiograph is the best single investigation. Small bowel is recognized by its central location, valvulae conniventes and by exclusion of the large bowel. A diameter of greater than 2.5 cm indicates obstruction. An erect abdominal film may confirm the diagnosis by the presence of multiple fluid levels but this finding can also occur in a non-obstructed patient after a curry or a few fizzy drinks. A single dilated small bowel loop may indicate strangulation. |

| Treatment | The decision to adopt surgery rather than conservative therapy (nasogastric aspiration with fluid and electrolyte replacement) depends upon the development of the features suggesting strangulation or the presence of increasing small bowel diameter on serial radiography. An incarcerated hernia will demand earlier surgery. Patients with disseminated peritoneal malignancy should be spared the indignity of a laparotomy. |

Large bowel obstruction

Common causes of large bowel obstruction are carcinoma, pseudo-obstruction, chronic diverticulosis and volvulus. A caecal size of greater than 10 cm indicates large bowel obstruction and often preceeds caecal rupture. Closed-loop large bowel obstruction (a competent ileocaecal valve) is more serious implying imminent caecal perforation. Pseudo-obstruction is inferred by the finding of a 'ballooned' rectum on rectal examination. Many unnecessary laparotomies have been performed for suspected carcinoma when pseudo-obstruction was found at operation. Differentiation between these conditions should be made first with an instant barium enema.

| Sigmoid volvulus | Sigmoid volvulus occurs most frequently in underdeveloped countries. In Europe and the USA, it occurs in the psychiatrically and mentally ill, and the senile. Predisposing |

conditions include a long, narrow mesocolon, laxative abuse and a high-fibre diet. Radiological appearances are characteristic: an ahaustral loop, coffee bean in shape, with its convexity to the right. The caecum is often seen in the right iliac fossa thereby distinguishing the condition from caecal volvulus. Emergency deflation with a flatus tube passed down the shaft of a sigmoidoscope is often an effective manoeuvre. A sigmoid colectomy is the usual treatment.

Caecal volvulus

Caecal volvulus is rarer than sigmoid volvulus because the caecum is usually retroperitoneal. Obstruction occurs at the terminal ileum which is why some purists classify the condition under small bowel obstruction. Radiologically, a large coffee bean-shaped loop of a haustral bowel is seen to occupy most of the abdomen with its major convexity under the left hemi-diaphragm. The right iliac fossa and the left colon are free of any gas pattern. A right hemicolectomy is the usual treatment.

Further reading

White H, Stacey MC, Bell RF, Burnand KG. The peritoneum, the mesentery, the greater omentum and the acute abdomen. In: Burnand KG, Young AE (eds) *The New Aird's Companion in Surgical Studies.* Edinburgh: Churchill Livingstone, 1992; 922–39.

Related topics of interest

IRRITABLE BOWEL SYNDROME

This constitutes a mixed collection of symptoms including abdominal pain, abdominal distension, alteration in bowel habit, sensation of incomplete evacuation, relief of abdominal pain on opening bowels, and dyspeptic symptoms. The motions often alternating between periods of constipation and looseness. Symptoms may be exacerbated by stressful events, and are recurrent, but there are no worrying features such as loss of weight or appetite, or bleeding per rectum. Associated symptoms may include chronic lower back pain, fatigue, lethargy, urinary problems or depression.

Individually, the abdominal symptoms may suggest underlying pathology. However, patients with irritable bowel syndrome will have many of these symptoms together, and the diagnosis can usually be established following a normal full clinical examination including a sigmoidoscopy. It may be wise to arrange either a barium enema or a colonoscopy in older patients to exclude colonic pathology.

Any age group may be affected, although it is most commonly diagnosed in the third and fourth decades. The aetiology is unknown, but it is probable that there is an element of overactivity of colonic musculature. This is based on the nature of the pain, which is usually lower abdominal and cramping, and the fact that antispasmodic medication often relieves it.

Management	The patient should be told they have irritable bowel syndrome and that this is caused by an overactive colon. The association between the symptoms and stress should be reinforced, as stress-avoidance may lead to an improvement.
	Frequently, patients already suspect the diagnosis, and reassurance that there is no serious pathology and a positive diagnosis of irritable bowel syndrome is all that is required. However, a trial of an antispasmodic drug or stool-modifying agent is usually necessary.
Pharmacotherapy	*1. Antispasmodic drugs.* The predominant symptom is usually abdominal pain and a variety of antispasmodic agents are available that may have an effect. The simplest is peppermint oil, which is available in capsules. This has a direct action on intestinal smooth muscle, and one or two capusles are taken three times a day. Other agents acting directly to inhibit smooth muscle are mebeverine hydrochloride (135 mg tds) and alverine citrate (60–120 mg tds).
	2. Anticholinergic drugs. These will reduce motility, with a dry mouth and difficulty with near vision as unwanted effects. Anticholinergic drugs that may be of use include hyoscine butylbromide (20 mg qds) and dicyclomine hydrochloride (10–20 mg tds).

3. Stool-modifying preparations. If the predominant bowel symptom is constipation, then a bulk-forming laxative such as Fybogel may be prescribed. Dietary modifications may be required to ensure a high-fibre diet. Antidiarrhoeal agents may be of use should there be a tendency towards loose motions; foods aggravating the diarrhoea may be identifiable and should be avoided.

Resistant cases

Psychotherapy and hypnotherapy may be of help. Referral to a psychiatrist is unhelpful in the absence of a psychiatric disorder such as depression. Should symptoms persist despite reassurance and courses of antispasmodic agents, then the possibility of a diagnostic error should be considered. Rare causes of abdominal pain may need to be excluded, particularly if symptoms worsen.

Related topics of interest

JAUNDICE – INVESTIGATION

The jaundiced patient must be investigated urgently. A complete history and examination are mandatory and may distinguish obstructive (or cholestatic) jaundice from haemolytic or hepatic causes. Passage of dark urine and pale stools is indicative of obstructive jaundice. Biliary obstruction caused by gallstones and malignancy, the two most common causes, may also be differentiated clinically.

History

Some hepatic disorders may cause intrahepatic cholestasis producing an obstructive picture; however, most cases of obstructive jaundice result from obstruction of the extra-hepatic biliary tree. Intermittent jaundice suggests common bile duct calculi, whilst progressive jaundice points to an underlying malignancy causing biliary obstruction. Jaundice associated with pain suggests calculous disease, and painless jaundice suggests malignancy. There are exceptions: carcinoma of the pancreas causes back pain if posteriorly related structures are invaded, and some tumours obstructing the common bile duct can necrose and diminish in size, temporarily relieving obstruction and jaundice. Weight loss and loss of appetite suggest malignancy.

Examination

General examination may show stigmata of chronic liver disease, pointing to a hepatic rather than obstructive jaundice. Charcot's Triad suggests cholangitis (pyrexia and rigors, jaundice and an enlarged, tender liver), which is rare in malignant but common in calculous biliary obstruction. Cachexia suggests a malignant cause. Spontaneous migrating superficial thrombophlebitis (thrombophlebitis migrans or Trousseau's sign) may indicate an underlying pancreatic carcinoma. Rectal examination may reveal malignant infiltration of the pelvic peritoneum, palpable as a mass jutting backward above the prostate (rectal shelf of Blummer), from transcoelemic spread of pancreatic carcinoma. Stools are typically putty coloured in obstructive jaundice. The superimposition of melaena produces a silvery 'gun-metal' stool, which is rare but suggestive of ampullary carcinoma causing both blood loss and obstructive jaundice. The abdominal examination may reveal ascites, hepatomegaly from metastases, a pancreatic mass, or a palpable gallbladder caused by biliary dilatation.

Courvoisier's Law

This states that in the presence of jaundice, if the gallbladder is palpable, then the jaundice is unlikely to be due to gallstones. This is because calculous gallbladders are usually small and fibrotic and impalpable. However, the gallbladder may be palpable if a mucocoele arises following impaction of a stone in the neck of the gallbladder.

Blood and urine tests

FBC, U&E, liver function test and a clotting screen are mandatory. In the presence of hepatic disease or obstructive jaundice, urinalysis will detect conjugated bilirubin in the urine. If urobilinogen is detected in the urine, then the jaundice cannot be obstructive, because conjugated bile cannot enter the intestine through an obstructed biliary system, and thus there is no conversion to urobilinogen for reabsorbtion and urinary excretion.

Liver function tests

These provide a useful picture of the underlying hepatobiliary disorder. Jaundice can become clinically evident if serum bilirubin exceeds approximately 60 mg/dl. The association of a raised alkaline phosphatase and a raised gamma glutamyl transferase points to the hepatic alkaline phosphatase isoenzyme (as opposed to the bone or gastrointestinal isoenzymes), and this is the usual pattern in both hepatic and obstructive jaundice. Obstructive jaundice is often associated with a greatly raised alkaline phosphatase and high levels of bilirubin. In hepatocellular disorders, the transaminases are usually grossly elevated, but the bilirubin may only be mildly raised.

Ultrasound

The intrahepatic bile ducts become distended before the extrahepatic biliary tree if there is a distal biliary obstruction. The maximum diameter of a normal common bile duct is 8 mm but distension rapidly occurs if there is distal obstruction. Following a cholecystectomy the common bile duct frequently dilates, and this can cause confusion if a complete medical history is not obtained. Gallbladder calculi are easily seen on ultrasound, but calculi are rarely seen in the common bile duct due to overlying gas in the duodenum. However, common bile duct calculi usually result in biliary dilatation on ultrasound. The liver is scrutinized for metastases, and the pancreas is examined for the presence of tumour.

ERCP

A side-viewing gastroscope is used to identify and cannulate the ampulla of Vater. Contrast is injected and radiographs outlining the biliary tree are obtained. The pancreatic duct is usually also outlined. A sphincterotomy can be performed, through which bile duct calculi may be extracted. Pancreatic or distal bile duct malignancies may be biopsied. Stents may also be placed to relieve obstructing lesions. If available, ERCP is the investigation of choice following an ultrasound in jaundiced patients.

PTC	A needle is inserted into the hepatic parenchyma. A dilated intra-hepatic biliary radicle is entered, and contrast is injected. The views obtained of the biliary tract are as good as with ERCP, although the pancreatic duct is not seen, and biopsies cannot easily be taken. PTC may be used for insertion of temporary and permanent biliary stents and drains. A guidewire can be inserted into the dilated duct system, and an external biliary drain is passed over it. Obstructed bile may be drained internally by placing a stent over the guidewire and across the obstruction.
Intravenous cholangiography	This concentrates contrast in the extrahepatic biliary tree, and may be used to assess biliary obstruction. It is a rather dangerous procedure with a recognized incidence of fatal hypersensitivity reactions. For this reason, a test dose is always given. It will not succeed in the presence of jaundice, as the hepatocytes will fail to excrete the contrast.
Radioisotope scans	HIDA and technetium scans may be used to assess both the hepatic parenchyma and bile ducts. The radiolabelled molecules are excreted by the liver into the bile even in the presence of mild jaundice.
Liver biopsy	Primary hepatic disease, or secondary malignant infiltration may require biopsy for confirmation of the diagnosis. This may be performed under ultrasound or CT control, or as a 'blind' procedure, or under general anaesthetic using a laparoscope. The latter allows a particular hepatic lesion to be targeted, and may be the procedure of choice if the liver is not diffusely infiltrated. The liver may also be biopsied via the transjugular route. A fine biopsy wire is passed through a cannula in the right internal jugular vein and the right heart is traversed to enter the hepatic veins under image intensifier control. The hepatic vein wall is breached, and the liver parenchyma can be biopsied.

Further reading

Cuschieri A, Bouchier AD. The biliary tract. In: Cuschiere A, Giles GR, Moosa AR (eds) *Essential Surgical Practice*, 2nd Edn. London: Wright, 1988; 1020.
Howard ER, Peel ALG. Surgical studies. In: Burnand KG, Young AE (eds) *The New Aird's Companion in Surgical Studies*. Edinburgh: Churchill Livingstone, 1992; 1129.

Related topics of interest

LOWER GASTROINTESTINAL HAEMORRHAGE

Bleeding may occur from any part of the gut. Blood loss may be chronic and occult resulting in anaemia. Overt blood loss varies widely in presentation. The lower gastrointestinal tract is less commonly a source of frank haemorrhage than the stomach or duodenum.

Clinical examination

Blood originating from the sigmoid colon or distally may be dark or usually bright red and copious; that from more proximal sites in the colon or in the distal small intestine is usually dark red or black, although it does not have the sticky consistency or typical offensive smell of partially digested blood that characterizes the melaena of upper gastrointestinal bleeding. Occasionally, upper gastrointestinal haemorrhage may be brisk enough to cause the passage of unaltered blood per rectum, thus mimicking a colonic bleed.

There may be a history of previous episodes, or patients may be known to suffer from haemorrhoids or ulcerative colitis. Clinical examination is usually unremarkable in terms of localizing the source of the bleed. A digital rectal examination is essential, as this provides the best clue to the origin of the bleed. Tachycardia may be the only sign, though haemorrhagic shock may be present in extreme cases.

Causes

1. Haemorrhoids. These may bleed profusely. The blood is bright red and there is usually a history of blood passed per rectum after passing a motion. First-degree (non-prolapsing) haemorrhoids are impalpable and present with bleeding only, and thus a rectal examination may be entirely normal apart from blood staining of the glove. The bleeding will usually cease, and the diagnosis can be established by proctoscopy, at which time the haemorrhoids can be injected with 3% phenol.

2. Colitis. This is an important cause of bleeding per rectum. Any cause of colitis may result in blood loss, including ulcerative, infective or ischaemic colitis. Infective colitis with *Campylobacter* species often presents with lower abdominal pain and the passage of frank blood per rectum. Ulcerative or Crohn's proctitis or colitis will result in diarrhoea, which may be blood stained. Ischaemic colitis, which usually affects the splenic flexure, may present with blood passed per rectum. The blood tends to be dark, and represents the sloughing of the mucosa resulting from the ischaemia. Rarely, radiation enteritis may cause bleeding. If this is so, then there will be a clear history of radiotherapy, usually for a pelvic malignancy like cervical or prostatic carcinoma. Innocent bowel may be inadvertently irradiated, and this results in increased vascularity.

3. Diverticular disease. A diverticulum can bleed when it is not inflamed. The perforating blood vessels penetrate adjacent to the neck of the diverticulum, where they can easily be eroded by impacted faecoliths. If there is inflammation, bleeding does not result, as mural oedema distances the vessels from the impacted faecoliths. The bleeding may be brisk and bright red, and there are usually no symptoms or signs in the abdomen. Diverticula at any site of the colon may bleed.

4. Angiodysplasia. The colonic mucosa may have small flat patches of telangiectatic vasculature, rarely greater than one centimeter in diameter. These are termed angiodysplasia, and they probably account for the majority of cases of acute and chronic colonic bleeds. They are often multiple and are most commonly found in the right colon, but may occur at other sites in the gastrointestinal tract.

5. Meckel's diverticulum. A Meckel's diverticulum may be the site of ectopic gastric mucosa. This will produce gastric acid, and whilst the acid-tolerating mucosa within the diverticulum will be relatively protected, the adjacent ileal mucosa will be intolerant, and a peptic ulcer may develop next to the neck of the diverticulum. This ulcer may bleed, like its counterparts in the duodenum, and will present with the passage of (often copious) dark blood per rectum.

6. Tumours. Carcinoma of the colon very rarely presents as frank haemorrhage, but frequently causes anaemia from chronic occult blood loss. However, the passage of dark blood per rectum may indicate this. Colonic polyps also present with the loss of dark blood per rectum. Lymphomas, leucomyomas and haemangiomas of the small bowel or colon may bleed.

7. Bowel ischaemia. Intestinal ischaemia, including ischaemic colitis, results in intraluminal blood, and may present with dark blood passed per rectum. Causes include mesenteric arterial or venous infarction or mesenteric embolism. Ischaemia as a result of bowel strangulation or obstruction may result in blood loss, as seen with intussusception. Acute hypovolaemic shock may cause sloughing of the intestinal (usually colonic) mucosa, resulting in blood per rectum.

Investigations

The pulse rate and blood pressure are measured hourly, and if possible, the central venous pressure is measured. Blood is sent for haemoglobin estimation and cross matching.

1. Endoscopy. Patients suspected of having a lower gastro-intestinal tract bleed must undergo proctoscopy and sigmoidoscopy. These may be difficult to perform during the bleeding, as the blood will tend to obscure the field of view. Occasionally, one can 'get above' the bleeding point, and blood no longer obscures the view, suggesting that the origin of the bleed is distal to that site. Proctocolitis may be evident and biopsies confirm the diagnosis. It is rare for colonic carcinoma to result in frank haemorrhage, though polyps are more likely to do so, and if these are present in the rectum, sigmoidoscopy will provide an occasion to biopsy these and to establish a diagnosis. Angiodysplasia may be seen on colonoscopy as bright red patches of dilated vessels in the colonic mucosa, and they may be treated by colonoscopic laser or diathermy.

2. Radiolabelled red cell scanning. Patients actively bleeding may be investigated using a radioabelled red blood cell scan. An aliquot of the patient's own blood is returned after labelling of the red blood cells with technetium-99. The patient is scanned by gamma camera and the site of any pooling of the isotope is seen as a 'hot spot' on the scan. Sites of blood loss as low as 0.1 ml/min may be identified.

3. Selective mesenteric angiography. Continued dramatic bleeding in the absence of a known cause warrants mesenteric angiography. The femoral artery is cannulated, and, in sequence, the coeliac axis, superior and then inferior mesenteric arteries are selectively cannulated and injected with contrast. The site of bleeding can be accurately located if blood loss is at least 1 ml/min, and surgery may be confidently undertaken. Selective mesenteric arteriography will also detect angiodysplasia.

Management

Generally, bleeding from the lower gastrointestinal tract ceases spontaneously, and thus most cases can be managed conservatively by blood transfusion and close observation of vital signs. Proctosigmoidoscopy should be performed, and unless an obvious lesion to account for the blood loss is seen, colonoscopy should be requested the following day. If bleeding continues, a radiolabelled red cell scan should be undertaken, though this is not available out of normal hospital hours. If this test fails to demonstrate the source, or frank bleeding continues, mesenteric angiography should be performed.

Should bleeding be copious and with no available diagnosis, 'blind' emergency surgery may be necessary. This is a most unfortunate scenario, as the bleeding source is rarely evident at laparotomy. The patient will almost certainly end up having had either a right hemicolectomy on the suspicion of caecal angiodysplasia, or a sigmoid colectomy on the suspicion of diverticular bleeding, or possibly a sub-total colectomy if no clues at all are encountered intraoperatively. Furthermore, a proportion of those who end up with a 'blind' bowel resection continue to bleed.

Further reading

Ambrose NS, Wedgewood KR. Bleeding from the lower gastrointestinal tract. *Surgery*, 1990; **85**: 2027–33.

Related topics of interest

LYMPHOEDEMA AND THE SWOLLEN LIMB

Lymphoedema is swelling of the tissues as a result of tissue fluid accumulation caused by abnormalities of the lymphatic system. The legs are affected principally (80%) but the arms, genitalia and face can be affected.

Differential diagnosis of the swollen leg

Causes of leg swelling other than lymphoedema are common and should be excluded before lymphoedema is diagnosed. Heart, renal and liver failure all cause leg oedema which is usually bilateral. Allergic conditions, angio-oedema, obesity, venous obstruction, lipodystrophy, factitious oedema and gigantism should be considered.

Primary lymphoedema

Abnormal lymphatic drainage is the mechanism but the underlying cause remains obscure. Having excluded other causes of leg swelling and lymphoedema, a clinical diagnosis of primary lymphoedema may be made. Primary lymphoedema may be classified according to its time of onset (congenital, praecox, tarda), or its lymphographic appearance (aplastic, hypoplastic, megalymphatics). Patients with distal swelling of the foot, ankle and lower leg tend to have distal, obliterative, aplastic lymphatics, whereas those with lymphatic vesicles and associated chylous ascites or chylothorax tend to have megalymphatics.

Secondary lymphoedema

Secondary lymphoedema is much commoner and usually the result of either malignant infiltration of regional lymph nodes or damage to lymph nodes as a result of surgery or radiotherapy, or both. Arm involvement is much commoner than in primary lymphoedema. Worldwide, infection with the *Wuchereria Bancrofti* worm and silica infiltration of the lymphatics, both causing chronic inflammatory changes in the lymphatics, are of far greater significance.

Clinical features

Swelling of one lower leg is the commonest presentation and in the early stages this usually pits. Fibrosis occurs with chronicity and the swelling may no longer pit. The ankle contour is lost at an early stage and, if the toes are involved, they adopt a square profile and develop lichenified filiform fronds, particularly on the dorsal surface. The increased fluid and protein content of the skin and subcutaneous tissues renders affected limbs more prone to cellulitis, which may be severe. Such episodes destroy residual lymphatics and may exacerbate swelling. In gross lymphoedema, the swelling may affect the thigh such that walking may become difficult.

Investigation

In many cases the diagnosis of lymphoedema can be made clinically. Where doubt exists, investigations to exclude other causes of oedema (renal, liver and cardiac function tests) should be performed.

1. Isotope lymphogram. This should be performed where the nature of the oedema remains unclear. The rate of isotope uptake by the groin lymph nodes is measured by gamma emission. Levels diagnostic of venous oedema and lymphoedema are established by individual laboratories.

2. Contrast lymphangiogram. This is no longer required to define the lymphatic abnormality in each case of lymphoedema but should be performed if isotope lymphography indicates an isolated lymphatic block at the groin or pelvic nodes. This will indicate whether mesoenteric lymphatic bypass is possible.

Treatment

1. Elevation, massage and compression stockings. The great majority of patients are best treated by mechanical means to reduce the oedema. Elevation reduces the intravascular and lymphatic hydrostatic pressure, whilst grade III graduated compression stockings increase the extravascular hydrostatic pressure, reducing the pressure gradient across the micro-circulation. Massage milks the oedema proximally and can be performed by pneumatic compression devices having chambers which inflate from distal to proximal. Massage with aqueous cream or light vegetable oils helps to keep the skin in good condition. Skin care to avoid the ingress of bacteria resulting in cellulitis is important and early treatment of cellulitis with elevation, hydration and antibiotics is vital. Diuretics are generally unhelpful.

2. Reduction operations. Most patients with lymphoedema do not require surgery. Where the leg becomes un-manageable by conservative means, a debulking procedure may be considered. If the skin is in good condition, Homan's operation may be performed. Flaps are raised and a central strip of skin and subcutaneous tissue is excised. The flaps are then sutured back together. This is usually performed on the medial side of the leg first, but may be repeated on the lateral side if further debulking is required. Above and below knee procedures may be performed.

Where the skin is in poor condition, Charles' operation is more suitable. All of the skin and subcutaneous tissue is excised. Split skin grafts are applied to the deep fascia.

3. *Ileal mesoenteric bridge operation.* This is the only successful lymphatic bypass operation, but it is suitable only for a small number of patients who have an isolated lymphatic block in the groin or pelvic nodes. Only 50% of these patients have a good result. A segment of ileum is taken out of circuit on its mesentery and the proximal and distal free ends anastomosed to restore bowel continuity. The isolated segment is opened along its long axis and stripped of its mucosa to expose the rich network of submucosal lymphatics. This segment is then tunnelled into the pelvis or groin where the lymph nodes just distal to the obstruction are bivalved. The segment of bowel is sewn on to the lymph nodes and lymphatic connections between the two surfaces form.

Lympho-lymphatic and lymphovenous anastomoses have been attempted but results are disappointing.

Further reading

Kinmonth JB. *Lymphatics, Surgery, Lymphography and Diseases of the Chyle and Lymph Systems*, 2nd Edn. London: Edward Arnold, 1982.
Wolfe JHN. Lymphoedema. In: Burnand KG, Young AE (eds) *The New Aird's Companion in Surgical Studies*. Edinburgh: Churchill Livingstone, 1992; 415–23.

Related topics of interest

MECKEL'S DIVERTICULUM

A Meckel's diverticulum is congenital, involving all three coats of the bowel wall, and is frequently described as being present in 2% of the population, 2 feet (approx. 60 cm) from the caecum and 2 inches long. In contrast to jejunal diverticulae it is present on the antimesenteric border and, just like the appendix, has its own artery. It is the commonest congenital anomaly of the small bowel, being a remnant of the vitellointestinal duct or omphalomesenteric duct. Ectopic gastric mucosa or pancreatic tissue is commonly found within the diverticulum. A Meckel's diverticulum can produce a wide range of complications, most of which occur in children. In adults, the commonest presentation is its presence as an incidental finding at laparotomy and the commonest complication is intestinal obstruction.

Historical	Johann Friedrich Meckel, the younger, 1781–1833, Professor of Anatomy and Surgery, Halle, Germany, first described this condition. He is also responsible for naming Meckle's cartilage, a remnant of the first branchial arch. Meckel, the older, identified himself with the fold of dura housing the gausserian ganglion situated at the floor of the middle cranial fossa: Meckel's cave.
Inflammation	An inflamed Meckel's presents with features indistinguishable from acute appendicitis. A narrow lumen with a long diverticulum predisposes to this complication. A Meckel's diverticulum should always be sought during the course of an operation for suspected appendicitis if the appendix is not at fault. In the presence of obvious appendicitis (not just serosal inflammation) the probability of a second acute pathology is extremely rare and it is best not to draw out several feet of small bowel to search for a Meckel's. This only spreads contamination and covers the small bowel with sticky inflammatory exudate. When this is then returned into the peritoneal cavity orientation becomes difficult and its new position could precipitate obstruction.
Peptic ulceration	Peptic ulceration from a Meckel's is a common cause of rectal bleeding in children. In 15% there is ectopic gastric mucosa within the diverticulum itself but the areas of ulceration usually occur at the base or on the mesenteric border of the ileum. Males are eight times more likely to develop these peptic ulcers than females. Adults present with post-prandial pain localized around the umbilicus. A pertechnetate technetium-99m scan is useful in localizing ectopic acid-secreting mucosa. Isotope uptake can be enhanced by pentagastrin stimulation.

Intussusception

Intussusception occurs usually when the heterotopic mucosa at the base of a diverticulum becomes inflamed and projects into the lumen. Reduction is achieved by milking the intussusceptum proximally through the intussuscipiens and not by distraction of both ends of the bowel. When maximal reduction is achieved, a short ileal resection is necessary. A Meckel's should never be invaginated like an appendix stump because this can precipitate an intussusception.

Perforation

A Meckel's can perforate from peptic ulceration, acute inflammation or foreign body entrapment resulting in generalized peritonitis.

Obstruction

A fibrous band, the remnant of the vitellointestinal duct or the vitelline vessels, is occasionally present running from the apex of a Meckel's to the umbilicus. Small bowel can twist around this causing a volvulus or the band itself may kink a loop of bowel. If a Meckel's diverticulum is found in a femoral or inguinal hernia, it can incarcerate, obstruct, strangulate or perforate. This is known as a Littre's hernia.

Neoplasia

A carcinoid tumour is the commonest neoplasm found in association with a Meckel's. These lesions characteristically cicatrize from the intense fibrosis typical of carcinoids in general. Intestinal obstruction is the usual presentation.

Incidental

If a Meckel's diverticulum is found incidentally at operation the decision to excise or leave alone is based on whether the morbidity of an intestinal anastomosis is greater or less than the natural history of a Meckel's developing a complication. The following factors are a guide favouring excision.

- Age under 40.
- Presence of ectopic mucosa.
- Scarring or induration.
- Base less than twice the length.
- Undiagnosed rectal bleeding.

Resection

Resection, if indicated, should be performed without narrowing the ileum. In some cases this involves complete excision, together with a segment of ileum, and an end-to-end anastomosis. In those which possess a narrow base, simple amputation, without invagination, is all that is necessary.

Further reading

Leijonmark CE, Bonman-Sandelin K, *et al*. *British Journal of Surgery*, 1986; **73**: 146–9.
The small and large intestines. In: *Bailey and Love's Short Practice of Surgery*. London: HK
    Lewis & Co., 1988; 1033-5.

Related topics of interest

MINIMAL ACCESS SURGERY

Diagnostic and therapeutic coelioscopy have been commonplace in gynaecological and urological practice for many years, but even diagnostic laparoscopy was not widely practised by general surgeons until the first laparoscopic cholecystectomies were performed in 1988. Since then laparoscopic surgical practice has exploded with surgeons learning and practising the techniques at a hitherto unseen rate. Demand for the new techniques was driven by public demand, although this was latterly tempered by several well publicized complications and deaths that emphasized inherent problems with the new two-dimensional, tactileless techniques, together with deficiencies in training and the regulation of minimal access surgery.

Minimal access surgery involves endoscopic and coelioscopic surgical procedures performed via an endoluminal or intracavitary route through multiple small incisions. The avoidance of a long abdominal wound seems to be the single most important factor in facilitating a rapid recovery. Minimal postoperative discomfort, a reduced hospital stay and early return to full activity are the principal advantages. Techniques such as endoscopic sphincterotomy, injection of bleeding ulcer and varices have been practised for some years, but with the evolution of video and instrument technology have developed cholecystectomy, thoracoscopic sympathectomy, appendicectomy, hernia repair, peptic ulcer surgery, repair of hiatus hernia, colonic resection, nephrectomy, splenectomy and adrenalectomy in general surgical practice. The techniques have been introduced in a wave of enthusiasm and largely without the benefit of randomized controlled trials. Many techniques remain controversial and only laparoscopic cholecystectomy and thoracoscopic sympathectomy are generally recognized as preferable to the open operations at present. Laparoscopic surgery lends itself more to excisional procedures than reconstructive procedures. Current indications suggest that conventional open techniques are unlikely to become obsolete for many years although technology and techniques are evolving rapidly.

General principles

Intracavitary abdominal procedures require the creation of a pneumoperitoneum using either a Verres needle to introduce carbon dioxide or the direct introduction of a cannula under vision through which carbon dioxide is introduced. A 0° or 30° laparoscope is introduced and subsequent trocars must all be introduced under direct vision. Basic instruments include fine grasping forceps for retracting, suction/irrigation cannulas, curved dissecting forceps and diathermy scissors or hook. Electrocoagulation is generally preferred to laser as the overshoot phenomenon, which can damage distant tissues, is avoided. Various clip devices are used to ligate small vessels and ducts and more sophisticated staple devices are available to close bowel and perform anastomoses. Roeder slip-knots can be used to ligate vessels and ducts. Instrumentation to extend the armamentarium of coelioscopic techniques is developing rapidly.

Complications

- Diagnostic laparoscopy: mortality < 0.03%, major complications 0.6%, minor complications 4%.
- Abdominal wall/omental emphysema.
- Circulatory/respiratory collapse from tension pneumoperitoneum.
- Trocar puncture of bowel or bladder.
- Trocar puncture of major vessel (aorta, iliac vessels, cava).
- Carbon dioxide embolus.
- Diathermy, laser, clip injury (e.g. to bile duct).
- Haemorrhage.

Specific general surgical procedures

1. Biliary surgery. Cholecystectomy remains the most widely practised and acknowledged procedure. Management of the common bile duct varies from ignoring the possibility of duct stones to endoscopic retrograde cholangiopancreatography or perioperative cholangiography routinely or selectively. Bile duct stones may be cleared laparoscopically using a fine-bore flexible choledochoscope, baskets and balloon catheters. Bile duct injury is the most significant complication and there is evidence that this occurs more commonly than in the open operation.

2. Appendicectomy. Laparoscopy can be used to verify the diagnosis, particularly in young women. Where acute appendicitis is confirmed, laparoscopic or laparoscopic assisted appendicectomy is logical. A good view of the peritoneal cavity is obtained allowing diagnosis of other causes of acute abdominal pain. The operation often takes longer than the conventional procedure and involves three or four trocar sites.The necessary equipment and appropriately trained staff must be available for emergency operating. Several large series have reported satisfactory results.

3. Hernia repair. The laparoscopic procedure changes a simple body wall operation that can be performed as a day case under local anaesthetic to an intra-abdominal or properitoneal procedure performed under general anaesthetic. A mesh is placed over the hernial defect from within providing a tension free repair. Early recurrence rates were unacceptably high, but the technique is evolving.

4. Antireflux surgery. The Nissen procedure has been developed for laparoscopy. Early results appear comparable to those for the open operation with low morbidity and mortality. The procedure is time-consuming and a high degree of operator expertise is required.

5. Sympathectomy. Thoracoscopic sympathectomy is a welcome alternative to the open operation performed via the difficult anterior supraclavicular or the transaxillary routes. Palmar hyperhidrosis is the prime indication. Unilateral or bilateral procedures can be performed. The thoracoscope is introduced through the fifth intercostal space in the anterior axillary line. The risk of Horner's syndrome is substantially lower than in the supraclavicular operation. Compensatory hyperhidrosis of the trunk or thighs occurs to some extent in 50% of patients and is commoner after bilateral operations.

6. Peptic ulcer surgery. Posterior truncal vagotomy with anterior seromyotomy is currently the preferred technique for the treatment of patients with refractory duodenal ulcer disease. Patching of perforated duodenal ulcer and gastroenterostomy can also be performed. Very few patients now require elective peptic ulcer surgery and few large series have been performed.

7. Colectomy. Series of resections for benign and malignant disease have been reported. Early results indicated that hospital stay and complications were not significantly reduced by using laparoscopic techniques. The possibility of inadequate clearance of malignant disease and the occurrence of port site metastases have tempered enthusiasm for the use of laparoscopic techniques in the treatment of bowel cancer, but resections for inflammatory bowel disease can be performed effectively.

Further reading

Rosin D (ed.) *Minimal Access General Surgery.* Oxford: Radcliffe Medical Press, 1994.

Related topics of interest

Appendicitis (p. 38)
Endoscopy (p. 124)
Gallstones and their complications (p. 139)
Gastro-oesophageal reflux (p. 151)
Inguinal hernia (p. 176)
Peptic ulceration (p. 236)

MONITORING OF THE CRITICALLY ILL PATIENT

Vital functions are monitored in the intensive care unit (ICU) to assess progress, identify impending organ failure and, as a consequence, to sustain organ function. The main systems monitored are the cardiac, pulmonary, renal and cerebral. Arterial and venous blood tests are performed regularly and the results are charted to demonstrate trends. A chest X-ray is performed daily.

Cardiovascular monitoring

The ECG is continually monitored. The CVP is measured following insertion of a teflon cannula into the superior vena cava via the internal jugular or subclavian vein. This enables a simple and rapid assessment of right heart filling pressure, and this CVP value directly reflects the cardiac preload. It also affords a simple measure of the state of tonicity of the circulation. Hypovolaemia, which may be actual or relative, and fluid overload can be identified. However, cardiac function is not reliably measured by means of a CVP line. Pulmonary ventilation may elevate CVP readings, and the right heart filling pressures do not reflect the pumping function of the left side.

The function of the left side of the heart is monitored by recording systemic arterial pressure, pulmonary artery wedge and occlusion pressures, and by measuring cardiac output. Arterial pressure is monitored from a teflon cannula usually located in the radial artery. Systolic and diastolic values are transduced, and mean arterial pressure can be calculated. When connected to a multipurpose monitor, the arterial pressure wave is represented. Hypovolaemia may be revealed by an excessive dip in arterial pressure as the patient inhales. Left atrial filling pressure is a better indicator of cardiac function than right heart filling pressure, but this cannot be measured directly. A good approximation is obtained using a Swann–Ganz catheter inserted via a large neck vein, and passed through the right side of the heart into a branch of the pulmonary artery. When the catheter is occluding the lumen of the pulmonary artery branch, the pressure at the catheter tip reflects the left atrial pressure (pulmonary artery wedge pressure), and an assessment of left ventricular preload can be made. Cardiac output may be measured using intracardiac temperature sensitive catheters.

Renal monitoring

Urine output via urinary catheter is measured continually and expressed in millilitres output per hour. Normal hourly urine output ranges widely, but levels lower than 30 ml/hour are highly suggestive of renal underperfusion. If this is allowed to continue, acute tubular necrosis and renal failure may ensue. This is characterized by a period of anuria, which may last up to 24 hours, followed by oliguria as the kidneys regain their function. This is common in the surgical patient with haemorrhagic or septic shock. If urine output drops, prerenal failure is best prevented by first ensuring adequate volume replacement (maintaining the right-sided cardiac pressures) and, if necessary, selectively vasodilating the renal vessels (thus maintaining renal perfusion) by infusing low-dose intravenous dopamine.

Respiratory monitoring

Not all patients on the ICU need ventilation, but many of the surgical patients emerging from theatre requiring intensive care will be electively ventilated to avoid respiratory depression and pulmonary atelectasis from heavy analgesia, thus ensuring optimal arterial and tissue oxygenation. Elective postoperative ventilation requires infused sedatives i.v. and full ventilatory support through an endotracheal tube. Patients being weaned off the ventilator with difficulty may need selective intermittent mandatory ventilation (SIMV) which demands respirations from the patient at intervals. Patients with pulmonary atelectasis or infection, both common in the surgical setting, may need extra ventilatory pressure to ventilate collapsed alveoli and this is achieved in the non-sedated patient using continuous positive pressure ventilation (CPAP) through a face mask, or intermittent positive pressure ventilation (IPPV), if the patient is intubated. Patients requiring prolonged ventilation (greater than 1 week) require a tracheostomy to protect the upper airway from prolonged laryngeal intubation, and to aid nursing and physiotherapy staff to suction the tracheobronchial tree.

All patients with respiratory difficulties need regular estimations of their arterial blood gases. An arterial line facilitates collection of arterial blood. The many parameters measured indicate both pulmonary and metabolic function. Poor PaO_2 despite a high percentage FiO_2 is indicative of parenchymal pulmonary disease, commonly ARDS, gross pulmonary collapse or consolidation. A base excess reducing progressively from -2.0 indicates a metabolic acidosis.

Cerebrovascular monitoring

Head-injured patients may have traumatic cerebral oedema or diffuse brain injury, and no evidence of a surgically correctable abnormality. These need the ICU for ventilation to avoid hypercapnia and reduce cerebral vasospasm, and maintain cerebral perfusion to counter increased intracranial pressure (ICP). Increasing the ICP reduces the cerebral perfusion pressure (CPP), and this is best monitored by the insertion of an extradural pressure bolt through which the ICP may be transduced. Continuous electroencephalography may be used to monitor cerebral activity.

Further reading

McCrirrick AB, Nevin M. Intensive care monitoring of the surgical patient. *Current Practice in Surgery*, 1994; **6**: 202–6.

Related topics of interest

Burns (p. 64)
Head injury (p. 161)
Multiple organ failure (p. 208)
Nutrition in the surgical patient (p. 213)
Organ support in the intensive care unit (p. 223)
Trauma management – principles (p. 301)

MULTIPLE ORGAN FAILURE

Multiple organ failure (MOF) is the leading cause of death in the surgical ICU. It was first recognized in 1973. It can be defined as the result of a severe physiological insult which leads to the failure of several organs not necessarily involved in the original insult. The realization that the organs involved become hypermetabolic rather than actually failing has led some to change the name to the multiple organ dysfunction syndrome (MODS). Similarly, the host response of disseminated inflammation to the powerful physiological insult has been termed the systemic inflammatory response syndrome (SIRS).

Aetiology

MOF typically occurs after shock, infection, massive tissue injury, and in the presence of large amounts of necrotic tissue. Depending on the physiological reserve of the organs concerned the order of failure commences with pulmonary, followed by hepatic, intestinal and, lastly, renal failure. There is a direct relationship between the number of organs failing and the length of time the patient is in organ failure with the mortality of the patient. Unfortunately, there remains a grey area where it is impossible to predict which patients will develop MOF prior to the insult and to predict with accuracy the outcome. This problem of patient assessment is a major factor limiting the value of various therapeutic trials. To date, IL-6 levels appear to be the best single predictor of outcome in the MOF syndrome.

Pathogenesis

The current hypotheses of MOF include a persisting focus of infection, uncontrolled generalized inflammation (SIRS), gut mucosal failure, reticuloendothelial system failure and the production of oxygen free radicals. The contribution of each of these to MOF will be examined.

Sepsis

The observation that the organs which fail are often remote from the disease process led to the suggestion that an endogenous or exogenous circulating factor acts as a mediator. Whilst in the majority of patients infection is the initiating cause, in a third of patients with MOF there has been no evidence of an infective focus. The concept of an empiric laparotomy to identify this infective focus is now outdated as these operations rarely discover occult sepsis that has been missed on less invasive investigations like ultrasound and CT.

Inflammatory mediators

The similarity between systemic infection and a septic state in which no infection has been identified suggests that common mediators are responsible. These have been isolated and include bacterial endotoxin, TNF-α, IL-6, IL-1 and oxygen free radicals. The injection of TNF-α or endotoxin into healthy human volunteers can accurately reproduce the septic response. TNF-α, specifically, is believed to participate in the muscle proteolysis that accompanies sepsis and it is enhanced by glucocorticoids.

Gut mucosal barrier

Recent interest has implicated the gut, with its reservoir of bacteria, as the driving force behind MOF. Loss of the gut mucosal barrier leads to the translocation of Gram –ve bacteria and endotoxin into the portal circulation, which is believed to initiate MOF. This situation is potentiated if the natural defences of the gut (the intestinal microflora, a host immune response and adequate functional enterocyte mass) are compromised, which is a common feature of a septic patient. Sepsis encourages immunosuppression and antibiotic regimes displace the normal intestinal flora with an overgrowth of potentially pathogenic flora. The upper intestinal tract becomes colonized if medication is given to reduce gastric acidity. Parenteral or hyperosmolar enteral feeds lead to disuse atrophy of the mucosa, further decreasing the gut's defence against invasion. If healthy human volunteers receive a single dose of enterotoxin, they develop a hypoalbumenaemic and capillary leak syndrome. The intestines become oedematous, form an ileus and exhibit increased permeability to bacteria.

Intestinal ischaemia

Impaired oxygen delivery to the gut occurs in shock, and its associated alteration in mesenteric blood flow. During reperfusion, injury occurs and macrophages are activated with release of IL-1, IL-6, TNF-α and free radicals, which further increase intestinal permeability and encourage endotoxin and bacterial translocation.

Reticuloendothelial system

The next barrier to a generalized septic state is the liver and the spleen. Bacteria can be cultured from these organs, the portal circulation and the intestinal lymph nodes after massive physiological insults. If the state of the reticulo-endothelial system in the liver is healthy, it should be effective in neutralizing a moderate bacterial and endotoxin load. If the liver is impaired, Kupfer cell malfunction occurs and endotoxins and bacteria are released into the systemic circulation.

Free radicals

Oxygen free radicals also contribute to MOF by damage to the microvascular circulation. They are generated during reperfusion when oxygen reacts with hypoxanthene, a metabolic product of ATP that accumulates during ischaemia, and is converted into the superoxide anion. The intracellular antioxidants are not capable of neutralizing this massive free radical load with consequent endothelial damage. This attracts neutrophils and encourages them to degranulate with the release of many inflammatory mediators, all of which play a role in the SIRS.

Further reading

Buchman TG. Multiple organ failure. *Current Opinion in General Surgery*, 1993; 26–31.
Deitch EA. Multiple organ failure. *Advances in Surgery,* 1993; **26**: 333–56.

Related topics of interest

NON-SPECIFIC ABDOMINAL PAIN

Fifty per cent of patients initially presenting to hospital with acute abdominal pain do not have a definitive diagnosis. This is still the case in 30% of patients admitted. In the absence of evidence of surgical, gynaecological or medical disease, these patients may be termed as having 'non-specific abdominal pain' or 'abdominal pain of unknown origin'. Approximately half of those initially diagnosed will leave hospital having been told they have dyspepsia, constipation, dysmenorrhoea, mesenteric adenitis or gastroenteritis. These are not absolute diagnoses, and therefore the percentage of cases of acute abdominal pain that remains 'non-specific' is probably between 40% and 50%.

The diagnosis has been entertained at all ages, but the implications may differ. In up to 30% of children with the diagnosis it is recurrent, and many will be submitted to appendicectomy, though in eight out of 10 such cases the appendix will be normal. However, in children it is important to rule out acute appendicitis, which is potentially disastrous if missed, and is eminently treatable as the next most common cause of acute abdominal pain presenting to hospital.

This diagnosis, however, should only be a diagnosis of exclusion in those aged over 50, as over 10% of those presenting (a higher proportion than expected) will develop a malignancy within the next 3 years. Additionally, 10% of the over 70s will develop ischaemic heart, abdominal aortic or mesenteric vascular disease over the same time period.

Symptoms and signs

- Acute onset of abdominal pain; may be diffuse but usually in the right iliac fossa.
- Vomiting and anorexia are absent.
- Rarely signs of systemic ill-health such as pyrexia, flushing or tachycardia.
- No signs of peritonism or peritonitis.
- Symptoms usually self-limiting, often disappearing after one night in hospital.

Differential diagnosis

In children and young adults, the chief differential is acute appendicitis. Patients with non-specific abdominal pain more commonly undergo appendicectomy, but have been shown not to have a greater incidence of acute appendicitis.

In those of school age this must be differentiated from the so-called 'functional abdominal pain'. There is often a classical history, and apparently severe pain that thoroughly outweighs any abdominal signs present. This has a basis in psychiatric illness and is very difficult to treat.

Women may have endometriosis, causing abdominal pain in the absence of discrete abdominal signs. A full gynaecological history must be taken, and, if indicated, a thorough pelvic examination must be performed otherwise tubo-ovarian disease may easily be missed.

Though the middle-aged patient with non-specific abdominal pain is at no greater risk of developing peptic ulceration or cholelithiasis, these are common conditions, and it may be advisable to screen for those in this age group.

While an elevated WBC may suggest the presence of a focus of inflammation, a normal count is no guarantee of diagnosis.

Management   A positive diagnosis precludes the need for surgical exploration for treatment or diagnosis. The correct management involves a positive diagnosis of non-specific abdominal pain, reassurance that there is nothing seriously wrong, and discharge from the emergency setting. If a surgical diagnosis cannot be excluded and the patient is admitted, a correct diagnosis may be made upon review the next morning, by which time the symptoms may have resolved. Adults may be given an appointment for a biliary ultrasound scan to exclude gallstones, or an endoscopy to exclude peptic ulceration, and be reviewed in the out-patient clinic.

The elderly should not be diagnosed as having non-specific abdominal pain. It is likely that there is some pathology detectable to account for the pain and even if no cause is apparent they should be followed-up in the out-patient clinic.

Further reading

de Dombal FT. Diagnosis and prognosis of patients with non-specific abdominal pain (NSAP). *Current Practice in Surgery*, 1994; **6**: 186–9.

Related topics of interest

Appendicitis (p. 38)
Assessment of the acute abdomen (p. 42)
Irritable bowel syndrome (p. 187)

NUTRITION IN THE SURGICAL PATIENT

Nutrition plays a vital role in wound healing and collagen maturation, and it boosts the energy reserves of the body. The combination of infection and injury (surgery or trauma) particularly predisposes to malnutrition. These additional stresses inhibit the ketotic response to starvation and encourage the preferential mobilization of muscle protein. The immune response to infection also becomes downregulated and T cell, B cell and macrophage function deteriorates.

Indications

Usually one week without nutritional support during the perioperative period provides no real problems so long as full intestinal recovery occurs. The indications for nutritional support include:

- Protracted postoperative recovery. Sepsis is the usual cause.
- Intestinal failure. For example, peritonitis or enterocutaneous fistulae.
- Profound requirements. For example, large burns or major trauma.
- Pre-operative malnutrition. For example, carcinoma of the oesophagus.
- Unconscious patient. Most long-term surgical patients in the ICU receive parenteral nutrition. Head-injured and ventilated patients usually need nutritional support.

Consequences of surgery

Abdominal operations result in a degree of gut dysfunction, the extent of which depends upon the severity of the disease pathology and on the type and trauma of the surgery. The sequence of intestinal recovery after a laparotomy is often predictable, small bowel recovering first followed by the stomach and then the colon. If enteral nutrition is withheld, functional gut mass reduces, the enterocytes decline in number and the villi flatten. The mucosal barrier then weakens which encourages bacterial translocation into the portal circulation. Endotoxins can be released from these Gram −ve bacteria and lead to endotoxic shock and circulatory failure.

Nutritional route

The preferred nutritional route is oral or enteral rather than parenteral. Hospital food is unappetizing so relatives are often advised to bring in tasty nutritious snacks. Oesophageal carcinoma produces complete dysphagia when a severely narrowed lumen is obstructed by a pellet of food. Clearance of this by endoscopy and subsequent dilatation can allow for the passage of a fine-bore nasojejunal tube.

Correct placement is determined radiologically, by the aspiration of bile or by listening for an abdominal gurgle when the tube is inflated with air. This is an ideal way to provide pre-operative nutrition in such patients.

Enteral feeding

Specialized enteral feeds come in two varieties.

1. Elemental. This consists of the L-amino acids and sugars. This diet is non-antigenic and can be as effective as steroids in inducing remission in children with IBD. The main disadvantage is the high osmolarity which often produces a profound diarrhoea.

2. Defined. This is based on milk protein and consists of peptones, medium chain triglycerides and polysaccharides.

All enteral feeds should commence at a quarter or half strength to allow for adaptation. If diarrhoea remains a problem the addition of tapioca starch may firm the stools.

Percutaneous endoscopic gastrostomy (PEG)

Other methods of enteral feeding should be considered before rushing to parenteral nutrition. The PEG is an ingenious way of placing a gastrostomy. It is achieved by incising over the illuminated tip of the endoscope whilst it is in the stomach and then rail-roading a feeding tube through the gastric and abdominal puncture hole. Most indications for this procedure are neurological: stroke, motor neurone disease, head injury, bulbar palsy. Complications are few but can be serious, like feeding tube displacement or colonic puncture.

Feeding jejunostomy

A feeding jejunostomy can be positioned at the time of surgery if nutritional support is anticipated postoperatively. Unfortunately, there is no satisfactory indicator of malnutrition pre-operatively. Reduced albumen or transferrin levels and a diminished absolute lymphocyte count is as good an indicator as clinical judgement. A purse-string suture is first sewn over a jejunal loop and the feeding tube is then inserted with a trocar into the lumen via a 4 cm submucosal tunnel. The purse-string suture is then carried on to the underside of the abdominal wall in order to keep the jejunum flush with the parietal peritoneum. Unfortunately, these tubes often fall out if not adequately secured. Regular flushing is required to prevent blockage.

Total parenteral nutrition (TPN)

The daily nutritional requirements are 14 g of nitrogen (this must include the essential amino acids), 2000 non-nitrogen calories (including the three essential fatty acids), with added vitamins and minerals (magnesium, selenium, zinc, copper, chromium and manganese are essential trace elements). The three essential fatty acids, arachidonic, linoleic and linolenic acid, are required for cell membrane structure and prostaglandin synthesis. This cocktail is usually given by a single 3-l bag into a central vein.

Complications of TPN

TPN, as well as being non-physiological, has a substantial complication rate and occasional mortality.

1. Access. Attempts at subclavian or internal jugular cannulation can produce a pneumothorax, thoracic duct or arterial puncture, or a brachial plexus injury. Advocates of peripheral venous feeding avoid this problem but cannulae need to be changed daily to avoid the irritant nature of a hyperosmolar and low pH solution which readily causes a thrombophlebitis. Other complications include central vein thrombosis, air embolism and catheter tip embolism.

2. Infection. Infected lines need to be removed, the tips cultured and the cannulae resited after 24 hours, preferably on to the other side. The responsible organisms are usually *Staphylococcus epidermidis* or *S. aureus* but fungi may also be cultured. Diagnosis is made inspecting the site, excluding other sources of infection and taking blood cultures through the line itself. Infection risk is minimized by using a tunnelled line (Hickman line), insuring insertion under sterile conditions, avoidance of several side-arm ports and keeping bag changes to a minimum.

3. Metabolic. A multitude of metabolic derangements are common. Daily urea, electrolytes with regular blood (glucose) monitoring (BM) stix and twice-weekly liver function tests are mandatory. Alkaline phosphatase and bilirubin levels rise to a plateau after a few days from the cholestasis that TPN produces. Glycosuria, hyperglycaemia and hyperkalaemia indicate glucose intolerance and require the gradual introduction of insulin into the regime.

Further reading

Grant JP. Total parenteral nutrition. *Current Practice in Surgery*, 1991; **3**: 38–43.
Moran BJ, Jackson AA. Perioperative nutritional support. *British Journal of Surgery*, 1993; **80**: 4–5.

Related topics of interest

OESOPHAGEAL CANCER

The outlook for patients with oesophageal cancer is poor, the overall survival rate at 5 years remaining about 5%. The primary therapeutic aim is prompt and lasting palliation from dysphagia. The condition is twice as common in men, occuring in middle age or the elderly. Northern China has a particularly high incidence at 35 per 100 000 (over eight times that seen in Europe and USA), where the disease is seen in younger patients.

Pathology

Most are squamous cell tumours; the 4% which are adeno-carcinomas are thought to arise from Barrett's metaplasia. Nearly all cardial lesions are gastric adenocarcinomas and will be considered under Gastric cancer (p. 144). Oat cell (small cell undifferentiated) and signet ring types have a particularly poor prognosis. Spread is usually direct along submucosal lymphatics causing occasional satellite nodules to appear. Lymphatic spread is to oesophageal and regional nodes, and haematogenous spread is mainly to the liver and lungs. The length of the tumour, depth of invasion, circum-ferential and longitudinal resection margins, and node status are the best determinants of survival.

Aetiology

Smoking, heavy alcohol consumption and a diet high in nitrosamines are associated with an increased risk of developing the disease. The following conditions predispose to the development of oesophageal cancer, possibly by promoting stasis.

Condition	Increased risk
Achalasia	7x
Barrett's oesophagus	30x
Lye stricture	22x
Post-cricoid web	9x
Peptic stricture	6x

Presentation

The most common presenting symptom is dysphagia. It is relentlessly progressive, starting with solids, then liquids and then the patient's own saliva. Weight loss and wasting are common. Unusual presentations include a cervical node, left recurrent laryngeal nerve palsy, overspill pneumonia, pre-prandial coughing (tracheo-oesophageal fistula) and massive haemetemesis (aorto-oesophageal fistula). In Northern China, screening by exfoliative cytology with a net balloon is used to detect early disease.

Examination	Clinical examination consists of a general nutrition assessment (e.g. wasting, cachexia) and the detection of secondary disease (clinical staging), such as a knobbly liver, cervical node or lobar collapse. Fitness for surgery should also be assessed.
Diagnosis	Diagnosis is essentially with a contrast (low ionic) swallow or an upper gastrointestinal endoscopy. The former provides better visualization and a record of the problem with demonstration of the suitability of the stomach for reconstruction. Endoscopy yields material for histology and is better at assessing smaller lesions and lesions of the cardia.
Assessment	By the time of clinical presentation, cure is almost impossible and the therapeutic aim is to prevent death from dysphagia. If surgery is considered, assessment of stage, resectablity and the patient's general condition is carried out. Chest X-ray, haemoglobin and liver function tests are mandatory. Abdominal spread is detected by ultrasound, CT or laparoscopy. Bronchoscopy or CT may be required for upper two-third lesions to exclude direct pulmonary invasion or azygous vein and major vessel involvement. A CT scan often exaggerates the extent of local spread. Care should be exercised in precluding such patients from surgery on the basis of apparent advanced local disease. Abstinence from smoking and pre-operative chest physiotherapy all contribute to an improved postoperative recovery.
Nutrition	Full nutritional resuscitation with a high protein liquid diet, supplemented with vitamins and minerals, is advisable. If dysphagia is complete, the obstructing food bolus can occasionally be removed with endoscopy, allowing the placement of a fine-bore feeding tube.
Surgery	There are four main surgical approaches.

1. Ivor–Lewis–Tanner procedure. In this procedure the stomach is mobilized through a midline incision. The lesion is approached via a right thoracotomy and the anastomosis (usually, jejunal–oesophageal) takes place in the chest.

2. McKeown three stage. This technique involves the addition of a cervical incision to the last procedure. A cervical anastomosis (usually, gastric–oesophageal) is achieved.

3. *Ong trans-hiatal dissection.* In this procedure the thorax is not directly entered. The entire operation is performed via a laparotomy and neck incision. The tumour is dissected free with a hand introduced into the posterior mediastinum.

4. *Abdomino-thoracic oesophago-gastrectomy.* A laparotomy is performed through an upper abdominal incision parallel to the right costal margin and extending to the left costal margin at the level of the 7th interspace. The stomach is then mobilized and the incision is extended right across the chest to gain access to the tumour. A jejunal loop is anastomosed to the remaining oesophagus. This exposure is excellent for lesions of the cardia.

Choice of approach

The advantage of an intrathoracic operation is that direct tumour dissection can be carried out, a necessary requisite for a radical operation. A cervical anastomosis has the obvious advantage that, if it leaks, fatal mediastinitis is less likely. Blunt trans-hiatal dissection can be hazardous if major vessels are inadvertently torn (e.g. the azygous vein). If the integrity of the thorax is preserved, postoperative respiratory complications are reduced. Resection should involve at least 5 cm of macroscopic clearance.

Continuity

Gastrointestinal continuity is usually restored with stomach after its mobilization on the right gastroepiploic artery. A pyloromyotomy is usually performed at the end of the operation to encourage early gastric emptying because the vagus nerves have been necessarily divided. Reconstruction with free jejunal transfers or colonic mobilization procedures increases the risk of anastomotic failure. The 30-day operative mortality rate approaches 10%.

Complications

Atalectasis, pneumonia and respiratory failure frequently occur. Specific postoperative complications include left recurrent laryngeal nerve palsy, phrenic nerve injury and thoracic duct injury. A contrast swallow should be performed at 7–10 days to ascertain anastomotic integrity before oral intake commences.

Palliation

Non-surgical palliative treatments are divided into endoscopic techniques to relieve obstruction and radiotherapy. Chemotherapy has no established place in treatment. Non-surgical procedures are indicated for advanced disease, the infirmity of old age and disabling concomitant medical conditions.

1. Endoscopy. Intubation remains the most commonly used method. It should always be performed endoscopically and is the treatment of choice for tracheo-oesophageal fistula or external compression. Tubes (e.g. Celestin) provide satisfactory palliation in most patients but they can be displaced or perforate the oesophagus. Obstruction can occur with a food bolus, tumour encroachment or hypomotility from submucosal spread. If placed too low, incapacitating reflux ensues. They cannot be sited for upper-third tumours. Recently, self-expanding stents made of nitinol, an alloy malleable at body termperature, have been deployed across a stenosis. These stents are more 'comfortable' and are reported to remain open for longer. Exophytic lesions are most suitable for laser therapy, with the neodynium yttrium–aluminium–garnet (YAG) laser, which recannalizes by vaporization. Multiple treatment sessions are necessary. Similar results have been achieved with bipolar diathermy. Endoscopic injection of absolute alcohol is under trial.

2. Radiotherapy. This offers a chance to inhibit the primary growth. It can be given traditionally by external beam or by an intracavity source (brachytherapy). Squamous cell carcinomas are more radiosensitive then adenocarcinomas. Chemotherapy alone has no place in treatment.

Further reading

Griffin SM, Robertson CS. Non-surgical treatment of cancer of the oesophagus. *British Journal of Surgery,* 1993; **80**: 412–3.
Hennessy TPJ. Oesophageal carcinoma. *Current Practice in Surgery,* 1991; **3**: 207-11.

Related topics of interest

Gastric cancer (p. 144)
Nutrition in the surgical patient (p. 213)

OESOPHAGEAL DYSMOTILITY

Oesophageal dysmotility disorders usually present with dysphagia in patients in whom a mechanical cause has been excluded or with angina-like chest pains. The dysphagia is characteristically intermittent and worse for liquids than solids. This aids in the differential diagnosis from an obstructing lesion when the dysphagia is progressive and worse for solids. The chest pain may occur on swallowing (odynophagia) or be retrosternal and crushing in character.

Classification

Classification is into primary, when only the oesophagus is involved, and secondary, when the oesophagus is involved as part of a systemic condition.

Primary	Secondary
Cricopharangeal spasm	Cerebrovascular accident
Pharyngeal pouch	Connective tissue disorder
Plummer–Vinson syndrome	Presbyoesophagus
Diffuse oesophageal spasm	Diabetes mellitus
Nutcracker oesophagus	Myaesthenia gravis
Achalasia	Chagas' disease

Investigation

Investigation is by barium swallow, endoscopy and oeso-phageal manometry.

1. Radiology. The salient radiological features include barium filling of a pharyngeal pouch, the corkscrew oesophagus in severe oesophageal spasm, the mega-oesophagus in Chagas' disease and the 'rat-tail' narrowing at the distal oesophagus in achalasia with 'flocculation' of barium above the food residue. Fluoroscopic screening with barium or barium-coated marshmallow provides a greater visualization of disordered peristalsis.

2. Endoscopy. Endoscopy is helpful in excluding an obstructing lesion, such as carcinoma or stricture, by unhindered passage of the scope into the stomach. It can also provide tissue samples for histology.

3. Manometry. The advent of oesophageal manometry has allowed direct measurement of oesophageal motor function and is essential for an accurate diagnosis. To produce a manometric tracing pressure, transducers are placed 5 cm apart along the oesophagus (25 cm long). Resting sphincter pressures are recorded with manometric profiles during swallowing. Abnormal features include high resting sphincter pressures, inadequate sphincter relaxation and incoordination of sphincter activity. Non-propagated peristalsis, peristaltic velocity and the normal 'after-contraction' of the lower oesophageal sphincter can also be recorded. The primary peristaltic wave normally travels at 2–4 cm/sec, lasts 4 sec at any one point and produces an occlusive pressure of 30–120 mmHg. Distension of the lower oesophagus results in a secondary peristaltic wave.

Cricopharyngeal spasm

Cricopharyngeal spasm presents in the elderly with the feeling of a lump in the throat. Occasionally, external compression from cervical adenopathy or thyroid enlargement may present in this way. The diagnosis is made by manometry when a high resting upper oesophageal sphincter pressure, sphincter incoordination and impaired sphincter relaxation may be recorded. If severe, treatment by endoscopic dilatation or cricopharyngeal myotomy should be considered.

Pharyngeal pouch

A pharyngeal pouch (Zenker's diverticulum) is a true pulsion diverticulum occurring at the pharyngo-oesophageal junction (Killian's dehiscence). It is due to an overactive upper oesophageal sphincter. The pouch gradually enlarges until food starts to collect within it and this compresses the upper oesophagus to produce the clinical symptoms of latent regurgitation, nocturnal aspiration and a palpable lump (usually on the left). Squamous carcinoma occurs in 10% of cases. Diagnosis is made by barium swallow because pouch perforation is a recognized complication of endoscopy and manometry is difficult. Treatment is by pouch excision and primary closure through a lateral cervical incision. Dissection is carried out between the lateral lobe of the thyroid and carotid sheath to identify the pouch, which is then traced to its origin and excised. A cricopharyngeal myotomy over 2–3 cm is then performed.

Post-cricoid web

The Plummer–Vinson syndrome was first described by Blankenstein in 1893. The syndrome encompasses dysphagia from an upper oesophageal web with iron deficiency anaemia, splenomegaly and a smooth atrophic tongue, and occurs in edentulous women between 30 and 50 years of age. A post-cricoid carcinoma can arise in an area of leucoplakia within the web. Treatment is by dilatation or endoscopic web division with correction of iron deficiency.

Diffuse oesophageal spasm

Diffuse oesophageal spasm presents with dysphagia and chest pain and is precipitated by eating and anxiety. A barium swallow can diagnose extreme cases by demonstrating the characteristic 'cork screw' oesophageal appearance. Manometry is essential for diagnosis when a high resting pressure with several nonpropagatory, simultaneous, multiphasic contractions are recorded. Treatment is with glycerol trinitrate, calcium channel blockers, oesophageal dilatation or a long oesophageal myotomy in extreme cases. A nutcracker oesophagus is a severe form of the condition when very high peristaltic pressures of long duration are recorded.

Achalasia

Achalasia (cardiospasm) is a functional obstruction at the lower oesophageal sphincter characterized manometrically by a high resting sphincter pressure with failure of relaxation and impaired oesophageal body peristalsis. Histologically, there is a reduction in the number of ganglion cells in Auerback's myenteric plexus. The condition affects both sexes equally and presents with a long history of intermittent dysphagia. An erect chest radiograph may demonstrate a widened mediastinum, an air/fluid level, aspiration pneumonitis and absence of the gastric air bubble. The 'rat-tail' appearance of the lower oesophagus after a barium swallow is characteristic. Pharmacological treatment with anticholinergics, nitrites or calcium antagonists is mostly unsatisfactory. Controlled pneumatic dilatation under radiological screening with a balloon passed over a guidewire is successful in over 75% of patients. Surgery is the most effective management and involves a single anterior myotomy at the cardia (Heller). The longer the oesophageal myotomy the greater the incidence of postoperative reflux which is why a 'generous' myotomy should be covered with a partial fundoplication. In advanced cases resection may be necessary.

Further reading

Watson A. Oesophageal function and motility disorders. *Recent Advances in Surgery*, 1993; 16: 63–86.

Related topics of interest

ORGAN SUPPORT IN THE INTENSIVE CARE UNIT

Specific therapy directed at every major organ system should commence whilst they are still healthy because as soon as one organ system fails, inflammatory mediators are released which encourage other organs remote from the primary insult to fail also (MOF). The pulmonary, cardiovascular, hepatoenteric, renal and cutaneous systems will be discussed in turn with reference to preventing their deterioration and supporting their function in established failure.

Prevention

General factors are the most important in preventing organ failure. These include the rapid treatment of haemorrhagic shock, the immediate definitive treatment of injuries and fixation of long bone fractures, the debridement and exclusion of necrotic tissue from the systemic circulation, the prevention of bacterial contamination by meticulous surgery, the specific antibiotic treatment of surgical sepsis, and the drainage of any postoperative fluid collections that could act as a nidus for infection.

Pulmonary support

Adult respiratory distress syndrome (ARDS) is one of the commonest clinical problems in the ICU. It occurs in response to a major physiological insult like sepsis, burns or trauma and is initiated by inflammatory mediators. In this syndrome, the pulmonary microcirculation becomes permeable (leaky) and the lungs become oedematous and rigid requiring high inflation pressures to maintain adequate ventilation. This results in hypoxia, increased shunting and patchy atelectasis. Specific pulmonary support consists of mechanical ventilation with positive end expiratory pressure (PEEP). This prevents atelectasis and improves oxygenation by limiting the areas of ventilation/perfusion mismatch. When hypoxia has continued, in spite of PEEP, other methods of ventilation have been helpful, such as continuous positive airways pressure ventilation (CPAP), high frequency jet ventilation and reversing the inspiratory-to-expiratory ratio, although these have not been shown to be superior to conventional techniques. Extracorporeal membrane oxygenation (ECMO) is a new technique which may improve survival in patients with ARDS. PGE_1 is a potent vasodilator of the pulmonary microcirculation. It has been given experimentally and clinically to improve pulmonary function by increasing arterial oxygenation. Fibreoptic bronchoscopy with lavage is effective at removing obstructing plugs of mucus.

Cardiovascular support

The hypermetabolism that accompanies the ICU patient results in a state whereby oxygen consumption is directly related to oxygen delivery. Under normal conditions, if oxygen delivery decreases, a compensatory mechanism arises to increase oxygen extraction from the blood by the tissues. However, in the hypermetabolic state, when tissue demand is greater, the limit at which there is maximum tissue extraction is exceeded, and oxygen delivery becomes supply dependent. The net result of this is that areas of underperfusion occur in parenchymal organs with consequent patchy necrosis and eventual failure. Oxygen delivery can be maintained by improving the cardiac output and oxygen saturation, and maintaining haemoglobin at 10–11 g/100 ml. Diagnosis of supply-dependent oxygen consumption is made by making serial measurements of oxygen consumption whilst increasing oxygen delivery. Cardiac output can be increased by ensuring enough fluids are given to maintain the preload, and then adding an inotropic agent such as dobutamine or adrenaline. Oxygen saturation should be maintained over 90% with a PaO_2 greater than 60 mmHg. The values to aim for in a high risk patient are: a cardiac index at or above 4.5 l/min/m², oxygen delivery at 600 ml/min/m² and oxygen consumption at 170 ml/min/m². Oxygen demand is reduced by assisting ventilation, preventing excessive feeding and treating elevations in temperature with rectal paracetamol and tepid sponging.

Hepato-enteric support

The gut mucosal barrier is appreciated by many as being contributary to the MOF syndrome by allowing the release of bacteria and endotoxin into the portal circulation. Once these have passed the hepatic reticuloendothelial system, generalized release into the systemic circulation occurs. Inflammatory mediators circulate and act on the gut to produce an ileus and leaking capillaries, which further encourage endotoxin and bacterial translocation, and so on. This cycle of events can be prevented by maintaining enterocyte mass, reducing the upper gastrointestinal microflora and maintaining the normal commensal lower intestinal microflora. Early enteral feeding with the addition of glutamine, the major respiratory fuel of intestinal enterocytes, provides intraluminal bulk and maintains enterocyte mass. The addition of specific nutrients and growth factors to encourage enterocyte proliferation further is still at an experimental stage. Gastrointestinal ileus is not a contraindication to enteral feeding since the stomach can be aspirated hourly before each feeding session. Coagulation factor deficiencies are corrected with vitamin K and FFP. Plasma oncotic pressure may be maintained with 20% albumen or hydroxyethylstarch (HESPAN) infusions.

Ulcer prophylaxis

H2 receptor antagonists and antacids, frequently used in the ICU, are administered to prevent stress-induced ulceration and bleeding. They also neutralize gastric pH, encourage upper gastrointestinal colonization and increase the incidence of nosocomial pneumonias in ventilated patients. Recent evidence suggests that stress ulcer prophylaxis is best achieved with sucralfate, which coats the gastric mucosa but does not effect its pH. In the same way, early enteral feeding may abolish the need for stress ulcer prophylaxis. Hypopharangeally applied non-absorbable antibiotics are an alternative way to reduce the incidence of nosocomial pneumonias.

Renal support

The commonest causes of renal failure in the ICU are prolonged periods of shock as part of the MOF syndrome or the uncontrolled administration of renotoxic drugs. As there is a direct relationship between renal bloodflow and renal failure, support is aimed at maintaining renal perfusion. This is achieved by optimizing oxygen delivery and administering low-dose dopamine (2–5 µg/kg/min), especially if inotropes are given which cause periods of renal vasoconstriction. Aminoglycoside levels should be actively monitored and other damaging substances, like myoglobin, removed. Oliguric renal failure has twice the mortality of polyuric renal failure. Frusemide, mannitol and dopamine are given in an attempt to encourage the conversion into polyuric failure. Established renal failure is treated with haemodialysis or, more recently, extracorporeal continuous arteriovenous haemofiltration (CAVHF) or continuous arteriovenous haemodialysis (CAVHD) which are not associated with the same cardiovascular instability as traditional dialysis. The eventual goal would be to develop a dialysis system which removes endotoxin and inflammatory mediators from the circulation.

Cutaneous support

Maintenance of skin care is of prime importance if the patient is immobile and ventilated. Prolonged sacral pressure (only 2 hours), malnutrition and urinary soiling will inevitably lead to an infected necrotic pressure sore which places a considerable physiological stress on a sick patient.

Regular turning (a trochanteric decubitis ulcer is preferable to a sacral ulcer), catheterization and adequate protein nutrition are minimum requirements in prevention.

Further reading

McCrory DC, Rowlands BJ. Septic shock syndrome and multiple system organ failure. *Current Practice in Surgery*, 1993; **5**: 211–15.

Related topics of interest

Multiple organ failure (p. 208)
Nutrition in the surgical patient (p. 213)

PANCREATIC CANCER

Carcinoma of the pancreas is a highly malignant growth of the acinar cells of the exocrine pancreas. It affects about 10/100 000 population, and the incidence is rising. Two males are affected for every female. It is rare before the age of 45, and thereafter the incidence rises progressively with age. Aetiological factors include smoking, which approximately doubles the risk, and possibly an elevated dietary fat intake and diabetes mellitus.

Pathology

Sixty per cent of pancreatic carcinomas occur in the head of the gland. Spread rapidly occurs to draining lymph nodes and local structures. The common bile duct is frequently invaded and obstructed, causing obstructive jaundice. The pancreatic duct is also invaded, and acute pancreatitis may result. Carcinomas of the head may spare the common bile duct but invade the duodenum and obstruct it, resulting in gastric outlet obstruction. Whether the common bile duct or duodenum is obstructed first, such is the rapid progression of the tumour that obstruction of the other frequently occurs.

Clinical examination

Thirty to sixty per cent of patients present with obstructive jaundice. Pain occurs in 50% and is usually felt in the back. This is usually indicative of a particularly poor prognosis, suggesting that the malignancy has eroded into posteriorly related prevertebral structures. Abdominal pain may, however, be the only presenting feature. Loss of weight is rapid and progressive, and occurs in 80% of cases. Less typical symptoms include: diarrhoea, general malaise, abdominal distension, nausea and vomiting. Trousseau's sign is migrating superficial thrombophlebitis (thrombophlebitis migrans) and this may occur in occult pancreatic carcinoma.

Clinical examination rarely identifies an abdominal mass. However, in the presence of painless jaundice, a palpable gall bladder suggests that the jaundice is not due to gallstones, but rather is due to to a malignant obstruction of the common bile duct, usually a pancreatic carcinoma (Courvoisier's law). Transcoelomic spread may occur, resulting in ascites, and spread to the liver may cause hepatomegaly, which may be easily palpable in an emaciated abdomen.

Investigations

- Ultrasound is used to confirm a dilated extrahepatic biliary tree, and may visualize a mass in the head of the pancreas.
- CT scanning should be performed to enable the size of the tumour to be assessed, along with the liver for

metastases, and spread to local structures that would affect the resectability of the tumour, such as the portal vein. Tumours in the body or tail of the pancreas can be confirmed by CT scanning.

- A histological diagnosis is essential to guide further management, as occasionally, chronic pancreatitis may present with obstructive jaundice or cause a localized pancreatic mass. Rarely, tumours in the pancreas may be benign. CT- or ultrasound-guided percutaneous fine needle aspirate or biopsy usually provides a diagnosis.
- ERCP may be used to obtain samples for cytology from the pancreatic or common bile duct.

Treatment

The aim of the above staging procedures is to assess the tumour with a view to resection, which is the only chance of cure. Tumours greater than 2 cm in diameter and those that have spread to the liver or lymphatics are not curable by surgery. The operation to resect a carcinoma of the pancreas is a radical Whipple's procedure for tumours in the the head or body, and distal pancreatectomy with splenectomy for tumours in the tail. If resection is not possible, or if the patient is unfit for major surgery, the prognosis is dismal. Frequently, despite adequate pre-operative investigations, a tumour is found to be unresectable only after an exploratory laparotomy with a trial of dissection of the pancreas. This may be due to invasion of vital local structures, or the presence of hitherto unknown lymphatic involvement. Ultimately, less than 10% of cases are amenable to surgical resection, and a cure may be achieved in less than 1%.

Prognosis

The mean survival after diagnosis is 6 months without resection, with only 10% of patients still alive at 1 year. Following resection, the 5 year survival is 4%, but there is a 10–20% operative mortality rate.

The prognosis is much better if the carcinoma is found to arise from the ampulla of Vater. This presents in an identical fashion to carcinoma of the head of the pancreas, and if treated conservatively has the same appalling prognosis, but if it is resected, the survival rate after 5 years is 15%.

Surgical palliation

Surgery has a role in the palliation of symptoms. Jaundice is relieved by means of a biliary bypass, best achieved using a loop cholecystojejunostomy or a choledochojejunostomy fashioned as a Roux-en-Y. As many patients later additionally develop duodenal obstruction, the stomach is bypassed prophylactically by means of an antecolic gastrojejunostomy. The afferent and efferent limbs of the loop of jejunum used in the biliary bypass may be anastomosed to avoid small bowel contents passing to the biliary tree.

Obstructive jaundice may also be satisfactorily relieved by stenting the malignant biliary stricture. This can be performed at ERCP, or as a radiological procedure using a percutaneous transhepatic route through dilated biliary radicles, gaining entry into the common bile duct from above. Stents offer excellent palliation in the short term, but may become blocked, and may migrate. They can, however, be replaced. The procedures used to place them are performed under local anaesthesia under sedation. They may be used as a temporary measure to relieve a patient of severe jaundice while surgery is planned. Transhepatic stenting offers an advantage in that an external biliary drain may be left *in situ* to decompress the biliary tree, and this may be useful should oedema occur at the stented site inhibiting free drainage, or as access for cholangiography or for further procedures.

Other pancreatic tumours

Tumours derived from endocrine cells and which are therefore active endocrinologically are insulinoma, glucagonoma, VIPoma (vasoactive intestinal polypeptide) and gastrinoma. Rarer tumours derived from exocrine portions are cystadenoma and its malignant form cystadenocarcinoma. Tumours of the ampulla of Vater are usually malignant, however, rarely, benign adenomyomas are encountered.

Insulinomas produce insulin and present with features of hyperinsulinaemia often referred to as Whipple's Triad. This comprises syncopal episodes during which there is proven hypoglycaemia, the episodes being reversed by the administration of glucose, and the reproduction of the same syncope by fasting. Though most insulinomas are benign, there is a malignant potential, and these tumours are best treated surgically. In some cases, a malignant insulinoma may already have metastasized at presentation, or possibly no tumour can be localized at all. Then surgery has little to offer, and medical treatment with diazoxide is started.

Glucagonomas are usually benign and present with diabetes mellitus and weight loss due to the overproduction of glucagon. They also produce a peculiar but typical circular erythematous truncal skin rash. Symptoms may be controlled with insulin. VIPomas produce vasoactive intestinal polypeptide, and present with profuse, watery diarrhoea. The inhibitory intestinal peptide somatostatin, or its synthetic analogue octreotide can be used to control the diarrhoea, or the tumour can be localized and resected. Gastrinomas present with recurrent peptic ulceration. Sixty per cent of these are malignant, and they are best resected. However, up to 30% of gastrinomas lie outside the pancreas, and localization may prove very difficult.

Further reading

Glazer G, Coulter C, Croyton ME. Controversial issues in the management of pancreatic cancer. *Annals of the Royal College of Surgeons*, 1995; **77**: 111–22, 174–80.

Rothmund M. Localization of endocrine pancreatic tumours. *British Journal of Surgery*, 1994; **81**: 164–6.

Watanapa P, Williamson RCN. Surgical palliation for pancreatic carcinoma. *British Journal of Surgery*, 1992; **79**: 8–20.

Related topic of interest

Jaundice – investigation (p. 189)

PENILE CONDITIONS AND SCROTAL SWELLINGS

Penile conditions

Phimosis

This condition is due to a narrow preputal meatus. It occurs in children when it presents with recurrent balanitis, ballooning on micturition, UTIs and smegma retention, and in adults when it is usually secondary to chronic balanitis. Occasionally, the opening in the foreskin can be like a pinhole causing urinary outflow obstruction. Foreskin fissuring and pain is common during intercourse.

Paraphimosis

This condition occurs when a tight foreskin is retracted behind the glans and causes progressive glandular engorgement. It may follow masturbation, intercourse or retraction during urination. A phimosis predisposes. Emergency treatment involves reduction by glandular pressure using the thumbs and by rolling the foreskin over the glans with the remaining fingers.

Balanitis xerotica obliterans (BXO)

This condition is equivalent to lichen sclerosis et atrophicus. It manifests as a chronic balanitis, often involving the urethral meatus, and is characteristically a fibrous plaque welding the foreskin to the glans.

Circumcision

The medical indications for circumcision are phimosis, paraphimosis, and chronic balanitis. Contraindications are hypospadias and other conditions where the foreskin can be used as a urinary conduit (urethral stricture). The procedure involves complete separation of the foreskin from the glans by division of all congenital or inflammatory adhesions to beyond the coronal sulcus. The foreskin is removed by direct dissection leaving an adequate cuff of 'mucosa'. All vessels are either ligated or cauterized with bipolar diathermy. There is no medical indication for neonatal circumcision, but it should be performed for religious reasons to prevent unsupervised circumcision 'at home'. A plastibell dome is placed between the separated glans and foreskin. A ligature is then tightened around the foreskin at its base. After 7–10 days, 'natural' separation occurs. Hydrocortisone cream or paraffin gauze are the best postoperative dressings because they reduce inflammation and they are less likely to fall off.

Carcinoma	Squamous cell carcinoma of the penis occurs in uncircumcised men with a poor standard of hygiene. Circumcised Jews rarely, if ever, develop the disease. Spread is direct, and to inguinal nodes. Presentation is often late since the lesions are hidden behind the foreskin. Treatment involves external beam radiotherapy with partial amputation of any recurrences. Occasionally, radical excision is indicated with complete genito-scrotal removal leaving a permanent perineal urostomy.
Erythroplasia of Queyrat	This presents as a deep red lesion over the whole surface of the glans. Histology reveals carcinoma-*in-situ*. Treatment with topical 5-fluorouracil is usually curative.
Penile warts	They are also known as condylomata lata, are due to infection with the HPV and are transmitted by sexual contact. Glandular or foreskin warts can be treated topically with 5-fluorouracil cream, podophyllin or scissor excision. Urethral warts and warts hidden within the navicular fossa require urethroscopic excision or diathermy.
Priapism	This condition is associated with sickle cell anaemia, leukaemia, spinal cord injury, dialysis patients and pelvic malignancy. Typically, the corpora cavernosa remain erect and the glans and corpus spongiosum remain flaccid. Initial detumescence therapy is achieved by aspirating the black blood directly from the shaft of each corpus cavernosum, via a trans-glandular approach, and by irrigating them with heparinized saline. Periodic inflation of a paediatric blood pressure cuff is also helpful. In resistant cases, a corpora-saphenous shunt using a mobilized portion of saphenous vein (still attached to the saphenofemoral junction) anastomosed directly to the base of the corpora is usually successful with a 50% incidence of retained potency. Constricting rings applied to the base of the penis in order to achieve erection can produce persistent tumescence progressing to strangulation unless the ring is removed.
Peyronie's disease	This condition is associated with retroperitoneal fibrosis, desmoid tumours, Dupuytren's contracture and Reidel's thyroiditis. It may also occur after an acute 'fracture' of the penis. A fibrous plaque is responsible for producing the dorsal or lateral curvature when erect making intercourse difficult. Diagnosis is established by palpation of the scarred corpora and by requesting that the patient provides a Polaroid snapshot of his problem. Surgical treatment involves producing an artificial erection with intracorporeal

saline injections and either excising the plaque or plicating the opposite side with reefing sutures (Nesbitt's operation).

Impotence

The cause is usually psychological, vascular or neurological. Excessive alcohol consumption, anxiety or diabetes often result in impotence and should be ascertained at any consultation. Early morning tumescence suggests a psychological cause. A full neurological assessment with bulbocavernous and cremasteric reflexes, and a full vascular assessment with penile Doppler pressures often localize the problem in difficult cases. Surgical procedures like pelvic dissection, abdominal aortic aneurysm repair, para-aortic node dissection and radical prostatectomy may lead to impotence and all patients undergoing such procedures should be forewarned of this complication. Intracorporeal papavarine or prostaglandin injections or inflatable prostheses are of benefit in a minority of patients.

Scrotal swellings

Hydrocoele

This is classified into four types which all involve abnormal fluid collections associated with the processus vaginalis or tunica vaginalis.

1. Vaginal hydrocoele. A fluid collection within the tunica vaginalis. It is the commonest type of hydrocoele. It can also occur secondary to a tumour, orchitis, torsion or after a hernia repair. Aspiration therapy is simple but associated with inevitable recurrence. Definitive surgical treatment involves several differing operations: hydrocoele excision, Jaboulay's operation of sac eversion, the bloodless operation of Lord which involves sac incision and plication, and Wilkinson's operation where the testis is placed outside the tunica. Meticulous haemostasis is mandatory after all scrotal operations to avoid haematoma formation.

2. Congenital hydrocoele. A patent processus vaginalis. This hydrocoele is often intermittent, and increases in size and turgor with increases in intra-abdominal pressure. It is really an inguinal hernia presenting in infancy or early childhood with only fluid filling the sac.

3. Infantile hydrocoele. The processus vaginalis is obliterated at the deep ring leaving a fluid collection in front of the testis and cord. It may be confused clinically with an incarcerated inguinal hernia.

4. *Hydrocoele of the cord*. A portion of the processus vaginalis has separated leaving a discrete fluid collection that is palpable along the cord. It is separate from the testis, one can get above it, and it descends with traction upon the testis.

Epididymal cysts

These are often multiple arising from the head of the epididymis. If they contain milky fluid they are termed spermatocoeles. A spermatocoele can also occur after a vasectomy. Large size or specific pain, arising from the offending cyst, is the indication for removal. Epididymectomy is occasionally required to prevent multiple recurrences.

Torsion

This condition peaks in incidence during the teens and is rare after 35 years of age when epididymitis becomes a commoner cause of scrotal pain. It is commoner on the right, in patients with incompletely descended testes, and it is due to a high investment of the tunica vaginalis which allows the testis to lie as a bell clapper. The type of torsion ('true' torsion) where the testis twists off the epididymis is rare. Patients present with sudden pain, often with similar previous episodes, and an extremely tender testicle. Colour duplex sonography can confirm the diagnosis if there are no flow signals detected from the testicular artery. Emergency exploration is required for all suspected torsions. A midline incision confirms the diagnosis and allows fixation of the opposite testis (orchidopexy). Testes of doubtful viability should be left *in situ*. Gangrenous testes are removed.

Varicocoele

This is a condition occurring around puberty and is caused by a dilatation of the pampiniform plexus of veins which surround the lower spermatic cord. Ninety-eight per cent occur on the left because of the anatomical drainage of the testicular vein into the left renal vein. The terminal venous valve of the left testicular vein is frequently absent, suggesting an aetiological factor. Presentation is with a scrotal mass which expands on standing or the val-salva manœuvre to give the appearance of a 'bag of worms'. They are associated with infertility and rarely a left renal cell carcinoma. Surgical treatment, if indicated, involves exposure of the testicular artery by the high retroperitoneal approach and ligation of its surrounding veins (Palomo operation). Selective testicular vein embolization is a radiological alternative to surgery.

Further reading

Paltrey E. The urethra and penis. In: Burnand KG, Young AE (eds) *The New Aird's Companion in Surgical Studies*. Edingburgh: Churchill Livingstone, 1992; 1333–52.

Whelan P. The scrotum, testes and epididymis. In: Burnand KG, Young AE (eds) *The New Aird's Companion in Surgical Studies*. Edingburgh: Churchill Livingstone, 1992; 1353–71.

Related topics of interest

PEPTIC ULCERATION

A peptic ulcer is the final morphological result of the interplay between the aggressive acid-peptic forces and the mucosal resistance to ulceration. Whilst acid attack is a marked feature of duodenal ulcer (DU), impaired mucosal resistance appears to be more important for gastric ulcer (GU). The discovery of *Helicobacter pylori* has dramatically changed the management of uncomplicated ulcer disease.

Duodenal ulcer

Epidemiology

DU disease has declined in prevalence because of improvements in living standards, the introduction of H2 antagonists and proton pump inhibitors, and effective therapy against *Helicobacter*. DUs are now occurring in a progressively older population. In 1977, H2 receptor antagonists became available and resulted in a dramatic change in the indications for operation such that whereas previously half of all operations performed for DU were done for pain, now over 98% are performed as an urgent intervention for complications: perforation, massive haemorrhage or obstruction. Mortality rates for emergency surgery have been static for 20 years despite an increase in the overall age of the patient at emergency operation. *H. pylori* infection is transmitted by close personal contact and is associated with low social class and poor living conditions.

Risk factors

Cigarette smoking, stress, NSAIDs, corticosteroids and infection with *H. pylori* are risk factors for DU development. NSAIDs deplete endogenous mucosal prostaglandin making the mucosa more susceptible to ulceration. Smoking impairs ulcer healing, accelerates gastric emptying, increases acid secretion and decreases pancreatic bicarbonate secretion. The exact mechanism by which *H. pylori* produces ulceration is not known. Over 90% of patients with a DU have this organism present. Most people with *H. pylori*, however, do not develop ulcers.

Physiology

Duodenal ulceration is associated with higher mean basal acid and maximal acid outputs often with reduced bicarbonate secretion by the duodenal mucosa. Gastric emptying is usually rapid and the total parietal cell mass is enlarged.

Medical treatment

Cessation of smoking and the intake of NSAIDs and alcohol, a change to a less stressful lifestyle, and a period of bed rest are general measures proven to be effective for healing ulcers. H2 antagonist therapy was considered equivalent to a proximal gastric vagotomy (parietal cell vagotomy, highly selective vagotomy), and it has virtually replaced the need for this operation. Omeprazole is a powerful inhibitor of acid secretion. It acts upon the proton pump causing almost complete acid suppression. Its introduction has rendered obsolete the need for operations against ulcer pain. It is now established beyond reasonable doubt that peptic ulceration is primarily due to *H. pylori* infection. Irradication of this organism with triple therapy (Tinidazole 500 mg b.d., Clarithromycin 250 mg b.d., Omeprazole 20 mg b.d.) heals the ulcer with rates better than those of H2 antagonists and considerably reduces recurrence.

Surgical treatment

In a patient with a resistant ulcer, who does not comply with medical advice or is dependent on NSAIDs a good argument can be made for a vagotomy as an additional procedure at the time of surgery for the complications of the disease.

1. Truncal vagotomy. This procedure results in extensive parasympathetic denervation of the gastrointestinal tract and may produce long-term problems such as gallstones and diarrhoea. A truncal vagotomy requires a gastric drainage procedure (gastroenterotomy or pyloroplasty) which in itself may promote bilious vomiting, chronic gastritis, stomal ulceration and an increased risk of gastric adenocarcinoma. Increased gastric emptying may also predispose to diarrhoea and the early (osmotic) and late (hypoglycaemic) dumping syndromes.

2. Selective vagotomy. This operation preserves the coeliac and hepatic branches. A drainage procedure is still required because the gastric nerves (anterior and posterior nerves of Latarjet) are divided.

3. Highly selective vagotomy. This procedure was performed for intractable pain and is now almost obsolete. It preserves the terminal branches of the gastric nerves which are relaxant to the pylorus, thereby avoiding the need for a drainage procedure. Care must be taken to ensure complete denervation of the lower 6 cm of the oesophagus because the nerves in this area are secromotor to the fundus (criminal nerves). The mortality from a highly selective vagotomy is low (0.1–0.3%) since there are no anastomoses which could leak. Performed in experienced hands ulcer recurrence rates can approach those with truncal vagotomy and drainage (5–15%) but complications are much fewer. Lesser curve necrosis following a highly selective vagotomy is rare and can be minimized by invaginating the lesser curve. Posterior truncal vagotomy with anterior seromyotomy is a simpler operation than, and reports equivalent results to, a highly selective vagotomy, and it avoids complete lesser curve devascularization. This operation can now be performed laparoscopically.

Complications

1. Perforation. Sudden onset of pain with peritonitis is the usual emergency presentation but these symptoms are masked in the elderly or patients on steroids or immunosuppressives. Subdiaphragmatic air is present on an erect chest radiograph in over 75% of patients. Maintenance of the upright position 10 min prior to taking the film further increases the detection rate of a perforation. A right lateral decubitus film or a water-soluble contrast swallow may also aid diagnosis. Management involves fluid resuscitation, antibiotics and surgery. Simple ulcer closure, omental patch placement and a thorough abdominal lavage is the commonest procedure. A partial gastrectomy is required if the ulcer is huge and closure would result in duodenal stenosis. Sixty-six per cent of ulcers persist or recur on long-term follow up indicating that further anti-ulcer therapy is required. Patients with a definitive aetiology (NSAIDs) or those not previously taking H2 antagonists should have appropriate postoperative anti-ulcer advice and therapy.

2. Obstruction. DUs may cause outlet obstruction by scarring, oedema or impaired gastric motility. Diagnosis of fixed scarring is difficult so initial management should involve H2 antagonist therapy and nasogastric decompression for 3–5 days to allow any oedema to settle. Failure to re-establish motility and the presentation of a severely malnourished patient are indications for surgery. A partial gastrectomy or gastroenterostomy is usually required.

3. Haemorrhage. This is discussed elsewhere (see Upper gastrointestinal haemorrhage, p. 313).

Gastric ulcer

Epidemiology

Gastric ulcers were commoner in young women before the 1970s and presented with perforation. Now they are relatively uncommon and present in the elderly with bleeding. The role of surgery is almost exclusively limited to the complications of the disease.

Risk factors

These include tobacco, alcohol, cocaine and *H. pylori* infection. Ten per cent of people taking NSAIDs have an acute gastric ulcer (H2 receptor antagonists should be taken concomitantly with NSAIDs). GUs frequently develop in degenerate and aged gastric mucosa. They are most frequently found near the incisura on the lesser curve in close approximation to an atherosclerotic left gastric artery. Pre-pyloric ulcers behave like DUs but are ineffectively treated by operations for DU. Differentiation from a malignant ulcer is essential. At endoscopy all such ulcers require four-quadrant biopsy. At surgery, if possible, the ulcer should be excised and appropriate anti-ulcer medication prescribed.

Complications

1. Perforation. All perforated GUs require operative intervention. Ulcer excision, or at least biopsy, is recommended with oversewing of the ulcer over an omental patch (Graham closure). The lesser sac should always be explored in patients where no site for peritonitis is discovered because posterior GUs can be missed. Excision or closure is frequently difficult with large ulcers and a partial gastrectomy may be necessary.

2. Obstruction. GUs obstruct by producing gastric atony. They also cause severe malnutrition, general ill health and anaemia. They are often large and heal slowly. Antrectomy with inclusion of the ulcer is the preferred operation for obstruction. Reconstruction is usually achieved with a Billroth II anastomosis.

3. Haemorrhage. This is discussed elsewhere (see Upper gastrointestinal haemorrhage, p. 313).

Further reading

Johnson AG. Management of peptic ulcer. *British Journal of Surgery,* 1994; **81**: 161–3.
Stabile BE, Passaro E. Surgery for duodenal and gastric ulcer disease. *Advances in Surgery,* 1993; **26**: 275–306.

Related topics of interest

PILONIDAL SINUS

Pilonidal disease (lit. nest of hair) is a persistant focus of sepsis, with granulation tissue and giant cells, due to the presence of unwanted hair. The breach in the dermis caused by the hair allows the influx of bacteria to deeper tissues. Males are predominantly affected (4:1) and the disease occurs from puberty to the age of 40. The natal cleft is the site mostly affected and the stereotypical person prone to the disease is depicted as an overweight, hirsute, dark-haired man with poor personal hygiene driving a jeep or lorry. Pilonidal sinuses can also occur in the umbilicus, the axilla, the pits of the anal canal and the interdigital clefts of barbers and sheep shearers. As well as buttock hair, head hair, non-autologous human hair and animal hair have been discovered within these sinuses.

Pathology

Sacrococcygeal pilonidal disease usually consists of one or more midline pits from which primary tracks lead into a cavity lined by granulation tissue. From this cavity a secondary tract may arise and erupt on to the surface away from the midline. The primary tract orifice is lined by cutaneous epithelium and may contain hair, but no hair follicles or sweat glands have been identified. The secondary tracks are lined with granulation tissue which spills on to the buttock surface.

Pathogenesis

The exact mechanism of hair entry into the pit and primary pit formation is unknown. There are two postulates.

1. Acquired theory. The pathogenesis probably involves direct penetration of healthy skin by hair. If a human capital hair is rolled between both palms it will travel progressively, root forward, which is analogous to a deep natal cleft contour subjected to repetitive buttock friction. Directly a broken or dried hair enters base first, the barbs on the hair shaft prevent it from being expelled. Hair occasionally enters tip first which is witnessed when a neighbouring hair follicle has its hair curving across with its tip buried into a pilonidal pit. Midline sweat gland or hair follicle orifices may enlarge from the shearing forces imposed upon them and form a primary pit.

2. Congenital theory. This postulates that sacrococcygeal cell rests, identified histologically, develop into pilonidal sinuses. It no longer holds much favour. Radical removal of all tissue overlying the sacrum in order to remove all embryonal remnants should not be regarded as essential to treatment. Pilonidal sinuses still occur within the flaps following a radical excision and a subsequent plastic rotation procedure.

Presentation

Clinical presentation is either with acute abscess formation or a chronic discharging sinus. The inguinal lymph nodes may be enlarged. In 7% of cases, the tract runs caudally, where it may present as perianal sepsis, or even communicate with the anal canal.

Management

There is no shortage of reports recommending the best treatment for pilonidal disease. Statistical results must be interpreted with caution since extensive disease usually demands more radical treatment and excludes patients from simple outpatient procedures. The ideal therapeutic aim is to achieve healing without risk of recurrence, avoid hospital admission and general anaesthesia, and minimize patient inconvenience and time off work.

1. General advice. This should be directed at weight reduction, improvement in personal hygiene and shaving the sacrococcygeal area, or by making use of depilatory creams.

2. Acute abscesses. These are formed from pre-existing pilonidal granulomas. They should be deroofed surgically. The risk of subsequent sinus formation is about 50% but early excision of the pit and primary tract at the time of drainage, or soon after, reduces the recurrence rate to 15%.

3. Outpatient therapy. Lord in 1965 recommended a local anaesthetic outpatient procedure which involved excision of the midline pits, removal of any discovered hairs and curretage of the tract with brushes or phenolization. This achieved over 90% success but involved frequent outpatient attendances and strict adherence to the aforementioned general advice.

4. Surgery. The two main surgical strategies for pilonidal sinus disease consist of either wide excision to include all infected tracts or simple laying open of all the tracts. Following wide excision, the wound can be left open to granulate or marsupialized by suturing the skin edges to the pre-sacral fascia. If the wound is closed, this can be achieved with a midline scar, an asymmetric scar or a rotation flap. The recurrence rates and healing times are tabulated below.

Operation	Recurrence (%)	Time to heal
Wide excision and midline closure	15	2 weeks
Wide excision and asymmetric closure	7	2 weeks
Wide excision and no closure	13	3 months
Wide excision and marsupialization	4	5 weeks
Laying open for tract drainage	10	6 weeks

Recurrence

Recurrence rates can be minimized with procedures that reduce buttock friction (excision procedures to flatten the natal cleft) and by displacing any scars away from the midline (asymmetrical primary closure). Care must be taken with primary closure techniques to ensure meticulous approximation of deep tissue layers so that any potential cavity is obliterated. Laying open of all the tracts can be a time-consuming method and involves a suitably wide excision to ensure adequate tract drainage.

Further reading

Allen-Mersh TG. Pilonidal sinus: finding the right track for treatment. *British Journal of Surgery*, 1990; **77**: 123–32.

Related topic of interest

Fistula-in-ano (p. 133)

PORTAL HYPERTENSION

Pathology

Chronic hepatic disease may lead to obstruction of the intrahepatic veins, raising the portal venous pressure above its usual limit of 10 mmHg. Common causes include alcoholic liver disease and chronic viral (B, C or D) hepatitis. Increased portal venous pressure results in the distension of existent, usually microscopic, portasystemic venous anastomoses. These occur at numerous sites, most importantly in the wall of the lower oesophagus where the left gastric (portal) and azygous (systemic) veins communicate. These become oesophageal varices, and they frequently cause life-threatening haemorrhage.

The severity of the causative hepatic disease is classified according to Child's classification, or its modification as proposed by Pugh, according to five parameters: serum bilirubin, albumin, the presence of ascites, encephalopathy and the nutritional state (Child) or prothrombin time (Pugh).

The patient is graded into one of three classes, A, B or C. These are commonly used in the assessment of prognosis, fitness for anaesthesia or requirement for surgery.

Clinical features

Portal hypertension may carry the stigmata of chronic liver disease, with clubbing of the nails, liver palms, spider naevi, ascites, peripheral (hypoproteinaemic) oedema, leuconychia, and wasting of the muscles, particularly if the cause is alcohol. An enlarged liver may be present, although the spleen is more likely to be enlarged. Cutaneous portasystemic anastomoses may be evident, such as the 'caput medusae' around the umbilicus (which is usually not completely circumferential), or around abdominal scars or stomas. Jaundice, liver flap and encephalopathy may be features of acute hepatic failure.

Variceal haemorrhage

Oesophageal varices bleed torrentially and result in 50% of deaths from gastrointestinal bleeding. Occasionally, gastric varices bleed. The diagnosis may be considered on the history of liver disease or alcohol abuse, or may be detected clinically through the above-mentioned signs. However, the diagnosis should be confirmed by gastroscopy, particularly as varices are best treated endoscopically in the first instance.

1. Endoscopic treatment. This involves the intravariceal injection of a vascular sclerosant, usually ethanolamine.

Alternative materials are cyanoacrylate glue or thrombin, which works best on bleeding gastric fundal varices. Repeated injections may be necessary, but cannot be repeated more than twice on successive days. Although the immediate success is of the order of 90%, recurrent bleeding is common, with about 40% of patients requiring emergency treatment in the future.

2. Drug treatment. If an emergency endoscopy service is not available, the patient may be treated with drugs. Intravenous vasopressin causes generalized and splanchnic vasoconstriction. Systemic vasoconstriction is less with terlipressin. Intravenous octreotide also reduces portal flow. Drug treatment is not as effective as variceal injection. Twenty-five per cent will require further treatment, and vasoconstrictors should be used is as a temporary measure whilst a patient is transferred to a specialist unit.

3. Balloon tamponade. Oesophageal intubation for balloon tamponade is more effective than medical treatment. This is achieved using a Sengstaken–Blakemore tube. This is a wide-bore tube with four external ports: two to allow inflation or deflation of oesophageal and gastric balloons, and two ports for oesophageal and gastric suction. The Minnesota tube is a similar device that lacks the oesophageal balloon. The tube is passed via the nose into the stomach and 300 ml of air is used to inflate the gastric balloon. The tube is withdrawn until the balloon impinges on the gastric cardia, and tension is kept on the tube to maintain pressure on the cardia. This effectively prohibits portal blood from filling the oesophageal varices. Inflation of the oesophageal balloon is not always required. Suction is necessary to prevent aspiration from the oesophagus, and absorption of an excessive protein load from gastric luminal blood which may precipitate encephalopathy.

4. Surgery. If conservative measures do not arrest haemorrhage, emergency oesophageal transection and gastric devascularization must be undertaken. Emergency portacaval bypass may help, but this is risky and may precipitate encephalopathy.

Long-term treatment of portal hypertension

1. Medical management. Spironolactone, the aldosterone antagonist potassium-sparing diuretic, may be prescribed to reduce ascites, which is at least in part due to secondary hyperaldosteronism in chronic liver disease. The beta-blocker propranolol may be given to reduce portal venous pressure. Alcohol is prohibited, whether or not the underlying cause is alcoholism.

2. Shunting of ascites. Gross and debilitating ascites may be shunted into the venous system by means of a peritoneal–jugular shunt. These tubular shunts are tunnelled subcutaneously from the peritoneal cavity to the internal jugular vein. Two devices are in common use, the LeVeen and Denver shunts, the former incorporating a one-way valve. These frequently become blocked by fibrinous deposits at their peritoneal end and their use in hepatic ascites is limited.

3. Repeated endoscopic sclerotherapy and banding. Oesophageal varices may be endoscopically banded. This is not as effective as injection sclerotherapy for bleeding varices, but may be a better elective treatment. Repeated treatments are usually necessary.

4. Portasystemic shunting. Many patients relapse following initial or repeated successful conservative management. Surgery may be effective in reducing portal venous pressure by means of a portocaval bypass. In those unfit for surgery, TIPS, as outlined below, may be of use. If the patient is fit for anaesthesia, a distal lienorenal shunt or a portacaval shunt may be performed. Rarely, portal hypertension may be due to thrombosis of the splenic vein, causing left-sided or sectorial portal hypertension. This may be treated by splenectomy.

5. Liver transplantation. The non-alcoholic patient with severe chronic liver disease may be suitable for hepatic transplantation, though this is not a therapeutic option in the emergency treatment of variceal haemorrhage.

Transjugular intrahepatic portasystemic anastomosis (TIPS)

Portal hypertension may be relieved by the formation of an intrahepatic anastomosis between branches of the hepatic and portal veins. This is performed under radiological control via the right internal jugular vein, and is known as transjugular intrahepatic portasystemic anastomosis (TIPS). A catheter is passed into and through the wall of a hepatic vein until a wire can be passed into a branch of the intrahepatic portal vein. The resultant fistulous tract is dilated and self-expanding vascular stents are positioned within the fistula to maintain patency. The procedure is complicated by shunt stenosis or thrombosis, and may precipitate encephalopathy. This may be a useful minimally invasive procedure to reduce portal venous pressure in the short term, mainly in those too unfit for portocaval bypass surgery, or in those awaiting hepatic transplantation. TIPS is being evaluated in acute variceal haemorrhage.

Further reading

Copeland G, Sheilds R. Portal hypertension and oesophageal varices. *Surgery*, 1991; **98**: 2342–7.

Jalan R, Redhead DN, Hayes PC. Transjugular intrahepatic portasystemic stent. *British Journal of Surgery*, 1995; **85**: 1158–64.

Related topics of interest

Jaundice – investigation (p. 189)
Upper gastrointestinal haemorrhage (p. 313)

POSTOPERATIVE CARE AND COMPLICATIONS

Care

Immediate

Immediately following surgery the patient is placed on the recovery ward in the theatre suite, where vital signs are measured by a specialist nurse with anaesthetists in close attendance. Problems arising as a direct consequence of the surgery will be evident, and the patient's proximity to the operating theatre makes immediate re-exploration feasible.

Ward care

Patients are monitored for adequate pain relief and the development of postoperative complications. Drainage from wound drains and nasogastric tubes needs to be monitored.

Pain relief

Adequate analgesia is necessary to allow patients to breathe deeply and cough without undue pain. Continuous analgesic regimens provide excellent pain relief. Low-dose opiates (usually morphine) may be continually infused through an epidural catheter or intravenously. Patient-controlled analgesia (PCA) is safe and effective but requires close surveillance. Opiates may also be infused continuously subcutaneously.

Blood tests

FBC and U&E should be requested on the morning following surgery. A fall in haemoglobin may require a blood transfusion. Electrolyte imbalances may be addressed by modifying the intravenous fluid regimen. A rising urea and creatinine may signify impending prerenal failure, and intravenous fluids may need to be increased.

Nasogastric tubes and drains

Nasogastric tubes may cause difficulty in breathing and are best removed at the earliest convenience. Occasionally, the stomach becomes atonic, and there is a copious nasogastric aspirate. If this occurs, the tube should be left in place on free drainage. Drains should be removed at the earliest opportunity, usually if drainage has been minimal for 2 days, and certainly when they cease to drain anything.

Intravenous fluid requirement

The normal daily intake is between 2.5 and 3.0 litres of fluid, with approximately 100 mmol sodium and 60 mmol potassium per day. The postoperative patient is not a normal situation, however. Fluid requirement may be less over the initial day, due to the metabolic response to trauma, however, there will have been fluid losses incurred during surgery. A standard intravenous regimen is thus 2 litres of 5% dextrose and 1 litre of 0.9% saline per day, each litre containing 20 mmol potassium. It is important to note excess fluid losses from drains, tubes, stomas or fistulae and replace these amounts with potassium supplemented 0.9% saline. Patients may rapidly become dehydrated with large nasogastric aspirates or high output fistulae or stomas.

Oral fluids and feeding

If a patient has a nasogastric tube, there is no harm in allowing sips of fluid. Following abdominal surgery, a safe rule is that if bowel sounds are present, oral fluids may be started. When patients have passed flatus or faeces, they may take a light diet.

Complications

These are early, intermediate and late. Late complications are specific to the condition being treated. These occur after some months have elapsed, and are considered during follow-up. Complications arising on the ward occur early (days) and intermediate (weeks) after surgery.

Pulmonary collapse

This is a common cause of an early postoperative pyrexia which disappears as the patient coughs up mucus which has been plugging a subsegmental bronchus. However, patients with poor respiratory function with major bronchial plugging may develop respiratory distress, and arterial blood gases must be performed. The patient is put on oxygen and a chest X-ray is requested. Treatment options include chest physiotherapy, bronchoscopy and suction, and, if there is respiratory failure, admission to the ICU for ventilation.

Chest infection

Minor infections are common in smokers or those with chronic lung disease, and are often the cause of a persistent postoperative pyrexia. The patient will be coughing sputum which should be sent for culture. A frank pneumonia is unusual but may cause respiratory failure necessitating intensive care. Infections usually occur in collapsed pulmonary segments, and postoperative chest physiotherapy does much to clear the airways and avoid infection.

Aspiration pneumonia

Gastric contents may be aspirated into the right lower lobe where it may cause a severe pneumonitis and consolidation. This is a potentially serious complication that usually arises on induction or recovery from anaesthesia. It may be avoided on the ward by nasogastric intubation in those with an ileus or gastric stasis. However, early removal of unnecessary nasogastric tubes may actually prevent aspiration by facilitating coughing.

Deep venous thrombosis

This causes a painful swollen leg. Clinically there is calf tenderness. If suspected, the patient should have ascending phebography. A duplex scan may be sufficient to diagnose femoral or popliteal thrombosis, but may miss calf thrombosis. The patient is heparinized, and this is monitored by daily activated partial thromboplastin times. Warfarin is started simultaneously, and the heparin is stopped as soon as the prothrombin time is under control. If the patient cannot be anticoagulated and has a proximal thrombosis, or if there is a large free iliofemoral thrombus, a caval filter may be necessary to prevent pulmonary embolism.

Pulmonary embolism

This is responsible for 3% of all hospital deaths, despite routine prophylaxis with anticoagulants. 2.5% of pulmonary emboli are fatal, and recurrent emboli occur in 30% if untreated. It may result in sudden death, or present with pleuritic chest pain, haemoptysis and shortness of breath. Signs include elevation of the jugular venous pulse, tachycardia, hypotension, a pleural rub, and hypoxia on blood gas estimation. There may be no signs of a deep venous thrombosis. This is treated on suspicion with full heparinization. Despite this, recurrent emboli occur in up to 10% of cases. Pulmonary embolism may be confirmed with ventilation/perfusion lung scanning. Major pulmonary emboli causing severe cardiorespiratory effects may require intensive care, pulmonary thrombectomy or thrombolysis.

Haemorrhage

Primary haemorrhage occurs at the time of surgery. Reactionary haemorrhage occurs within hours of surgery from vessels that initially constrict but later bleed, or as a result of a slipped ligature. Secondary haemorrhage usually results from localized infection, ulceration or malignancy causing erosion of a vessel wall. It occurs 1 or 2 weeks after surgery, and may be torrential and life-threatening.

Anastomotic leak

A gastrointestinal anastomosis may break down giving rise to serious complications. Factors that contribute to anastomotic leaks or dehiscence include ischaemia or tension of the bowel ends, or local contamination at the time the anastomosis was fashioned. The leak must be drained, and the bowel ends exteriorized if possible, or a proximal diverting stoma may be created.

Wound dehiscence

The oozing of haemoserous fluid from an abdominal wound is an ominous sign. This may occur at around 1 week, and it indicates that the wound is coming apart or dehiscing. Localized dehiscence may result in strangulation of a knuckle of bowel. Full length dehiscence may result in evisceration. These constitute surgical emergencies, and resuturing is mandatory.

Wound infection

This is common after contaminated operations. Up to 20% of all wounds may become infected. A persistent, postoperative pyrexia must prompt examination of the wound. Infecting organisms are often Gram negative following bowel surgery. Wounds from clean operations that become infected usually harbour staphylococci. Minor infections respond to antibiotics. Small superficial collections usually drain satisfactorily after removal of two or three sutures. If a wound abscess results, formal drainage is necessary, and the wound is left open to heal by secondary intention.

Cardiac

Myocardial infarction and left ventricular failure with acute pulmonary oedema may occur in the postoperative period. An ECG and chest X-ray must be performed on patients who have chest pain or become short of breath. Acute pulmonary oedema responds well to intravenous diuretics.

Acute renal failure

Hypovolaemia or hypotension results in reduced renal perfusion. The urinary output may fall below the accepted lower limit of the acceptable range, which is 30 ml/hour. This should initially be managed by administration of intravenous crystalloid fluid. If the patient is adequately hydrated and still producing insufficient urine, a bolus dose or continuous infusion of frusemide is given. If this state of prerenal failure and oliguria is allowed to continue, acute renal tubular necrosis will ensue. This will result in an aneuric phase which may last for 2 days, representing tubular necrosis. The urea and creatinine rise, and there will be a metabolic acidosis. Following this there is a phase of polyuria as the kidney recovers. Both these phases need to be treated by careful fluid management. If the urea fails to fall or approaches 35 mmol/l, or if there is hyperkalaemia, haemofiltration or dialysis may be indicated.

Acute retention of urine

This is common in men after abdominal or bilateral inguinal hernia surgery. There is usually a history of bladder outflow obstruction. Urethral or suprapubic catheterization is required. The patient is referred to the urologists for cystoscopy and a TURP. This may, rarely, occur in a woman. There may be an underlying urethral stenosis, or a neurological cause, possibly multiple sclerosis.

Psychiatric

Acute confusional states are common in the elderly or alcoholics. The diagnosis in the latter is likely to be acute alcohol withdrawal, and is treated with intravenous or oral chlormethiazole. Vitamin B complex should also be administered. In the elderly, confusion may signify an underlying infection, anaemia, hypoxia or metabolic derangement. It is highly non-specific, and the patient must be fully investigated.

Paralytic ileus

This represents atonic small intestine, and some degree is common after any abdominal operation. The small bowel usually recovers within 24 hours, but occasionally this is prolonged, and the term paralytic ileus then applies. The patient remains distended, and there will be few bowel sounds. Vomiting may occur. Electrolyte imbalance, particularly potassium, predisposes to this. It is managed by continued nasogastric suction if there is vomiting, correction of electrolyte disturbances, and prohibition of oral intake.

Gastric stasis

The stomach may become atonic after abdominal surgery, and may take days to recover its function. This may require nasogastric suction, and prohibition of fluids. Acute gastric dilatation, which probably simply represents extreme gastric stasis, carries a high risk of aspiration and mortality. It may occur following any abdominal surgical procedure, causing discomfort, effortless vomiting, hiccoughs, and abdominal bloating. It is remedied by insertion of a wide nasogastric tube. Contributory electrolyte imbalances, particularly hypokalaemia, must be corrected.

Further reading

Smith JAR. *Complications of Surgery in General.* Oxford: Ballière Tindall, 1984.

Related topics of interest

Blood transfusion (p. 55)
Fluid replacement (p. 136)
Postoperative pain relief (p. 252)

POSTOPERATIVE PAIN RELIEF

Postoperative pain is generally inadequately recognized, inadequately monitored and inadequately treated. The introduction of minimally invasive surgery as a substitute for open surgery has resulted in a major decrease in the amount of postoperative pain and consequent prolonged admission for pain control. The establishment of an 'acute pain team' of trained clinicians may be an effective measure to minimize postoperative surgical pain.

Consequences of pain

Postoperative pain increases morbidity and mortality, delays mobilization and prolongs hospital stay. After thoracic or upper abdominal surgery, deep breathing and coughing are inhibited, functional residual capacity decreases and small airways close. Sputum retention leads to resorption collapse of alveoli (atelectasis) especially in dependent lung regions. Myocardial ischaemia in patients with ischaemic heart disease is increased in the presence of pain. Pain also increases the metabolic rate and oxygen demand.

Consequences of pain relief

Postoperative pain relief too has its problems. Opioids, such as morphine, decrease tidal volume and rate ventilation, and make breathing irregular. Carbon dioxide retention is encouraged with an increase in the number and severity of episodes of sleep apnoea. Morphine intoxication should be considered in any drowsy or unresponsive patient following major abdominal surgery. Treatment with 0.1 mg of Naloxone is rapid and effective but may need to be repeated since its half-life is much shorter than most opioids. Opioids suppress rapid eye movement sleep and encourage nausea with vomiting. Subsequent aspiration may be fatal. All patients should avoid smoking the week leading to surgery to improve baseline respiratory function. The pre-admission clinic is an ideal time to give this advice.

Advances

The main advances in postoperative pain relief have been the increased appreciation of patient-controlled analgesia and the administration of spinally applied opioids. The concepts of pre-emptive analgesia and psychoprophylaxis are now widely accepted and should be frequently applied.

1. Patient-controlled analgesia. Differing individual analgesic requirements at different times for different operations led to the development of patient-controlled analgesia (PCA). Two thirds of patients wait until severe pain develops before requesting analgesia and one third of nurses will not administer analgesics until a request is made by the patient. Once the patient is in control of the pain, anxiety is reduced and pain tolerance is increased. The system requires a rapid response if the patient is to feel in control of the pain. Directly a bolus of analgesia is delivered a 'lock-out' interval ensues to ensure the drug is appreciated before further demands are met. The usual regime is an intravenous 1 mg morphine bolus with a lock-out interval of 5 min. Before taking sole control of the intravenous or epidural delivery of analgesia the patient should be comfortable and told to titrate the drug to a level of tolerable discomfort rather than to total analgesia.

2. Spinally applied opiates. These can be given by the epidural or subarachnoid route, and produce a very effective and prolonged analgesia by acting upon the rich concentration of opiate receptors clustered in the dorsal horn of the spinal cord. Morphine is the most widely used drug. It is relatively lipid insoluble, being distributed in the CSF rather than to the cord, which is unfortunate because its effects are subjected to CSF movements. Any sudden change in position or straining can thereby induce respiratory depression. Consequently, such patients should be monitored with apnoea detectors and pulse oximetry in a high dependency area. The risk is further reduced by delivery with a slow infusion into the lumbar, rather than the thoracic, spine using a large volume of solvent. The combination of local anaesthetic and opioid enhances the effect and duration of both agents. Hypotension, urinary retention and leg weakness are the other main drawbacks of its use.

3. Pre-emptive analgesia. Pre-emptive treatment of pain with opiates reduces pain for much longer than the expected action of the drug. This is achieved by inhibition of the increase in sensitivity at the post-synaptic spinal cord neurone which painful stimuli produce. Phantom limb pain can be eliminated in this way by ensuring a pain-free interval prior to amputation. Local anaesthetics prolong the the pre-emptive effects of opiates. NSAIDS also reduce the need for opiates. They are particularly useful in day case surgery and are often given as a suppository at the conclusion of an operation.

4. Psychoprophylaxis. The ability to cope with pain depends upon individual personality, the perceived support from relatives, the level of distraction, the individual pain threshold and fear of the unknown. A pre-operative anaesthetic visit and an explanation of the surgical procedure both reduce anxiety, although a concise explanation is just as effective as a detailed explanation. Benzodiazepines, given as premedication, help to alleviate anxiety.

Local anaesthesia

Wound infiltration by local anaesthetic at the end of an operation successfully reduces the opiate requirements for most operations including inguinal herniorrhaphy and open cholecystectomy. Topical lignocaine gel can be applied to mucous membranes, split skin grafts or to the suture line following a circumcision. Local anaesthetic application by intercostal, paravertebral, rectus sheath, brachial or femoral cannulation alongside the appropriate nerve can provide long-lasting postoperative pain relief.

Further reading

Alexander JI. Post operative pain control. *Recent Advances in Surgery*, 1993; **16**: 1–19.
Justins DM. Anaesthesia and pain control. In: Burnand KG, Young AE (eds) *The New Aird's Companion in Surgical Studies*. Edinburgh: Churchill Livingstone, 1992; 221–42.

Related topics of interest

PRE-OPERATIVE ASSESSMENT

Clinical examination

A full current and past medical history will alert the houseman to possible problems that may need special attention, particularly for the anaesthetist (respiratory or cardiac disorders, glaucoma, epilepsy, cervical arthritis, drug sensitivity), but also for the surgeon (previous surgery) and for the postoperative period (past venous thromboembolism, prostatism, diabetes). The examination should be geared to assessing disorders picked up on the history, but also to detecting unknown disease, for example in the cardiovascular system, hypertension, cardiac murmurs, cardiac failure, arrhythmias, peripheral vascular disease.

Anaesthetic assessment

This will be performed by the anaesthetist, who should have been alerted to potential problems. The patient's fitness for anaesthesia is assessed and graded according to the American Society of Anethesiology (ASA) scale of 1 to 5. ASA 1 amounts to a fit and healthy individual, and ASA 5 is a moribund patient who is not expected to survive and is undergoing surgery as a last resort.

Blood tests

FBC and estimation of U&E is recommended in all patients. The haemoglobin and potassium levels are important considerations for the anaesthetic, and all the results will provide a baseline should postoperative problems occur. Severely unwell patients with metabolic complications should have arterial blood gases performed, as acidosis reduces cardiac function, and co-existing hyperkalaemia can cause arrhythmias. Patients from the West Indies and Africa must have a sickle-cell screen. Patients undergoing major bowel or arterial operations will need blood cross-matched according to the surgeon's requirement. It is prudent if serum is sent for a group-and-save from all patients having major surgery.

Cardiac

For anaesthetic purposes, an ECG is usually requisite in all patients over the age of 50. If patients are currently symptomatic, either with angina or heart failure, or if they have a history of severe cardiac illness, then the opinion of a cardiologist should be sought prior to a general anaesthetic as measurement of the left ventricular contractility or ejection fraction or an excercise ECG may be indicated. If hitherto unknown murmurs or arrhythmias are detected pre-operatively, these must be investigated first. Patients at risk of bacterial endocarditis should receive prophylactic antibiotics.

Pulmonary	Patients with current symptoms or signs, or a history of chest disease, and the elderly should have a routine pre-operative chest X-ray. Those with chronic airways disease must have simple spirometry and peak flow velocities measured as part of their work-up, and nebulized bronchodilators should be prescribed perioperatively. For surgery involving the thorax, including oesophageal or pulmonary resections, formal pulmonary function tests should be performed.
Nutritional	Chronically debilitating disorders, for example, in the gastrointestinal tract ulcerative colitis, high output gastrointestinal fistula, or gastro-oesophageal malignancies, result in hypoproteinaemia and electrolyte imbalances. These must be assessed by serum albumin, transferrin, haemoglobin and electrolytes, and potential problems must be addressed pre-operatively. Supplemental enteric or parenteral feeding may be required. Unfortunately, nutritional status is often only considered after its ill effects have become evident with cachexia, gross hypoproteinaemic oedema or poor healing.
Risk of venous thromboembolism	Factors with an increased risk of DVT include advanced age, obesity, cardiac failure, trauma, previous episodes of venous thromboembolism, malignant disease, and major abdominal or pelvic surgery. The last three constitute particularly high risks. Patients may be graded according to their risk of DVT. Patients with no risk factors having minor surgery with early ambulation may not require prophylactic anticoagulation, but ought to wear compression stockings perioperatively. However, all other patients should have prophylactic anticoagulation with either twice daily 5000 units of heparin or once daily low molecular weight heparin subcutaneously. Consideration for full anticoagulation or prophylactic caval filtration should be given to those at very high risk.
Patients on steroids	Long treatment with steroids necessitates intravenous hydrocortisone 100 mg qds to avoid an Addisonian crisis from adrenal suppression.
Day-case surgery	Patients for minor surgery under local anaesthetic need not be screened. Patients for general anaesthesia, and those for intermediate procedures under local anaesthesia, will need to be screened for medical conditions and social factors that are contraindications to day-case surgery. Initial screening must take place in the outpatient clinic. Clearly those with a

history of ischaemic heart disease or chronic lung disease or other medical conditions that may cause intra- or immediate postoperative complications will be unsuitable. Social considerations are also very important. Patients living alone, the elderly or those without a GP may not be suitable.

Further more detailed screening is performed in a pre-admission outpatient clinic. This is best undertaken by the trained nursing staff of the day-case unit who will screen the patient's hospital records (if any), and take a history and perform a clinical appraisal according to a clerking pro forma. Absolute and relative contraindications to day case surgery will become evident, these having been previously agreed by the anaesthetists responsible for the day case list.

Further reading

Cuschieri A. Preoperative, operative and postoperative cares. In: Cuschieri A, Giles GR, Moosa AR (eds) *Essential Surgical Practice*. London: Wright, 1988.
Powell M. Cardiopulmonary assessment of the surgical patient. *Surgery*, 1993; **11**: 361–7.
Reilly CS. Cardiac risk and its relevance to the preoperative assessment. *Surgery*, 1991; **97**: 2308–10.

Related topic of interest

Day case surgery (p. 114)

RENAL TUMOURS

Conditions which may give rise to a renal mass are listed below.

Benign	Malignant
Simple cyst, multiple cysts	Renal cell carcinoma
Polycystic kidney	Transitional cell carcinoma
Tubular ectasia	Squamous cell carcinoma
Dermoid	Nephroblastoma
Lipoma, angioma, leiomyoma	Sarcoma
Angiomyolipomata	Metastatic (lung, breast)
Tuberculosis	

Renal cell carcinoma

Renal cell carcinoma (clear cell, hypernephroma, Grawitz, adenocarcinoma) arises from the epithelial cells of the proximal convoluted tubule and is the commonest adult renal neoplasm. It is over twice as common in men and peaks in incidence between the 6th and 8th decade.

Risk factors   Polycystic kidneys and acquired cystic disease (common in patients on dialysis) both lead to an increased incidence. A familial tendency is present in the von Hippel-Lindau syndrome (cerebellar and retinal angiomas). Cigarette smoking and coffee drinking are associated with an increased risk.

Pathology   The tumours are characteristically yellow and demonstrate a clear cell pattern on microscopy due to the cholesterol- and lipid-rich cytoplasm. Venous microinvasion is commonly demonstrated.

Presentation   Classical presentation is with loin pain, haematuria and a palpable mass but this triad occurs in only 10% of patients. Loin pain is attributed to intratumour haemorrhage or 'clot colic'. Weight loss, fever and night sweats are usual accompaniments. Many earlier symptomless tumours are now detected due to improved imaging techniques. Other associated features include the sudden development of a varicocoele, caval obstruction and various hormonal and metabolic manifestations, as listed below:

1. Hypertension. Juxtaglomerular tumours often secrete renin.

2. *Hypercalcaemia.* This is due to the secretion of a parathyroid-like hormone.

3. *Erythrocytosis.* This is due to the secretion of an erythropoietin-like hormone.

4. *Hyponatraemia or a nephrotic syndrome.*

Investigations usually commence with an IVU, a chest radiograph, a renal ultrasound and a CT scan. MRI and PET scanning, if available, add diagnostic detail.

1. Intravenous urography. This may demonstrate the presence of a cortical mass, splaying of the calyces and a normal functioning kidney on the contralateral side.

2. Ultrasonography. This differentiates a cyst from a solid mass and can accurately establish the presence or absence of a tumour or thrombus within the vena cava in approximately 80% of cases. If the upper limit of the tumour extends above the diaphragm an echocardiogram is mandatory. Right atrial encroachment requires consultation with a cardiac surgeon so that bypass facilities can be used if resection is indicated.

3. Contrast CT. This may detect evidence of local invasion and caval involvement.

4. Chest radiograph. Metastatic spread can be detected by a chest X-ray or thoracic CT.

5. Bone scan. This can identify the occasional bone deposit.

6. Fine needle biopsy. This causes needle tract seeding, is seldom necessary, and is contraindicated if a phaeochromocytoma is suspected.

7. Selective arteriography. In the past, this was a commonly used investigation, often combined with renal artery embolization. This is rarely used now because the tumour readily develops an excellent collateral supply from adjacent tissues and the absence of renal artery pulsation can make pedicle location difficult at operation.

Prognosis

The main prognostic indicators include tumour stage and size. The Robson stage classification of the extent of local growth and distant spread is tabulated below.

Stage	Description
I	Confined within the capsule
II	Into perirenal fat (Gerota fascia intact)
III	Into renal vein (± perinephric/lymph node involvement)
IV(A)	Adjacent organ involvement (excluding adrenal)
IV(B)	Distant metastasis

Surgery

Tumours less than 3 cm long, which do not involve lymph nodes or adjacent organs, have a greater than 50% 5-year survival.

A radical nephrectomy is indicated for cure and for palliation. This involves removal of the perinephric fat, Gerota's fascia and the lymph nodes around the renal pedicle. The transverse, transperitoneal approach provides good access to the IVC and allows inspection of the opposite kidney. The thoraco-abdominal approach or the 12th rib bed approach is favoured by others. If extensive tumour thrombus is present in the IVC, cardiac bypass is required for its removal. Sudden isolation of a very vascular tumour can cause profound hypertension and heart failure. Gradual clamping and the use of peripheral vasodilators help to avoid this complication.

Advanced disease

Metastases are usually of the cannonball variety, solitary and large, and can occur in the bones, brain and lungs. Palliative removal of the primary tumour has frequently been reported to cause regression of these metastases. Medroxyprogesterone acetate is occasionally given to palliate advanced disease. Radiotherapy and chemotherapy have little to offer in improving survival, but the former can be useful to treat painful bony metastases.

Transitional cell carcinoma

Solid or papillary urothelial tumours can occur in the renal pelvis. They are 20 times less common than the bladder lesion. They are treated with a radical nephroureterectomy because recurrence can occur within the ureteric stump. Regular cystoscopic review is essential for follow up since around half will develop bladder recurrences.

Squamous cell carcinoma

Squamous cell carcinoma of the renal pelvis is rare. It is almost invariably associated with calculus disease and the prognosis is poor.

Other

Nephroblastoma

Nephroblastoma (Wilms' tumour), neuroblastoma and lymphoma are the commonest solid childhood malignancies (two thirds of childhood malignancies are solid). Wilms' tumours account for 12%, 5–10% occur bilaterally and most occur under 3 years. They are associated with other congenital abnormalities such as hypospadias and body hemi-hypertrophy. Clinical features include the finding of a large mass occupying the abdomen, weight loss and pyrexia. Differential diagnosis is usually from a retroperitoneal neuroblastoma. Bony deposits, haematuria and tumour lateralization favour a Wilms' tumour. Treatment should take place in a specialist centre and involves a radical nephrectomy, radiotherapy to the tumour bed and adjuvant chemotherapy. Over 80% can be cured in this way.

Angiomyolipomata

These are benign, frequently multiple and bilateral, and in 50% of cases are associated with tuberous sclerosis. They contain fat which allows a confident diagnosis to be made on CT scanning. Angiographic appearances are characteristic.

Further reading

Cumming J. Renal cell carcinoma. *Recent Advances in Surgery*, 1992; **15**: 137–51.
Tolley DA. The kidney and ureter. In: Burnand KG, Young AE (eds) *The New Aird's Companion in Surgical Studies*, Edinburgh: Churchill Livingstone, 1992; 1233–85.

Related topic of interest

Carcinoma of the bladder (p. 71)

RENOVASCULAR SURGERY

Renal artery stenosis is the most important renal vascular disorder that is amenable to surgical correction. Other rarer disorders include renal artery aneurysm, congenital arterial anomalies, and acute renal artery occlusion.

Renal artery stenosis

1. Pathology. Seventy per cent of cases are due to atherosclerosis and 30% to fibromuscular hyperplasia. Stenosis of a single renal artery can result in hypertension from stimulation of the renin–angiotensin system of that kidney. Angiotensin is a very potent systemic hypertensive hormone. As a result of the stenosis, the function of the affected kidney reduces and the kidney becomes smaller. If both renal arteries are involved, then hypertension certainly ensues, as does progressive renal failure.

2. Clinical indications. Systemic hypertension, often of sudden onset, is the most significant result of renal artery stenosis causing typical symptoms such as headache and epistaxis. Young males are most often affected. If symptoms of hypertension should start at an early age, or be particularly difficult to control with standard antihypertensive drugs, then renal artery stenosis should be considered. Approximately 2–5% of hypertensives have some degree of renal artery disease, but whether this is cause or effect is difficult to prove.

Renal artery stenosis is one of the rare but readily identified and treated causes of hypertension, along with, for example, coarctation of the aorta and phaeochromocytoma. Many other causes of chronic renal failure also result in hypertension, but these are rarely treatable surgically.

3. Diagnosis. The changes seen on an intravenous urogram are typical if one side only is affected. The kidney appears smaller, and there is delayed excretion of contrast compared to the normal side. Similar changes are seen on isotope renography. Intravenous digital subtraction arteriography may identify renal artery stenosis; however, this requires a large bolus of intravenous contrast which is nephrotoxic and may precipitate acute renal failure if both kidneys are involved and there is established renal impairment. Selective arteriography utilizes less contrast, and provides better quality films, although it requires a direct arterial puncture. The assessment of renal vein renin levels after selective catheterization is an alternative means of establishing diagnosis if doubt remains after the above tests.

4. Surgical procedures. In the elderly, medical treatment for hypertension is the optimal treatment. Surgery is best reserved for middle-aged or younger patients. The two main options are percutaneous transluminal angioplasty (PTLA) or surgical endarterectomy or bypass. The choice is usually governed by the aetiology of the stenosis, whether angioplasty has already been performed, and the length of the stenosis.

Most stenoses are short. Those caused by fibromuscular hyperplasia are usually treated by PTLA. Atheromatous stenoses are better treated with surgery than PTLA. However, if the lesion is in the main segment of the renal artery, then angioplasty is the best option, with an initial success rate of about 90%. If the stenosis is at the aortic ostium, then surgical bypass using autologous vein or a short polytetrafluoroethyolene graft from the aorta to the post-stenotic portion of the renal artery is performed.

These procedures will reduce systemic blood pressure but will not result in the recovery of lost renal function. Generally, results for both first-time PTLA and bypass are better for fibromuscular hyperplasia than for atheromatous stenoses. However, about half the patients having PTLA will need further treatment within two years. The benefit of PTLA over surgery is that it is far easier to repeat should this be required.

Other surgical options include vein patching or endarterectomy, or both as a combined procedure. A very long stenosis from the aortic ostium to the renal hilum may require a nephrectomy, with extensive patching of the stenotic segment of the renal artery with reimplantation on the iliac artery.

Other renal vascular disease

Renal artery aneurysms are rare. They are usually small and saccular, are more commonly seen in association with hypertension, and occur at bifurcations in the artery. The aetiology of these is usually atherosclerosis or medial necrosis. They are usually found by chance on an arteriogram performed for another reason, and they are best left alone as they rarely rupture.

Acute renal artery occlusion is rare but is an occasional cause of flank pain of sudden onset. Sudden occlusion of the renal artery is usually embolic, and a source for the embolism should be sought. This is not amenable to surgery.

Congenital renal vascular anomalies are common, but rarely important. They are usually arterial, and comprise aberrant polar arteries. These are only important when encountered during operations on the kidney, or when identified on arteriograms.

Further reading

Bredenberg CE, Sampson LN, Ray FS *et al.* Changing patterns in surgery for chronic renal artery occlusive diseases. *Journal of Vascular Surgery*, 1992; **15**: 1018–24.

Hansen KJ, Starr SM, Sands RE *et al.* Contemporary surgical management of renovascular disease. *Journal of Vascular Surgery*, 1992; **16**: 319–31.

SALIVARY GLAND CALCULI

Submandibular calculi are far commoner than parotid calculi. Various reasons postulated for this include: the uphill course of the submandibular duct, a higher mucous:serous acinar ratio resulting in thicker secretions and a larger duct diameter so that by the time the calculous obstructs it is more likely to be detected radiologically.

Anatomy

The submandibular duct (Wharton's duct) opens on one to three papillae on the floor of the mouth beside the frenum of the tongue. The parotid duct (Stenson's duct) opens on a papilla opposite the upper second molar tooth. Both ducts are 5 cm long. The calculi have a composition identical to that of dental tartar. They often occur in patients with good oral hygiene.

Submandibular calculi

Submandibular calculi are usually oval in shape and can be situated in a ductal, hilar or intraglandular location.

Diagnosis

They can occur at any age, though rare in infancy, and present with severe, sudden onset submandibular pain, lasting minutes to hours, which is precipitated by chewing food. Examination may reveal a tender gland and a stone may be felt by bimanual palpation of the gland and the floor of the mouth. Occasionally, pressure on the gland causes a foul taste to occur in the mouth and pus to appear from the duct orifice. In rare instances, several spherical secondary calculi may develop distal to an obstructed duct. Calculi can be demonstrated radiographically by a posterior oblique occlusal or submental view. The radiographic plate is held between the teeth and the X-rays are directed from underneath the lower jaw.

Ductal calculi

Ductal calculi are removed from the floor of the mouth. Under a general anaesthetic the tongue is distracted to the opposite side. A stay suture is placed around the duct proximal to the stone to prevent backward displacement. A longitudinal incision is made over the calculus which is teased away from the duct. The rent is not sutured because of the fear that a stricture may result.

Submandibular gland excision

Excision of the gland is indicated for hilar calculi and in the symptomatic patient with intraglandular disease. Care should be taken to avoid the mandibular branch of the VII nerve by placement of the incision two finger breadths below the mandible. Dissection should proceed close to the gland at all times to avoid injury to the hypoglossal and lingual nerves. The facial artery and vein are usually divided because they are intimately associated with the gland. The superficial part of the gland is then followed around the posterior border of the mylohyoid to the deep part. Both are removed with a length of duct leaving a short stump to drain into the mouth.

Parotid calculi

Parotid calculi are situated within the gland or duct. They are rare under 30 years and occur more frequently with increasing age. They can arise secondary to autoimmune gland damage from rheumatoid arthritis or Sjögren's syndrome. Over 70% of cases of recurrent unilateral parotiditis are due to calculi.

Diagnosis

Presentation is with sudden-onset pain occurring during chewing, lasting a few hours or days, and ceasing as abruptly as it arose often with a foul-tasting fluid gush into the mouth. Examination may reveal a global swelling in the parotid region with an oedematous and pouting papilla at the orifice to Stenson's duct. Massage of the gland or the introduction of lemon juice into the mouth may precipitate the pain or encourage a foul duct discharge. Occasionally, a palpable stone may be felt intra-orally along the duct. An anterior–posterior radiograph or an intrabuccal coned view, with the mouth held open, may reveal the offending stone. Parotid sialograms are often more helpful in the diagnosis of parotid calculous disease because stones are less often demonstrated with plain X-rays in this situation. Aqueous contrast medium (0.5 ml) is injected directly into the duct. Filling defects, a complete block or areas of stricture and distension may be revealed.

Duct disease

A stenosed ductal meatus can be caused by ill-fitting dentures, irritation from a sharp tooth or a careless bite. Treatment methods include a papilloplasty or direct duct repair using a sleeve of incorporated cheek mucosa. As with submandibular calculi, parotid stones may ulcerate through the duct and cause a salivary fistula. The majority of these require no specific treatment unless an area of stenosis results. Simple strictures may be excised or, alternatively the duct may be re-implanted at a more proximal level.

Superficial parotidectomy

Intraglandular calculi are treated with a formal superficial parotidectomy if they are symptomatic or there is evidence of damage from chronic infection. Histological features of chronic sialadenitis include acinar atrophy, periductal fibrosis and infiltration by masses of chronic inflammatory cells.

Further reading

Hobsley M. The salivary glands. In: Burnand KG, Young AE (eds) *The New Aird's Companion in Surgical Studies*. Edinburgh: Churchill Livingstone, 1992; 469–87.

Related topic of interest

Salivary gland tumours (p. 268)

SALIVARY GLAND TUMOURS

Approximately 80% of parotid gland tumours, 60% of submandibular tumours and 40% of sublingual salivary tumours are benign. Twenty per cent of malignant tumours have lymph node metastasis at the time of presentation. All these tumours have a characteristic capacity for local recurrence.

Classification

Classification into benign, low-grade, high-grade and non-salivary tumours is convenient for prognostic purposes.

Benign	Pleomorphic adenoma
	Adenolymphoma
Low-grade	Mucoepidermoid
	Acinic cell
High-grade	Adenoid cystic carcinoma (cylindroma)
	Adenocarcinoma
	Epidermoid carcinoma
	Undifferentiated carcinoma
	Carcinoma in a pleomorphic adenoma
Non-salivary	Lymphoma (parotid only)
	Metastatic deposit (lung, breast, kidney)
	Lipoma, neurofibroma, haemangioma

Pleomorphic adenoma

This tumour is a slow-growing lesion which enlarges over a period of many years. It is commoner in women and peaks in incidence at the 5th decade. The tumour surface exhibits many bulbar protrusions which abut on to the capsule causing its thinning and, in some places, complete capsular disruption with penetration into the surrounding normal salivary gland. Histology reveals many adenomatous areas within a mucoid or myxoid stroma that resembles cartilage. Three per cent undergo malignant change.

Adenolymphoma

The adenolymphoma or Warthin's tumour is the commonest of the monomorphic adenomas. It only occurs in the parotid gland because none of the other salivary glands contain lymphoid tissue. After complete excision there is little tendency to implantation recurrence but 5–10% of these tumours are multifocal or bilateral. Histology reveals a two-layered, eosinophilic staining epithelium. An inner columnar layer and an outer cuboidal layer line many cystic spaces which are rich in lymphoid stroma.

Mucoepidermoid

These tumours are the commonest parotid malignancies. Histologically, many serous secreting goblet cells are identified amongst sheets of epidermoid cells. Most grow slowly. Occasionally, aggressive behaviour occurs with metastasis to regional nodes. Seventy-five per cent of patients survive 5 years.

Acinic cell

These tumours arise from serous secreting acini and almost all are found in the parotid gland. They are rare, slow growing but may metastasize unexpectedly. Three per cent are multifocal. Seventy-five per cent of patients survive 5 years.

Carcinomas

The adenoid cystic carcinoma or cylindroma characteristically grows slowly and relentlessly. It invades perineural lymphatics and travels along periosteum for long distances. Invasion into the base of the skull is a common mechanism of death. Histology reveals sheets of ductal epithelial cells containing microcysts of basophilic material giving a cribriform or 'Swiss cheese' appearance. Twenty per cent of patients survive 5 years. The remaining carcinomas (adenocarcinoma, undifferentiated, those arising in a pleomorphic adenoma or epidermoid) usually produce obvious clinical signs of malignancy at an early stage.

Parotid gland anatomy

The parotid gland is divided into superficial and deep lobes by the facial nerve. The deep part of the gland is crossed by the external carotid artery and its terminal branches, and by the veins which drain into the posterior facial vein. The boundaries of the parotid gland should be appreciated because the majority of tumours develop in the periphery. Eighty per cent of all salivary tumours occur within the parotid.

Presentation

Most tumours present as a slow-growing localized swelling. Malignancy is inferred by rapid growth, facial palsy, fixation and pain. It is not usually possible to differentiate deep and superficial tumours clinically but those which project into the oropharynx on oral examination are most often deep lesions.

Diagnosis

Needle biopsy or Tru-Cut biopsy carries a high risk of tumour implantation. Fine needle aspiration is popular in Europe. If malignancy or deep lobe involvement is suspected a CT scan should be performed.

Surgery

The aim of treatment is complete excision with facial nerve preservation. Local excision without VII nerve identification produces good cosmetic results but the risk of local recurrence and permanent VII nerve damage is high. A superficial parotidectomy is carried out through a cervico-facial–mastoid incision. The trunk of the VII nerve is located between the mastoid process and the bony part of the external auditory meatus. As a guide, the depth of the nerve should be level with the plane of the posterior belly of the digastric muscle. Once identified, the trunk of the VII nerve is dissected forwards to reveal the upper and lower divisions and everything superficial to the nerve is taken. The main disadvantage of this approach is that, if the tumour capsule is breached, cells will be implanted directly on to the exposed nerve and make subsequent re-excision and VII nerve salvage impossible. VII nerve damage usually occurs by injudicious diathermy to venous oozing from the posterior facial vein or the stylomastoid artery. Intra-oral deep lobe tumours or posterior tumours involving the VII nerve or mandibular ramus require the assistance of an ENT or oral surgeon. A radical parotidectomy (VII nerve sacrifice) is carried out for malignant disease. If local lymph nodes are involved, an ipsilateral block dissection of the neck is considered.

Radiotherapy

Postoperative radiotherapy reduces the risk of tumour recurrence for malignant disease and is advocated by some for incomplete excision of benign disease.

VII nerve palsy

If the VII nerve is sacrificed during the course of a radical parotidectomy the nerve resection margins must be free of invasion. This may involve exploration of the middle ear. An inadvertently divided nerve may be sutured together directly with the aid of an operating microscope. Large gaps are bridged with a great auricular nerve graft. This nerve should always be identified during the approach to the parotid should its subsequent use become necessary. VII nerve palsy is usually temporary, lasting several months until complete neuronal regeneration occurs. A lateral tarsorrhaphy or plastic eye patch may be required in the interim. Plastic procedures like a facia lata graft can be incorporated into the face and used to 'hitch up' the outer canthus of the eye and angle of the mouth in patients with permanent VII damage.

Frey's syndrome

Frey's syndrome (gaustatory sweating) develops 6–9 months after resection in many patients. It is due to cross-regeneration of divided parotid parasympathetic secromotor fibres into cutaneous sympathetic fibre sheaths. Tympanic neurectomy or greater auricular nerve avulsion can cure some resistant distressing cases, but the use of antiperspirants is all that is needed in most patients.

Submandibular/ sublingual/minor

The submandibular gland and the minor salivary and sublingual glands harbour 20% of all the salivary tumours. About 40% are malignant and most of these are adenoid cystic carcinomas. Sixty per cent of submandibular gland tumours are pleomorphic adenomas and 40% of the sublingual and minor salivary tumours are pleomorphic adenomas.

Further reading

Gunn A. Salivary gland tumours. *Surgery*. 1989; **68**: 1623–9.
Hobsley M. The salivary glands. In: Burnand KG, Young AE (eds) *The New Aird's Companion in Surgical Studies*. Edinburgh: Churchill Livingstone, 1992; 469–87.

Related topic of interest

Salivary gland calculi (p. 265)

SEPSIS IN THE SURGICAL PATIENT

The term sepsis indicates a severe infection, usually. Sepsis suggests the presence of pus, or systemic infection usually with a bacterial organism. Surgical patients may present with sepsis, or it may complicate treatment. It may be localized or generalized, acute or chronic.

Generalized sepsis

Systemic infections may result from any infected focus. The transient presence of bacteria in the bloodstream is termed bacteraemia, and the persistence of a bacteraemia from a severe septic focus resulting in tachycardia, pyrexia, rigors and shock is septicaemia. Whilst these rarely complicate minor infections in healthy individuals, a trivial boil may result in an overwhelming infection in someone who is immunocompromised. Infected sources may also 'metastasize' to distant sites, and haematological spread may be the cause of osteomyelitis, cerebral and hepatic abscess, or necrotizing fasciitis.

Endotoxic shock and the sepsis syndrome

Generalized infection with Gram-negative bacilli may result in endotoxic shock. The bacterial walls of these organisms consist of lipopolysaccharide endotoxin, which is a potent stimulus to the humeral and cellular inflammatory response. There is an early rise in circulating levels of inflammatory cytokines, such as tumour necrosis factor-α and interleukin-1α and these initiate a cascade of events that ultimately comprise septic shock. This may be clinically diagnosed by the association of hypotension with peripheral vasodilatation (warm peripheries), which is readily distinguished from cardiogenic or haemorrhagic shock, which result in peripheral vasoconstriction ('cold and clammy' peripheries). Multi-organ failure may supervene. Endotoxaemia most commonly complicates biliary, urological or gastrointestinal tract-related infections, as these are most likely to be due to Gram-negative bacilli. Prompt diagnosis, correction of the relative hypovolaemia, and treatment with high dose broad-spectrum antibiotics active against the Gram-negative organisms may be life-saving.

Localized sepsis

The skin is a common site of sepsis, and the peritoneal cavity is of particular importance to the general surgeon. Chronic sepsis tends to be localized.

Cutaneous and subcutaneous sepsis

1. Lymphangitis and lymphadenitis. Lymphatic structures draining a source of infection may show signs of inflammation: lymphangitis is indicated by red, tender, subcutaneous streaks passing along a limb, and lymphadenitis amounts to painful, enlarged and tender draining lymph nodes.

2. Cellulitis, erysipelas and carbuncle. Infection with a pyogenic organism can result in the formation of abscesses or carbuncles (usually *Staphylococcus aureus*), or cellulitis or erysipelas (usually *Streptococcus pyogenes*). Underlying causes may be apparent, for example, a staphylococcal abscess may result from infection of an existant sebaceous cyst, resulting in a sebaceous abscess; cellulitis may result from minor wounds, possibly even unnoticed, on extremities, and is a common complication of lymphoedema of the lower limb. Up to 10% of surgical wounds become infected by *Staphylococcus* or Gram-negative bacilli. Infecting organisms are commonly multiple, for example, cellulitis is often secondarily infected by *Staphylococcus* species, and infected wounds often grow mixed coliforms. Local sepsis commonly occurs in diabetes and the immunocompromised.

3. Necrotizing fasciitis. Severe subcutaneous infections may lead to thrombosis of the vessels leading to the overlying skin, and cutaneous gangrene supervenes. This is necrotizing fasciitis, and tends to complicate cellulitis caused by group A streptococci or a mixed group of anaerobic and aerobic organisms, in which case it is called Meleney's synergistic gangrene. If this occurs in the perineum, it is termed Fournier's gangrene. The presence of devitalized tissue promotes infection by anaerobic organisms. This is seen particularly in ischaemic amputation stumps where gas gangene caused by *Clostridium welchii* might occur if patients are not prescribed prophylactic penicillin.

Surgical treatment of local sepsis

This follows basic surgical principles: the release of pus, and the debridement of devitalized tissue. Localized infections that have have not formed collections of pus (identified by the absence of fluctuation) are treated with antibiotics. Cutaneous abscesses and infected wound collections require draining. A wide opening to the cavity in a dependent (better draining) part of the collection is made. Abscesses are best drained under general anaesthesia. It is common practice to pack an abscess cavity with a gauze wick impregnated with an antiseptic compound. This is helpful if the cavity is bleeding briskly, but serves no other purpose. The packs are painful to remove the next day. If continued drainage from a

Intraperitoneal sepsis

cavity is envisaged, then a corrugated drain, cut to size, may be sutured in place.

Septic foci are common in the peritoneal cavity. A focus of bacterial infection within the peritoneal cavity may resolve with appropriate antibiotic treatment. However, an infection may progress to form an abscess if it is contained locally, or peritonitis if the purulent process spreads.

1. Intra-abdominal abscess. Septic foci can result in a localized abscess. Following peritonitis, or as a consequence of rupture of a localized abscess, collections of pus may occur within anatomical gutters or recesses of the peritoneal cavity. Peritoneal collections tend to occur in the pelvis, left or right subphrenic space, and paracolic gutters, or between loops of small intestine and the greater omentum. Intraperitoneal abscesses may be multiple. Patients with intraperitoneal septic foci are very unwell with swinging pyrexias, and localized signs in the abdomen. Treatment revolves around evacuation of pus and eradication of the cause. Simple collections may be dealt with by percutaneous drainage by insertion of a wide-bore drain under ultrasound or CT control. Whilst this is easily performed, the underlying cause must still be sought and treated.

2. Peritonitis. If there are signs of peritonitis, a laparotomy is required, at which time the cause may be identified and treated, and the peritoneal cavity may be washed out with warm saline (lavage). Portal pyaemia and multiple hepatic abscesses may develop as a consequence of the portal venous drainage of infected intraperitoneal organs. This is a serious complication that is now fortunately rare because of the use of antibiotics.

Chronic sepsis

1. Cutaneous. Some specific organisms may be responsible for chronic localized sepsis. *Mycobacterium tuberculosis* can cause localized collections of virtually sterile pus, the so-called 'cold abscess', which typically occurs on the neck. These may present as a small superficial collection which communicates with a larger collection deep to the investing cervical fascia, termed 'collar-stud abscess'. These usually complicate tuberculous cervical lymphadenitis. *Actinomyces* are Gram-negative filamentous bacteria that can cause localized sepsis, typically over the angle of the mandible and in the right iliac fossa from a terminal ileal fistula. Treponemal infection of the skin of the lower leg results in a chronic ulcer, and chronic osteomyelitis with discharging sinuses is another differential diagnosis of leg ulceration. The principle behind the treatment in these situations is to establish the correct diagnosis in situations where there may be doubt about the diagnosis, and to initiate the appropriate antibacterial treatment. It is best not to lay open a tuberculous abscess as chronic discharging fistulae may result.

2. Intraperitoneal. Chronic intraperitoneal sepsis usually complicates underlying chronic disease (pelvic inflammatory disease or Crohn's disease), or previous surgery, particularly of the bowel. The presence of a collection should be proved by ultrasound or CT scan. If the source is occult, as it frequently is in chronic sepsis, an indium-labelled leucocyte scan may help to localize the collection.

Further reading

Lucarotti ME, Virjee J, Thomas WEG. Intra abdominal abscesses. *Surgery*, 1991; **98**: 2335–41.
Molloy RG, Mannick JA, Rodrick ML. Cytokines, sepsis and immunomodulation. *British Journal of Surgery*, 1993; **80**: 289–97.

Related topics of interest

SKIN COVER

Although the skin is abundant, we are born with only just enough. Its main function, besides cosmetic, is in the provision of a barrier to infection and fluid loss. Skin is lost from burns, ulcers, pressure sores and after trauma or radical cancer surgery. It can be replaced by a variety of methods described below.

Graft

A skin graft is taken from one part of the body and transferred to a recipient site where it must establish its own blood supply. Autografts are transferred within the same individual. Allografts are carried out between animals of the same species and xenografts between animals of different species.

Flap

A flap remains attached by a pedicle which carries its blood supply. There are many varieties.

1. Random Pattern Flap. This is the traditional flap where the length is not allowed to exceed with width of the base.

2. Axial pattern flap. This is a modification on the previous flap which allows the flap to attain greater lengths by utilizing a known and dependable blood supply.

3. Axial island flap. This flap allows for greater mobility. The flap is detatched cutaneously from its origin and maintained on an isolated artery and vein.

4. 'Free' flap. The advent of microvascular surgery has allowed the transfer of 'free' flaps to remote regions by immediate arteriovenous anastomosis to a named recipient artery and vein.

5. Tube pedicle flap. This flap is now rarely used and has been replaced with other more suitable flaps. It is included for historic interest.

Split skin graft

1. Principle. Split skin grafts can be harvested at various thicknesses. In each case, the entire epidermis is taken with a variable proportion of the dermis. Unlike the epidermis, the dermis is not capable of regeneration. The quality of the established graft therefore depends upon the initial dermal thickness. Thicker grafts however require a greater blood supply and are harder to 'take'.

2. *Harvesting*. The donor site chosen to resurface extensive burns involves the use of all available areas including the scalp and the sole of the foot. Grafts are harvested with either a hand-held Humby knife or an electric or gas-powered dermatome. Thin grafts ensure rapid donor site re-epithelialization (7–10 days) and allow the same site to be used over and over again. Re-epithelialization from the undamaged keratinocytes of sweat glands, hair follicles and sebaceous glands occurs most rapidly in a moist sterile environment. Placement of an 'op-site' sheet over the donor site achieves both conditions. Common donor sites in most patients involve inconspicuous areas like the buttocks or inner thighs. The lateral thigh is preferred in the elderly as the dermis, here is thicker and dressing becomes easier.

3. *Technique*. The chosen donor site should be sterilized with chlorhexidine or Savlon (iodine preparations interfere with lubrication) and smeared liberally with paraffin. Wooden boards flatten the desired portion of skin whilst the operator of a hand-held knife harvests the graft with short frequent slicing movements. The technique involves a lateral movement rather than a forward progression, with an aim towards the advancing board.

Meshing

Split skin can be meshed and expanded up to a ratio of 6:1. Such widely expanded autografts are ideal for covering extensive areas. A major disadvantage however is the final 'string vest' appearance of these grafts. This is because the interstices heal by epithelialization alone whereas the actual mesh contains a thickness of dermis. Meshed allograft (from a related donor) can be applied over this, with considerable take, to cover the wound further (the sandwich graft). With smaller full-thickness defects it is often better to first allow wound contraction to occur which reduces the size of the defect. If split skin grafts are placed directly on to a wound, the cosmetic defect remains fixed at the larger original size.

Tissue expansion

The technique of tissue expansion is an effective method of providing full-thickness skin. Sialastic balloons are placed beneath the dermis and inflated weekly with saline through a subcutaneous access port. Directly sufficient skin has been developed the implant is removed and primary closure is then often achieved. This method is particularly valuable in post-burn alopecia.

Research

Recent advances in keratinocyte culture techniques can produce 2000 cm^2 of confluent sheets from just 1 cm^2 of split skin in 3 weeks. These grafts have no dermal element and consequently are very difficult to establish on a wound surface. Fibrin glue and isobutyl cyano-acrylate (super glue) have been tried to enhance take but with limited success.

Flap types

Below are a few of the commoner examples of various plastic techniques to cover wounds with full thickness skin.

Flap	Procedure	Example
Advancement	Undermining and advancement to cover defect	Scalp defects
V-Y Plasty	Special advancement flap	Terminal digit cover
Rotation	Semi-circular incision and undermining. Rotation to cover defect	Pressure sores
Rhomboid	Rhomboid-shaped flap to cover adjacent defect	BCC of face
Strap	Adjacent longer parallel incision. Lateral advancement to cover defect	Long elliptical limb defects
Bilobed	Raising a secondary smaller flap to cover the primary defect	Nasolabial BCC
Island	Island of skin dissected on its arteriovenous pedicle	TRAM flap or LD flap following mastectomy
Free	Microvascular arterio-venous anastomosis	Radial forearm flap (Chinese) used for jaw reconstruction

Further reading

Rossi LFA, Shakespeare PG. Recent advances in the treatment of burn injuries. *Recent Advances in Surgery*, 1991; **14**: 69–84.

Related topics of interest

SKIN TUMOURS

The skin is the largest organ of the body and harbours a multitude of pathological processes which involve every clinical speciality. The commonest skin tumour (taking the definition of tumour as being a swelling) to present to the general surgeon is the sebaceous cyst. This is not derived from sebaceous glands but either from the infundibular portion of the hair follicles, when it is known as an epidermoid cyst, or the hair follicle epithelium, when it is known as a trichilemmal cyst. A large trichilemmal cyst may ulcerate, and then it is known as a Cock's peculiar tumour. Pott's putty tumour is a diffuse oedematous swelling of the scalp over a patch of osteomyelitis.

Basal cell carcinoma (BCC)

The BCC or rodent ulcer is the commonest skin cancer. It presents as a pearly protruberance, often with a central depression, and is characterized with telangectatic vessels. Sun-exposed sites like the inner canthus of the eye or the nasolabial fold are frequent locations of these lesions. Histological appearances are of basiloid cell clusters with peripheral palisading. They can be nodular, cystic, pigmented, multiple or give a 'field-fire' appearance. BCC cells proliferate extremely rapidly but their rate of cell death is also high which gives the impression of indolence. They are locally destructive and metastases are rare. Treatment involves local excision or radiotherapy.

Squamous cell carcinoma (SCC)

Squamous cell carcinomas similarly develop in areas exposed to solar irradiation, like the upper lip. The are commoner in the immunosuppressed, within areas of actinic keratosis and in sites of Bowen's disease (carcinoma-*in-situ*). Malignant change in an area of ulceration (venous ulcer) is termed a Marjolin's ulcer. Histological appearances are of protruding tongues of dysplastic squamous cells into the deep dermis or subcutaneous fat. They are locally destructive, spread along peripheral nerves and involve regional nodes in 5–10% of cases. Therapy involves excision with a block dissection of the draining nodal basin if it is involved. These tumours are also very radiosensitive. Multiple early lesions can be coated with topical 5-fluorouracil to good effect.

Miscellaneous

Benign tumours may also arise from sweat glands (hidradenomas) and pilosebaceous follicles. The eccrine poroma arises from the intra-epidermal portion of a sweat duct and commonly occurs on the sole of the foot. A cylindroma or turban tumour occurs on the scalp and is a benign apocrine tumour. The benign calcifying epithelioma of Malherbe or pilomatricoma arises from the hair matrix, and most commonly occurs in the first two decades. A kerato-acanthoma (molluscum sebaccum) develops as an umbilicated mass, dries out and eventually heals within 6 months. Differentiation from an SCC can only be confidently made on histology.

Malignant melanoma

The incidence of malignant melanoma is doubling every decade such that, by the year 2000, 1 in 90 people will develop the disease. Queensland, Australia harbours the highest incidence.

Risk factors

Intermittent sun exposure (especially burning at a young age), fair skin, blue eyes, red or blond hair all predispose to an increase in risk. Other risk factors include the dysplastic naevus syndrome, albinism, xeroderma pigmentosum, a prior history of melanoma and congenital giant hairy naevi.

Detection

Detection of early disease is of paramount importance because early lesions are curative and advanced lesions have an appalling prognosis. Most melanomas develop in a pre-existing mole. Changes to recognize in a suspicious mole are: increase in growth, change in contour or colour, bleeding, ulceration, or itching.

Classification

Four types of malignant melanoma are recognized.

Type	Characteristic	Incidence (%)	Prognosis
Superficial spreading	Horizontal growth	70	—
Nodular	Vertical growth	10	Poor
Lentigo maligna	Flat, slow growing	7	Good
Acral lentigenous	Palms, soles, subungual, retina, genital	13	Poor

Truncal melanomas (commoner in men), melanomas occurring in the BANS region (Back, back of Arms, Neck, Scalp) and ulcerated melanomas have a poorer prognosis, stage for stage. The incidence of acral lentigenous melanomas is increased in Asian and black populations.

Microstaging

Tumour thickness (Breslow microstaging) is the single most important prognostic factor. It is measured histologically with an occular micrometer from the granular surface to the deepest penetration.

Breslow thickness and relative 5-year risks

Tumour thickness (mm)	Risk of local recurrence (%)	Risk of node metastasis (%)	Risk of distant metastasis (%)
<0.76	0.2	2	2
0.76–1.5	2	25	8
1.5–4	6	57	15
>4	13	62	72

The level of tumour invasion into the various subdivisions of the dermis forms the basis of the Clark microstaging.

Clark microstaging

Level	Description
I	Intraepithelial
II	Into papillary dermis
III	Papillary/reticular junction
IV	Into reticular dermis
V	Penetration into subcutaneous fat

Both methods are complementary but have their drawbacks. Ulcerative lesions and regressed lesions may be relatively thin yet have a poor prognosis. Similarly, a thick lesion on the sole or back may only reach Clark level I.

Biopsy

Diagnosis of a suspicious lesion is confirmed on an incisional or excisional biopsy. Excision biopsy is preferable and a good rule of thumb is that impalpable lesions require a 1 cm margin, just palpable lesions a 2 cm margin and obviously palpable or ulcerated lesions a 3 cm margin. Incision biopsy is favoured when the amount of skin loss is critical for cosmesis. If indicated, subsequent wide re-excision requires removal of all the underlying subcutaneous fat, inclusion of the scar and, on occasion, the fascia (especially if the underlying layer of fat is thin). Orientation of any elliptical incision, required for primary closure, should be along the axis of lymphatic drainage. Subungual melanomas require partial amputation with the level of bone section just proximal to the middle phalangeal head. Auricular melanomas are treated with wedge excision. Differentiation between a local recurrence and an 'in-transit' or satellite deposit is difficult and responsible for the varying 'local' recurrence rates after wide excision. Recurrence is more a function of tumour thickness than local excision margin.

Lymphadenectomy

Regional lymph node metastases, if palpable, should be treated by a regional block dissection for palliative and putative curative reasons. The performance of a prophylactic lymph node dissection for occult micrometastatic disease is controversial. Protagonists advocate the procedure for lesions between 1 and 4 mm. Thinner lesions have a slim chance of lymph node involvement and lesions greater than 4 mm have a high probability of systemic spread. Forty-two per cent of patients harbour micrometastasis in the removed lymph nodes (identified by extensive sectioning), and by catching the regional disease early, systemic involvement may be prevented. Antagonists state that node dissection causes excessive morbidity and no impact on survival has been demonstrated. A groin dissection has an incidence of lymphoedema at 25% and a wound problem rate of 75%. The corresponding figures for an axillary dissection are 1% and 25%, respectively. If doubt arises as to which group of nodes to remove, cutaneous lymphoscintigraphy with an intradermal injection of labelled colloid can demonstrate the draining lymph node basin.

Isolated limb perfusion

Isolated limb perfusion with alkylating agents, indicated for local recurrence and 'in-transit' disease, is effective at reducing lesion size and, on occasion, healing them completely. The procedure is usually combined with a modified lymph node dissection. Enthusiasts also use this technique as adjuvant therapy for primary lesions greater than 1.5 mm thick.

Malignant melanoma is refractory to chemotherapy but radiotherapy plays a major role in the treatment of symptomatic brain, bone and spinal cord metastasis. Single deposits, like peripheral pulmonary deposits or cerebral lesions, are often removed surgically to good effect. Immunotherapy using antimelanoma monoclonal antibodies conjugated with toxins (ricin), α-interferon, IL-2 or the latter two in combination is an ingenious idea but the results are usually disappointing.

Further reading

Ross MI, Balch CM. The current management of cutaneous melanoma. *Advances in Surgery*, 1991; **24**: 139–200.
Scott RN, Makay AJ. Elective lymph node dissection in the management of malignant melanoma. *British Journal of Surgery*, 1993; **80**: 284–8.

Related topic of interest

Skin cover (p. 276)

SMALL BOWEL TUMOURS

Less than 2% of all gastrointestinal malignancies occur within the small bowel. This is surprising because the mucosal surface area of the small bowel comprises 85% of the total gastrointestinal mucosal surface. Two thirds of small bowel tumours are malignant.

Small bowel malignancy	Incidence (%)
Adenocarcinoma	39
Carcinoid	29
Lymphoma	17
Sarcoma	14

The commonest small bowel malignancy is from invasion by peritoneal seedlings or a neighbouring carcinoma (e.g. stomach, ovary). Half of all patients who die of malignant melanoma have small bowel deposits demonstrated at autopsy. The poor prognosis of small bowel malignancy is related to delays in diagnosis. No lesion is truly benign unless it has been confirmed by excision biopsy. Benign lesions include lipoma, fibroma, leiomyoma, neurofibroma, adenoma, juvenile and hyperplastic polyps, and the Peutz–Jegher's hamartomas. Adenomas are commonest in the second part of the duodenum, often as part of a familial polyposis syndrome. Presentation is usually with obstruction, gastrointestinal haemorrhage or intussusception.

Diagnosis

Diagnosis is achieved with contrast radiology and endoscopy. The technique of enteroclysis involves inflation of a balloon proximal to an enteral catheter in order to occlude the gastroduodenal junction and thus prevent reflux. Introduction of barium into the duodenum in this way improves the detection rate of small bowel abnormalities. Endoscopy can be combined with endoscopic transduodenal ultrasonography or performed intraoperatively through a small enterotomy. The entire small bowel can be visualized from within and transilluminated. This technique is especially indicated if occult bleeding from a small bowel tumour is suspected.

Carcinoid tumour

Eighty-five per cent of appendicular neoplasms are carcinoid tumours, but 73% of malignant carcinoids occur in the ileum. Of all removed appendices, 0.5% have carcinoids in their tip. Some occur in extragastrointestinal sites like the bronchus. The tumour is typically a yellow, submucosal mass surrounded by an intense fibrotic reaction. The cells are identified histologically by the staining of their granules with silver preparations (argentaffinoma/chromaffinoma).

These tumours also form part of the amine precursor uptake and decarboxylation (APUD) biochemistry system. Appendiceal tumours less than 1 cm in size can be cured with an appendicectomy. Larger lesions require a right hemi-colectomy.

Carcinoid syndrome

Four per cent of patients with carcinoid tumours develop the carcinoid syndrome of flushing, bronchospasm and diarrhoea due to the secretion of 5-HT, bradykinin and histamine. Increased levels of the metabolic product, hydroxy indole acetic acid (5-HIAA), are found in the urine. This syndrome is a feature of advanced hepatic disease because the liver normally inactivates kinins before they are released into the systemic circulation. Kinins encourage intense fibrotic reactions and their release in the systemic circulation can result in right-sided cardiac lesions like pulmonary stenosis and tricuspid fibrosis. The amino acid tryptophan is required for nicotinic acid and 5-HT synthesis, and if supplies become depleted pellagra develops. Tumour debulking by hepatic resection, intrahepatic arterial chemotherapy, hepatic artery embolization or radiotherapy reduces the severity of carcinoid attacks. Antiserotonin therapy with Methysergide can also control the attacks pharmacologically. Octreotide, a recently introduced, stable analogue of the peptide somatostatin, acts on the somato-statin receptors of the tumour to palliate carcinoid symptoms in 80% of cases. Octreotide is also valuable perioperatively as prophylaxis against an intraoperative carcinoid crisis precipitated during tumour handling.

Adenocarcinomas

Fifty per cent of small bowel adenocarcinomas are duodenal and duodenal tumours comprise half of all small bowel malignancies. The carcinogenic potential of bile may play a causative role. Patients present with epigastric pain, weight loss, vomiting and, depending on the location, jaundice. Differential diagnosis is from periampullary tumours and carcinoma of the head of the pancreas. A CT scan is helpful in assessing these lesions. Pancreaticoduodenectomy (Whipple's operation) affords the only hope of cure. A palliative biliary or gut bypass is occasionally required. The 5-year survival approaches 20%.

Lymphomas

Small bowel lymphomas are usually multiple and diffuse. They can ulcerate causing anaemia or perforate with generalized peritonitis. Coeliac disease and diffuse nodular lymphoid hyperplasia predispose to lymphoma. A small bowel enema often demonstrates areas of abnormal mucosa and diffuse wall thickening. Although lesions are very radiosensitive they are best managed by chemotherapy. Perforation is a common complication of such treatment. Obstructing lesions are resected or bypassed.

Stromal tumours

Leiomyoma and leiomyosarcoma are stromal tumours. They tend to ulcerate the overlying mucosa and present with profuse gastrointestinal bleeding. A large round luminal filling defect is often seen on a barium meal. Central necrosis or fistulation suggests sarcomatous change. Kaposi's sarcoma occurs frequently in patients with AIDS.

Gastrinomas

Most gastrinomas are malignant and occur in the pancreas, but some are duodenal. They lead to the Zollinger–Ellison syndrome by secreting excess amounts of gastrin. A little less than 1% of all duodenal ulcer patients have a gastrinoma. Treatment is surgical although the proton pump inhibitor, omeprazole, is very effective in controlling symptoms.

Peutz–Jegher's syndrome

Peutz–Jegher's is an autosomal dominant condition characterized by circumoral mucocutaneous pigmentation and multiple hamartomatous polyps within the small intestine. The polyps develop during childhood and commonly present with intussusception. Histologically, they consist of a fibromuscular core covered with normal intestinal epithelium. Malignant change occurs in less than 3% of patients. The polyps are removed endoscopically through a single enterotomy at the time of surgery.

Further reading

Basson MD. Small bowel tumours. *Current Opinion in Surgery*, 1993; 219–24.

Related topic of interest

Pancreatic cancer (p. 227)

SOFT TISSUE SWELLINGS

Musculoskeletal

1. Ganglion. This is a cystic swelling arising from the synovial lining of a joint or a tendon sheath. They occur commonly around the wrist, on digits, and on the dorsum of the foot and can be excised under local infiltration if small, or under Bier's block if larger.

2. Bursae. These may develop into cystic swellings which may become acutely or chronically inflamed or infected (bursitis). They are frequently found around the knee (housemaid's knee if prepatellar, and parson's knee if infrapatellar) or over the olecranon. If they are symptomatic, they may be excised. Abscesses must be drained.

3. Baker's cyst. A cystic swelling in the medial part of the popliteal fossa in children and young adults is likely to be a semimembranous bursa. This is often called Baker's cyst, though the term should be reserved for inflammatory swellings in the popliteal fossa. These arise as a complication of arthritis of the knee from posterior rupture of inflamed synovium, or from a communicating existent popliteal bursa.

4. Synovial swellings. The synovium may be inflamed as a result of systemic disease, such as rheumatoid or sarcoidosis. Benign 'brown tumours' may occur, and rarely malignant synovioma may result.

Benign soft tissue tumours

1. Lipomas. These are are very common benign tumours of adipose tissue. They are classified according to their anatomical layer. They may be subcutaneous, extrafascial, subfascial, intramuscular, subperiosteal, extraperitoneal, subserosal, submucosal, or retroperitoneal. Malignant change to liposarcoma is a rare occurrence.

Lipomas are frequently lobulated by fibrous septa. They are soft and may feel fluctulant. The edge of a subcutaneous lipoma, the most common variety, can be displaced laterally under the examining finger. This 'slipping' sign is said to be typical.

Lipomas can easily be excised under local anaesthesia. Larger lipomas on the trunk are almost always related to deep fascia. They are often much larger than initially thought. These are best dealt with under a general anaesthetic. Multiple spontaneously painful subcutaneous lipomas is Dercum's syndrome, or adiposis dolorosa.

2. Neurofibromas, neurilemmomas and schwannomas.
These are neural tumours arising from supporting cells of
the sensory component of peripheral nerves. The three types
are differentiated on histological appearance. They present
as lumps, usually on a limb, which may cause altered
sensation distally. Clinically, they are fixed in the plane
parallel to the axis of the nerve, and are mobile
perpendicular to this. When palpated, tingling may be felt
along the distribution of the nerve.

3. Neurofibromatosis. This is Von Recklinghausen's
disease, comprising multiple (up to many hundreds) of
small, soft, sessile, cutaneous neurofibromas, freckling of
the axillary skin, and oval café-au-lait patches. It may be
associated with central nervous system gliomas, cranial
nerve neuromas, and phaeochromocytomas. Neurofibromatosis is a congenital disorder of the neuro-ectoderm, one
of a group called phakomatoses (others are Von-Hippel
Lindau and Sturge–Weber syndromes, and tuberose
sclerosis). Larger neurofibromas with a broad base and a
fissured surface may occur on the trunk or a limb girdle.
These are plexiform neurofibromas and should be observed
carefully for increase in size or the development of hard
areas which may signify sarcomatous change.

4. Neuroma. This may arise following trauma to a nerve.
Peripheral nerves regenerate if damaged, however the
regeneration may become disordered, and a tangled mass of
neuronal tissue can evolve. These are most often seen in
amputation stumps, or at the edges of surgical wounds. They
may be a source of constant pain and can be successfully
treated by injection of local anaesthetic. Permanent relief
may follow phenolic ablation if local anaesthetic infiltration
is successful.

5. Desmoid tumours and fibromatoses. These are rare and
sporadic but may be seen as part of the familial polyposis
coli syndrome. They are localized collections of well-
vascularized fibrous tissue which are not malignant, but
which often recur after excision. They commonly occur in
the abdominal wall where they are said to arise from
aponeurotic tissue. They may occur in the neck. Desmoid
tumours may respond to radiotherapy if they recur following
wide excision.

Desmoid tumours may occur as part of a diffuse fibrotic condition known as fibromatosis. This includes other fibrotic conditions such as Dupuytren's contracture of the palmar and plantar fascia, retroperitoneal and mediastinal fibrosis, Peyronie's disease of the penis, Reidel's thyroiditis and keloid scarring.

6. *Leiomyomas.* These can occasionally present as slow-growing subcutaneous lumps.

Malignant soft tissue tumours: sarcomas

The majority of sarcomas encountered arise from bone, cartilage or periosteum, however soft tissues may also give rise to malignancies. The incidence of soft tissue sarcomas rises with age, and peaks in the seventh decade. They present as painless masses that increase in size. They feel firm or rubbery, and their edge is indistinct. They may be warm to the touch, and there may be an overlying bruit. They spread by local invasion through tissue planes and via the bloodstream to the lungs.

MRI is the investigation of choice, although CT is adequate. The sarcoma appears as an encapsulated solid mass. The diagnosis may be obtained by core biopsy in 90% of cases. Definitive surgical resection entails wide resection beyond the sarcoma pseudocapsule, which frequently contains tumour. Adjuvant treatment in the form of radiotherapy to the tumour bed results in reduced recurrence rates. Chemotherapy may also be used, though it is often reserved for unresectable or recurrent tumours.

Sarcomas may be classified according to the tissue of origin. Varieties include fibrosarcoma, malignant fibrous histiocytoma, liposarcoma, rhabdomyosarcoma, Kaposi's sarcoma, lymphangiosarcoma, synovial sarcoma, malignant schwannoma, and malignant mesenchymoma.

1. *Liposarcoma.* These are rare malignant tumours arising from adipose tissue and mostly occurring in the region of the limb girdles and in the retroperitoneum. There is some debate as to whether larger lipomas can become malignant, but if a patient is thought to have a large lipoma, and clinically there are hard areas within it, this must be excised.

2. *Kaposi's sarcoma.* Also known as cutaneous haemorrhagic angiosarcomas, these tend to occur in particular races, especially the Eastern Europeans, Jews and sub-Saharan Africans. They are purple or red coloured cutaneous papules and tend to be multiple. They are

common in AIDS when they are often very small and may occur on any mucosal surface as well as the skin. Gastrointestinal Kaposi's sarcomas may bleed.

3. Rhabdomyosarcoma. These arise from skeletal muscle, and embryonal and mature histological types are described. The commonest sarcomas of childhood, they are found in the head and neck, genitourinary tract and, in older children, in the trunk and limbs.

4. Dermatofibrosarcoma protruberans. This is a skin tumour arising from subcutaneous elements of the trunk as a progressively enlarging smooth, bulbous, lobulated mass, often with ulceration of the overlying skin. It is of questionable malignant potential, recurring if it is not widely excised, but histologically typically having a high mitotic rate.

Further reading

Pittam MR, Thomas JM. Sarcomas of soft tissue and bone. In: Burnand KG, Young AE (eds) *The New Aird's Companion in Surgical Studies*. Edinburgh: Churchill Livingstone, 1992; 179.

Related topics of interest

Skin tumours (p. 279)
Vascular malformations and tumours (p. 336)

SUTURE MATERIALS

Suture materials are frequently classified according to their properties, size, structure and composition. The selection of an appropriate suture is essential to achieve effective wound closure and cosmesis.

Suture size and application

As suture diameter increases, the number decreases: 2/0 is a wider and more robust suture than 6/0. Sutures larger than 2/0 are 0, 1 and 2. The largest sutures in common general surgical practice are usually 0 and 1, and these are often used to close the abdominal wall after a laparotomy. The finest sutures are 10/0 and 12/0, used in microscopic repairs of small vessels and nerves, or in ophthalmic surgery.

Suturing the skin of the face requires 6/0 for ideal cosmesis. 5/0 may be used on the neck, 4/0 is ideal for use on digits, and 3/0 on the leg or arm. Suturing the skin of the trunk requires 3/0 or 2/0.

2/0 is an ideal size for sutures placed in subcutaneous tissues and fascial layers. For intestinal anastomoses, 2/0 or 3/0 is generally used. Aortic anastomoses require 2/0 or 3/0, with smaller sutures for distal anastomoses.

Needles for arterial suturing are round backed in cross-section to avoid tearing the vessel wall. Tougher tissues such as skin need to be sutured with cutting-edged (triangular cross-sectioned) needles.

Composition and properties

1. Synthetic sutures

(a) *Permanent.* Synthetic sutures that are non-resorbable are polyamine (nylon) and polypropylene (prolene). Nylon and prolene sutures combine strength with slenderness. Nylon stretches more than prolene, and thus prolene is the ideal suture for vascular anastomoses, and nylon is often the choice for closing the musculature of the abdominal wall. For skin closure, prolene is best for subcuticular running sutures, and nylon is ideal for interrupted sutures. Both need to be removed. Stainless steel sutures are occasionally used.

(b) *Resorbable.* Resorbable synthetic sutures are polyglycolic acid (dexon), polyglactin (vycril) and polydioxanone (PDS). Dexon and vycril are resorbed after about 3 weeks, PDS in 3 months. These are used internally, for example, all three can be used to anastomose bowel, and vycril and dexon are often used as ligatures. PDS lasts long enough to be used to close the abdominal wall, with the additional advantage of being resorbed.

2. Natural sutures. Silk is non-resorbable, catgut is totally resorbable and linen, which is often termed simply thread, is very slowly and only partially resorbable. Catgut is composed of sheep intestinal collagen. Plain catgut lasts only a matter of days unless treated to produce chromic catgut, which lasts for approximately 10 days. All these are used as ligatures. Catgut sutures are frequently used internally, including intestinal anastomoses. Silk sutures were once commonly used on the skin, though synthetic monofilament sutures are superior.

Suture structure

Sutures are monofilament or braided. Nylon, prolene and PDS are monofilaments. For extra strength, nylon is also available in a braided form (ethibond), and prolene and nylon are available as looped sutures. Monofilament synthetic sutures slip easily through tissues, and are thus ideal for skin closure. However, natural sutures have better handling qualities, and are usually preferred as ligatures. Silk is braided, and allows bacteria to flourish in its interstices, and thus minor degrees of infection are common when used on the skin.

Wound clips

Staples may be used to close wounds. These are quick to apply, and this is their main advantage over sutures. Care must be taken to ensure that the wound edges are everted during the application of the clips.

Steristrips and tissue adhesives

Steristrips are adhesive strips that can often be used to close clean, well opposed wound edges. They are ideal for use on the face and neck, and in children. They are often applied in addition to subcuticular sutures, to close any gaps that might be present. Tissue adhesives may be used to close skin wounds. This is methyl methacrylate (essentially superglue) and should be used with care.

Further reading

Eden CG. A classification of suture material and needles. *Surgery*, 1991; **91**: 2179.
Eden CG. Properties of individual suture materials. *Surgery*, 1991; **95**: 2271.

Related topic of interest

Wounds: healing and closure (p. 349)

TESTICULAR TUMOURS

Ninety per cent of testicular tumours can now be cured.

Classification

For the purposes of therapy, primary testicular germ cell tumours are classified into seminoma and non-seminoma. The non-seminoma group consists mainly of teratomas. The remainder includes Leydig cell, Sertoli cell, the choriocarcinoma or yolk sac tumour and the most primative tumour, the embryonal carcinoma. Secondary tumours (bronchus, prostate, kidney, colon) and adenexal tumours (rhabdomyosarcoma, leiomyosarcoma, epididymal) are rare. A testicular lymphoma is a stage IV lymphoma and it carries a poor prognosis.

Presentation

Men usually present in the third (teratoma), or fourth (seminoma) decade with a heavy, woody, insensitive testicle. Fifty per cent of patients wait for more than 3 months from the time of first symptoms, and in 40% of cases the primary clinician fails to establish the correct diagnosis. Sertoli cell tumours produce gynaecomastia in adult males. Leydig cell tumours produce precocious puberty in boys ('the infant Hercules') and gynaecomastia in adults. A thorough testicular examination is required in all patients with gynaecomastia of recent onset. Occasionally, aggressive tumours present with the features of secondary spread like back pain, sciatica, ascites and lymphoedema (hurricane type).

Investigations

Mandatory investigations at presentation include a chest radiograph and blood sampling for tumour markers. α-Feto-protein and human β-chorionic gonadotrophin are elevated in 90% of non-seminoma tumours and reflect the advancement of the disease and, later on, its response to treatment. Testicular ultrasound may reveal an impalpable intratesticular tumour with a false positive and false negative error of 10%.

Orchidectomy

All suspicious testicular lumps require surgical exploration. A groin incision is recommended to allow a soft bowel clamp to be placed on the cord before inspection and mobilization. The risk of haematogenous dissemination is thereby reduced and a cleaner removal of the testis can subsequently be performed. Although an inguinal incision is preferred, many studies have shown no increase in local or systemic recurrence rates after a trans-scrotal orchidectomy.

Insertion of a secured prosthesis is also preferable 'from above' since sloughing of a scrotal wound with extrusion of the prosthesis is an occasional problem. If doubt remains as to whether the testis is abnormal it can be bivalved, the contents inspected and the tunica albugina repaired (Chevassu's manoeuvre).

Testicular biopsy

Occasionally, surgeons advocate contralateral testicular biopsy because 3–5% of patients develop bilateral tumours and carcinoma-*in-situ* is known to develop into invasive cancer in 50% of cases. A stab incision is made into the tunica and the testis is squeezed to extrude a few seminiferous tubules which are subsequently excised with scissors. Biopsy is especially indicated in the contralateral testicle at risk identified by a history of infertility, cryptorchism or testicular atrophy. A short course of local radiotherapy prevents the progression of carcinoma-*in-situ*.

Staging

After orchidectomy the disease is staged by a thoracic and abdominal CT scan so that subsequent therapy can be deployed.

Stage	Description
I	Confined to the testis
II	Retroperitoneal or inguinal nodes:
IIa	less than 2 cm
IIb	between 2 and 5 cm
IIc	greater than 5 cm
III	Metastasis elsewhere

Grading

There are three types of seminoma: seminoma, spermocytic seminoma and anaplastic seminoma. Teratomas are classified according to their degree of differentiation, the presence of the least differentiated cell type being recorded. Primary tumour histology can identify groups which have an increased risk of recurrence. Lymphatic invasion, vascular invasion, the presence of undifferentiated cells and the absence of yolk sac elements each increase the risk of recurrence from 20% to 50%.

Surveillance

In the UK, surveillance is the standard management of stage I non-seminoma. Within 18 months, 33% relapse and most of these are successfully treated with chemotherapy. Patients with a high probability of relapse on histology or high initial titres of markers require adjuvant chemotherapy.

Surveillance for the low-risk group is by chest radiography, tumour marker estimations and thoraco-abdominal CT every 4 months.

Chemotherapy

Combination chemotherapy is indicated for metastatic non-seminoma (II, III) and advanced metastatic seminoma (III). Cisplatin has revolutionized treatment since its introduction over the last 20 years. The commonest regime is with BEP (bleomycin, etoposide and cisplatin) but each has a potentially serious side effect. Bleomycin can lead to irreversible pulmonary fibrosis, etoposide, reversible alopecia, and cisplatin is nephrotoxic and ototoxic and can cause a peripheral neuropathy. An analogue of cisplatin, carboplatin, is less toxic and is now the preferred drug.

Radiotherapy

Seminomas are extremely sensitive to radiotherapy. It is indicated as adjuvant treatment for stage I seminoma for the ipsilateral pelvic and retroperitoneal nodes. In stage II, seminoma relapse following radiotherapy is treated with combination chemotherapy. Side effects include peptic ulceration (5%), gastrointestinal upset and genotoxicity from scatter irradiation.

Lymphadenectomy

Retroperitoneal para-aortic lymphadenectomy is primarily indicated for residual active disease. Twenty-five per cent of patients harbour a residual retroperitoneal mass after cessation of chemotherapy. This should be monitored with CT and guided biopsy should be performed for those masses which cease to regress. The complication of permanent damage to sexual function can be avoided by preserving the lumbar sympathetic outflow.

Fertility

All men in whom treatment is likely to lead to irreversible damage to fertility should be offered cryopreservation of their semen. At presentation, however, only 25% of men have a sufficient quantity of good quality semen.

Further reading

Fordham M, Newlands ES. The management of testicular cancer. *Current Practice in Surgery*, 1990; **2**: 216–22.
Horwich A, Hendry WF. Treatment of testicular cancer. *Surgery*, 1993; 505–10.

Related topic of interest

Penile conditions and scrotal swellings (p. 231)

THYROGLOSSAL TRACT ANOMALIES

The thyroid gland develops from the thyroglossal duct (median bud of the pharynx) during the 4th embryonic week and passes ventrally from the foramen caecum at the back of the tongue to the pharynx, just below the position of the developing hyoid cartilage. This line of descent is called the thyroglossal tract. The thyroglossal duct thus formed usually degenerates, but its incomplete regression results in the following congenital abnormalities which are rarely evident at birth.

Thyroglossal cyst

May occur with patent or closed thyroglossal duct.

- May occur at any age, but 40% present in the age group 0–10 years.
- Incidence: male = female.
- Midline usually, but may deviate slightly.
- Commonest midline cervical tumour in infants.
- Does not usually transilluminate.
- Usually situated just above or below the hyoid bone.
- Moves up on protrusion of tongue.

It is lined by squamous or ciliated pseudostratified epithelium and may contain thyroid or lymphoid tissue which may be dysplastic in the wall.

Thyroglossal sinus

This is not congenital but results from infection in or inadequate excision of a thyroglossal cyst.

- Midline orifice with tract leading cranially.
- Crescentic fold of skin (concavity faces down) at skin orifice.
- Mucopurulent discharge.
- Recurrent infection.
- Lined by columnar epithelium.

Sistrunk's operation

This is the operation of choice for thyroglossal cyst and sinus. A transverse incision is made over the cyst (transverse elliptical incision around the mouth of a sinus) and the tract followed up between the strap muscles to the hyoid bone. The tract, duct, cyst or sinus is then excised with the central portion of the hyoid bone (or recurrence is likely). For suprahyoid cysts or sinuses, the tract should be followed to the base of the tongue.

Lingual and aberrant thyroid

A lingual thyroid gland results from failure of descent of part or all of the embryonic thyroid gland from the foramen caecum. In most cases, it represents the only thyroid tissue present. It may remain symptomless or develop any of the recognized thyroid abnormalities. Clinical problems occur most commonly in young women when physiological hypertrophy at the time of pregnancy occurs or an adenoma develops. Symptoms and signs include:

- Dysphagia.
- Speech impairment.
- Respiratory obstruction.
- Haemorrhage.
- Smooth, vascular dark red projection at the back of the tongue.

Symptomless glands should be left alone. If treatment is required, an iodine or technetium isotope scan should be performed to determine the presence of any other thyroid tissue. Glands may be reduced in size by antithyroid drugs, thyroxine or radioiodine. Excision is required if malignant change occurs.

Aberrant thyroid tissue may occur at any site along the thyroglossal tract and this may be the only thyroid tissue present. If a non-cystic mass is found during Sistrunk's operation, the procedure should be abandoned and an isotope scan performed subsequently to determine the site of all thyroid tissue.

The term 'lateral aberrant thyroid gland' is a misnomer, the thyroid tissue found in these lateral sites being cervical node metastases from a papillary thyroid carcinoma.

Further reading

Young AE. The thyroid gland. In: Burnand KG, Young AE (eds) *The New Aird's Companion in Surgical Studies*. Edinburgh: Churchill Livingstone, 1992; 633–60.

Related topics of interest

THYROID NEOPLASMS

Thyroid neoplasms may present as a solitary nodule, in common with many benign processes that affect the gland, 5% of Western populations having a palpable thyroid nodule. The incidence of thyroid malignancy is low but may be rising (1.5% of all malignancies, 4/100 000 per year).

Benign

1. *Follicular adenoma*
- The majority of benign neoplasms.
- Differentiation from malignant follicular tumours is difficult.
- Scintiscanning may show a 'solitary cold nodule'.
- Cytological distinction from follicular carcinoma is impossible.
- Treatment is by total hemithyroidectomy with frozen section to exclude malignancy.

2. *Teratoma*
- Rare.
- Arises from all three primitive germ layers.
- Benign in children.

Malignant–differentiated

1. *Papillary*
- 70% of all thyroid cancers.
- Peak incidence 20–40 years.
- Female-to-male ratio 3:1.

Tumours tend to be multifocal and unencapsulated, but there is a spectrum from occult intrathyroid tumours (< 1.5 cm diameter) to locally invasive and metastatic tumours. They invade lymphatics and spread to cervical lymph nodes early. Distant metastases rarely occur. The misnamed 'lateral aberrant thyroid' is invariably a cervical metastasis from a papillary tumour. Tumours may occur with a mixed papillary and follicular pattern, and should be treated as papillary tumours, even if the predominant element is follicular. Diagnosis is by FNAC.

Total lobectomy is satisfactory if the tumour is confined to a single lobe. A more extensive tumour necessitates total thyroidectomy, allowing subsequent diagnosis and treatment of metastases by radioiodine. Lymph node involvement should be treated by modified cervical block dissection or by 'cherry-picking' (removing nodes individually), particularly for node recurrence. Radioiodine should be given if the tumour extends beyond the thyroid capsule. Thyroxine suppresses residual tumour and is necessary after lobectomy and total thyroidectomy. External radiotherapy is of value where there is residual metastatic disease after radioiodine or where there is no iodine uptake, or if there is a large, unresectable tumour. The prognosis for intrathyroid tumours is similar to that of the normal population. The 10-year survival for patients with extrathyroid disease is 55%.

2. *Follicular*
- 15% of thyroid malignancies.
- Older age group than papillary tumours (mean age 45 years).
- Female-to-male ratio 3:1.
- Commoner in endemic goitrous regions.

These tumours are usually solitary, encapsulated and metastasize by haematogenous spread to lung and bone. Local lymph nodes are involved late. Malignancy is diagnosed by capsular invasion and vascular spread, and cannot be assessed by FNAC.

If the diagnosis is uncertain pre-operatively, total lobectomy should be performed, proceeding to completion total thyroidectomy if frozen section reveals malignancy. Where the frozen section is uncertain, completion total thyroidectomy is performed at a second procedure, if frank invasion is demonstrated by paraffin sections, enabling radioiodine to be given. Modified block dissection should be performed only if nodes are involved. Life-long thyroxine suppression/replacement is employed. Thyroglobulin is a marker for both recurrent papillary and follicular tumours.

3. *Medullary*
- Arises from the parafollicular cells (C-cells) which synthesize calcitonin.
- 5–10% of thyroid neoplasms.
- Wide age range.
- Most are sporadic, but 20% are familial, occurring both with and without the other features of multiple endocrine neoplasia MEN type II a or b.
- Lymph node metastases are present in 25%.

The tumours secrete calcitonin and carcinoembryonic antigen, and a range of other peptide hormones, causing diarrhoea in some patients. If a medullary tumour is suspected, other abnormalities of the MEN II syndromes should be sought. The diagnosis is made by FNAC.

Total thyroidectomy should be performed with ipsilateral modified block dissection regardless of node status, or bilateral if the disease appears multicentric. Calcitonin levels should be measured to monitor recurrence for which radioiodine, radiotherapy and chemotherapy are reserved. The 5-year survival is 90% and 50% in node-negative and node-positive disease, respectively.

4. Lymphoma
- Rare.
- Primary or secondary.
- Usually diffuse histiocytic. Must be distinguished from small cell anaplastic carcinoma.
- Occur in old age, affecting women more often than men.
- Usually a history of a rapidly growing goitre.

Pre-existing Hashimoto's disease is found in 30% (few cases of Hashimoto's thyroiditis progress to lymphoma). Primary lymphoma is treated by total thyroidectomy with postoperative radiotherapy. Secondary or recurrent disease is treated by chemotherapy. In primary disease, the 5-year survival is 85% falling to 40% for metastatic disease.

5. Squamous
- Very rare.
- Must be distinguished from squamous metaplasia of papillary tumours.
- Arise in embryonal remnants.
- Very aggressive.
- Treatment usually ineffective.

6. Sarcoma
- Very rare.
- Poor prognosis.

7. Teratoma
- In adults these are highly malignant.
- Few patients survive 1 year.

8. Metastatic
- Rare.
- Malignant melanoma, breast.

Malignant – anaplastic
- Peak incidence 60–70 years.
- Women are affected slightly more often than men.

- Commoner in endemic goitrous regions.
- Invariably a long history of goitre.

These extremely aggressive tumours usually arise from a differentiated carcinoma or, occasionally, a benign adenoma. There is usually a hard, fixed mass involving the trachea and adjacent structures. There may be stridor or hoarseness from recurrent nerve invasion.

Distinction from lymphoma is important and a biopsy rather than FNAC is usually required. Treatment by total thyroidectomy is seldom feasible, local debulking and tracheal decompression being the only option. The response to radiotherapy is usually poor. Chemotherapy (doxorubicin) may be useful in younger patients. Few patients survive 1 year.

The solitary nodule
- Clinical diagnosis unreliable.
- Malignancy suggested by male, young patient, cervical lymphadenopathy, hoarseness, pain or dysphagia.
- In children, the incidence of malignancy in a solitary nodule approaches 50%.

Ultrasound scanning should be performed to confirm the solitary nature of the nodule (50% are dominant nodules in a multinodular goitre), to determine whether it is cystic or solid. If needle aspiration resolves the cyst completely, no further treatment is necessary. If the nodule is incompletely removed or recurs, excision is necessary. If repeated FNAC indicates benign disease only, thyroidectomy is not required unless symptoms determine otherwise. If FNAC indicates a follicular nodule, total lobectomy should be performed with frozen section. Other tumours are dealt with as described above.

Further reading

Young AE. The thyroid gland. In: Burnand KG, Young AE (eds) *The New Aird's Companion in Surgical Studies*. Edinburgh: Churchill Livingstone, 1992; 633–60.

Related topics of interest

TRAUMA MANAGEMENT – PRINCIPLES

Trauma is the cause of 545 000 hospital discharges and 14 500 deaths annually in the UK. Road traffic accidents account for 850 000 hospital bed nights and in 1985 cost the British economy £2.8 billion.

Death from trauma has a trimodal distribution. The first peak occurs within seconds or minutes of injury and is caused by severe neurological, cardiac or vascular injuries. Few of these patients are salvageable. The second peak occurs within the first few hours following injury as a result of extra- or subdural haemorrhage, haemopneumothorax, splenic or hepatic injury, or severe haemorrhage (the period between the first and second peak is known as 'the golden hour'). Many of these deaths are preventable and it is hoped that the widespread adoption of the advanced trauma life support (ATLS) approach will improve the management and survival of such patients. The third peak occurs weeks or months following injury and is caused by sepsis or multisystem organ failure.

The location of designated trauma centres, the training of paramedics and the use of helicopters for transporting severely injured patients are currently under scrutiny. The adoption of American-style trauma centres in the UK now seems unlikely.

Triage and trauma scoring systems

Triage is the sorting of patients based on the need for treatment. Ideally, the number of patients and the severity of their injuries does not exceed available facilities. Injury severity should be assessed and an estimate of survival probability made so that management can be instituted with the appropriate degree of urgency and in the appropriate place. In general, the most severely injured patients are treated first. Where the number of patients and/or the severity of their injuries exceeds available facilities, those patients with the greatest chance of survival requiring the least expenditure of time, equipment and personnel should be treated first.

1. Injury severity score (ISS). In this system, injuries in six anatomical regions are scored on a 1–5 scale at death or discharge. The sum of the squares of the three highest values are taken (maximum score is 75). The ISS is an accurate predictor of mortality, time to death or discharge, and the degree of residual disability.

2. Trauma score (TS). This score is based on five variables: respiratory rate, respiratory effort, systolic blood pressure, capillary refill, Glasgow coma score. Patients with a score of 12 or less should be transferred to a trauma centre. Survival is closely related to the TS for blunt and penetrating injuries.

3. Revised trauma score (RTS). The Glasgow coma scale, systolic blood pressure and respiratory rate are recorded. Each measurement is assigned a coded value which is weighted according to regression analysis derived from the Major Trauma Outcome Study (26 000 patients). The RTS provides a more accurate assessment for triage than the TS.

4. Paediatric trauma score (PTS). A score between −1 and +2 is assigned according to the weight of the child, airway quality, systolic blood pressure, conscious level, type of fractures and extent of cutaneous injury. A PTS of 8 or less indicates potentially high mortality and morbidity, and the need for management in a trauma centre.

5. TRISS method. The RTS and ISS are plotted against each other for a given patient on a graph. A standard regression line on the graph indicates the division between patients expected to survive and perish. Unexpected deaths and successes can thus be identified for audit purposes.

Principles of management

A standard format for the management of severely injured patients is essential to ensure that all injuries are detected and treated correctly. The ATLS system is used here.

1. Primary survey. The primary survey is undertaken to identify life-threatening conditions. Management of these injuries should be simultaneous.

- Airway maintenance with cervical spine control. Assume cervical spine fracture and stabilize in patient with multisystem trauma.
- Breathing and ventilation. A bag-valve device should be used via a mask or endotracheal tube to deliver oxygen at an FIO_2 greater than 0.85. Tension or open pneumothorax and flail chest must be recognized and treated.
- Circulation. The state of consciousness, skin colour and pulse are valuable in rapidly assessing haemodynamic status. External bleeding should be controlled with direct pressure.
- Disability – neurological status. A rapid neurological evaluation to determine the level of consciousness: A, alert; V, vocal stimuli; P, painful stimuli; U, unresponsive. Good oxygenation should be achieved for the assessment.
- Exposure. The patient must be fully undressed and examined thoroughly.

2. Resuscitation. Oxygenation, control of haemorrhage and volume replacement are the priorities. Oxygen therapy is to achieve an FiO_2 greater than 0.85. Two large-bore intravenous catheters (16 gauge or larger) are sited and blood is withdrawn for cross-match, FBC, U&E. Two litres of crystalloid fluid should be infused initially and, if necessary, type-specific or low titre type-O blood may be used whilst cross-matched whole blood is prepared.

A urinary catheter and nasogastric tube should be inserted providing there are no indications of urethral rupture or cribriform plate fracture, respectively.

Regular monitoring of ventilation, pulse, blood pressure, arterial blood gases, electrocardiograph and urine output should be undertaken.

3. Secondary survey. The head, eyes, face and neck should be further examined for any undetected injuries. Any faciomaxillary trauma indicates the possibility of a cervical spine injury, and the neck should be immobilized until such an injury has been excluded.

The chest should be re-examined for pneumothorax, flail segment, haemothorax and cardiac tamponade. An erect chest radiograph must be obtained.

Frequent re-evaluation of the abdomen should be undertaken in the face of blunt trauma to exclude a visceral or vascular injury that may not be initially apparent. Rectal examination should be undertaken to detect blood in the bowel lumen, any rectal defect, anal sphincter laxity, a pelvic fracture or a high-riding prostate.

Extremities, the chest wall and pelvis should be examined for fractures and the presence of peripheral pulses noted. Appropriate radiographs should be taken at this stage.

A comprehensive evaluation of motor and sensory systems, a reassessment of the level of consciousness and pupils, and scoring on the Glasgow scale are performed.

Continuous re-evaluation of the patient is vital to detect emerging signs of injury.

4. Definitive care. Injuries detected should be treated and, where local expertise is unavailable, discussion with or transfer to a specialist unit should take place.

Further reading

ATLS Core Book. Chicago: American College of Surgeons, 1993.

Barros D'Sa AAB. Principles in the management of major trauma. In: Burnand KG, Young AE (eds) *The New Aird's Companion in Surgical Studies*. Edinburgh: Churchill Livingstone, 1992; 97–124.

Report of the Working Party on the Management of Patients with Major Injuries. London: Royal College of Surgeons of England, 1988.

Related topics of interest

ULCERATIVE COLITIS

This is an inflammatory condition of the colon of unknown cause that affects any age group, though the peak incidence occurs in the third and fourth decades. Females are affected more than males. Ulcerative colitis always involves the rectum and may involve a variable extent of proximal colon. The rectosigmoid is the only site of inflammation in 60% of cases, colitis up to the splenic flexure occurs in a further 25%, and there is total colitis in the remaining 15%. The colon is always affected in continuity, such that skip lesions characteristic of Crohn's disease are never seen.

Clinical assessment

Ulcerative colitis presents with diarrhoea with the passage of blood and mucus per rectum. Abdominal pain may occur, and the patient often feels generally unwell. The abdomen may be tender over the affected colon. There may be systemic signs characteristic of chronic inflammatory bowel disease. The patient may have oedema from hypo-albuminaemia and pallor from anaemia.

Ulcerative colitis can take one of a number of clinical courses. Acute colitis may occur once and not recur, but more often there are relapses, often with a background, persistent, low-grade colonic inflammation. Rarely, it is fulminant, with toxic dilatation of the colon necessitating emergency colectomy.

Investigation

- Full clinical examination and sigmoidoscopy will demonstrate typical changes including mucosal erythema, contact bleeding, granularity of the mucosa and luminal pus.
- Biopsy will confirm the diagnosis of colitis.
- FBC may show leucocytosis or anaemia.
- Disease activity may be monitored by ESR and C-reactive protein levels, both typically rising in acute episodes.
- Stool culture may exclude infective colitis.
- Colonoscopy or barium enema will assess the extent of the disease once the acute episode has settled.

Pathology

Macroscopically there is erythema of the mucosa and ulceration with ajacent areas of regenerating mucosa which appear polypoid (pseudopolyps). Histologically there is predominantly mucosal acute and chronic inflammation with some specific features, including paneth cell metaplasia and goblet cell depletion. Granulomata and transmural inflammation are not seen (this is important in differentiating ulcerative from Crohn's colitis). In severe ulcerative colitis, fissuring ulcers may be seen with inflammatory changes present deep to the mucosa, leading to diagnostic confusion with Crohn's disease. It may be impossible to determine the nature of colitis histologically, and the description indeterminate colitis may be used.

Complications

1. Dysplasia and malignancy. Ulcerative colitis predisposes to colorectal carcinoma. This does not arise as a consequence of the polyp–cancer sequence, but directly from dysplasia occurring in the colonic epithelium. Areas of dysplasia are usually not apparent macroscopically, and the diagnosis can only be established in multiple biopsies taken from different sites.

The risk of malignancy rises in proportion to the extent of the disease, the duration of colitis, and the degree of epithelial dysplasia. There is no risk of carcinoma until the duration of disease passes 10 years, and thereafter there is a steady rise in risk. Those with total colitis are at greater risk. The carcinomas are often poorly differentiated, plaque-like or stricturing, and more likely to be multifocal and locally advanced at presentation than sporadic carcinomas.

2. Toxic megacolon. This is severe, intractable, progressive acute colitis. Tachycardia, pyrexia, abdominal distension and tenderness result. The colon is seen to distend increasingly on sequential plain abdominal X-rays, which must be performed daily. A transverse diameter of 6 cm or greater is indicative of a toxic megacolon. Perforation and faecal peritonitis will ensue unless emergency colectomy is undertaken. It may complicate colitis of any cause, although it is most commonly associated with ulcerative colitis.

Medical management

1. Anticolitics. 5-Aminosalicylic acid (5-ASA) forms the basis of oral anticolitic drugs. The drug is formulated in different ways. 5-ASA bonded to the sulphonamide sulfapyridine is Salazopyrin, which has excellent anticolitic properties, but may cause infertility in males. The molecule is cleaved in the colon to release the active 5-ASA. Olsalazine is two 5-ASA molecules joined by a diazo bond. The molecule is cleaved by colonic flora and thus acts locally. Mesalazine is enteric coated 5-ASA. This may be of greater benefit in those with terminal ileal chronic inflammatory disease as the active molecule is liberated in the distal small bowel. These drugs should be continued to prevent relapses at lower doses.

2. Steroid preparations (hydrocortisone foam or prednisolone enemas). These may be instilled per rectum to treat acute episodes with good effect but must not be used on a long-term basis. Should 5-ASA and local steroid instillations not control symptoms, then oral or intravenous prednisolone should be started in high doses. This will improve severe colitis in most patients.

3. Antidiarrhoeal drugs. These may be prescribed to reduce bowel frequency, but they will not modify the course of the disease. Total alimentary rest and parenteral feeding via a tunnelled feeding line are indicated in severe colitis.

Surgical management

The indications for surgery are:

- Toxic megacolon.
- Failure of medical treatment to control symptoms.
- Presence of mucosal dysplasia.
- Development of carcinoma.

The operation in all these situations is essentially the same, amounting to at least a subtotal colectomy to the level of the rectum. The rectum and proximal ileal end are dealt with differently according to the circumstances.

1. Proctocolectomy and permanent ileostomy (panproctocolectomy). Dysplasia or carcinoma necessitates removal of all colonic mucosa (deemed to be unstable and premalignant). A proctocolectomy with formation of a permanent right iliac fossa spouted ileostomy (Brooke ileostomy) is required. The anus and adjacent rectum should be excised, and the perineal wound is closed as with an abdomino-perineal excision of the rectum. This is also the definitive operation for those who have failed medical treatment.

2. Sub-total colectomy mucous fistula, and permanent ileostomy. This is usually undertaken for toxic megacolon. The rectum is brought out as a mucous fistula, and a spouted end ileostomy is fashioned in the right iliac fossa. This allows the option of a later elective ileorectal anastomosis, ileorectal pouch, or proctectomy if symptoms persist from the retained rectum. Persistent rectal disease can usually be controlled with instillation of anticolitics or steroid.

3. Restorative proctocolectomy. Younger patients need to be considered for restorative proctocolectomy. This is a three-stage procedure that avoids a permanent ileostomy by the formation of a pelvic ileal reservoir acting as a neorectum. The first stage is a subtotal colectomy and end ileostomy. The second stage invoves the creation of the ileal reservoir. The residual rectum is denuded of its mucosa (mucosectomy) and the pouch is placed within the rectal muscle tube and anastomosed to the upper end of the anal canal. The pouch is defunctioned by a split (loop) ileostomy. The third stage is ileostomy reversal after confirmation of an intact reservoir and pouch-anal healing by contrast radiology.

Restorative proctocolectomy should only be performed if the patient is keen and well-motivated and accepts the possibility of complications or failure of the procedure. Success also depends on satisfactory anal tone, the length of the anal canal and a preserved anorectal angle, and patients should undergo anorectal physiological tests pre-operatively. Complications include continued inflammation ('pouchitis'), pelvic sepsis from anastomotic dehiscence, dehydration and electrolyte imbalance, and adhesion obstruction. Ten per cent of cases will continue to have mucus leakage, and the operation fails outright in approximately 5%. Over 75% of those operated will have satisfactory bowel evacuations up to six times a day with good control.

Other surgical options include sub-total colectomy with ileorectal anastomosis which has few indications since the development of restorative proctocolectomy and the ileorectal pouch. Patients have difficulty controlling their motions, and many require conversion to an end ileostomy. There is a risk of carcinoma developing in the rectal stump which must be screened at regular intervals.

The Koch continent ileostomy is an end ileostomy leading into an ileal reservoir, the two linked via an invaginated spout of ileum acting as a valve to maintain continence. The reservoir is emptied at intervals using a catheter.

Complications of ileostomy

Water, sodium and potassium depletion may easily arise from continued loss of small bowel fluid. This fluid and electrolyte imbalance can occur imperceptibly, and complications must be pre-empted by careful monitoring of ileostomy output volume.

Ileostomies may retract, prolapse, and develop parastomal hernias. The most common and troublesome complication is excoriation of the peristomal skin due to enzymatic digestion from contact with ileal effluent. This is minimized by the spouting of the ileostomy to direct the effluent into the stoma bag.

Further reading

Golligher J. Ulcerative colitis. In: *Surgery of the Anus, Rectum and Colon*, 5th Edn. London: Ballière Tindall, 1984.

Saga PM, Taylor BA. Pelvic ileal reservoirs: the options. *British Journal of Surgery*, 1994; **81**: 325–32.

Schofield PF. Inflammatory disease of the large bowel. *Surgery*, 1990; **85**: 2020–6.

Tjandra JJ, Fazio VW. The ileal pouch – indications for its use and results in clinical practice. *Current Practice in Surgery*, 1993; **5**: 22–8.

Related topics of interest

UNDESCENDED TESTES

Placing a testicle in its natural location within the scrotum may aid subsequent development. Orchidopexy is now performed much earlier than previously. The ideal age range is between 1 and 3 years. Anecdotal evidence suggests the incidence of malignant change and infertility will be consequently reduced.

Definitions

Confusion arises in the classification of this condition. An undescended testis is any testis that fails to descend into the scrotum, and it includes those which fail to descend along the normal path (incomplete or arrested descent) and those found in locations remote from the normal path (ectopic). Ectopic testes lie in one of four sites: superficial inguinal, base of penis, perineal or femoral (crural). An incompletely descended testis can be intra-abdominal, intracannalicular, emergent or high scrotal.

Development

The testis originates from the posterior abdominal wall mesoderm, the urogenital (Wolffian) ridge, and migrates into the scrotum via the inguinal canal. It is directed along this path by the gubernaculum (rudder). The accepted theory is that failure to follow the correct fibromuscular gubernacular strand leads to an ectopic testis and maldevelopment of the gubernaculum produces an incompletely descended testis.

Incidence

Undescended testes (cryptorchism) occur in 1–2% of males but 4–5% of males undergo orchidopexy. This suggests that retractile testis are inappropriately coming to surgery.

Complications

The complications of undescended testis are: an associated inguinal hernia (50%), trauma, infertility (40% if unilateral, 70% if bilateral), failure of development of secondary sexual characteristics (if bilateral and very immature) and malignant change (seminoma). The predisposition to malignancy and infertility is considered a secondary effect to the abnormal testicular location; however, there are testes which are dysplastic from the start. Returning a testis into its scrotum has not conclusively been shown to prevent these complications but the testis will become more accessible to screening (palpation and/or ultrasound). The increased risk of malignant change is 30-fold, which is equivalent in incidence to that of ovarian carcinoma.

Diagnosis

The diagnosis of cryptorchism is made by the exclusion of a retractile testis. The examination should take place in a warm room on a relaxed child by a competent clinician. The bony landmarks are first identified. With the flat of one hand the testis is milked into the scrotal neck whilst the other hand catches it and records the lowest limit it can be drawn. All retractile testis can be placed deep into the scrotum in this way. Loss of scrotal rugae suggests cryptorchidism.

Treatment

At 1 year, all testes should be palpable within the scrotum. If not, orchidopexy should be performed before 3 years of age. This is the age when secondary testicular degeneration is believed to be irreversible. An inguinal incision identifies the testis. The gubernaculum is divided well below the low lying vas and the inguinal canal is opened. The cord is mobilized up to the deep ring by division of peritoneal adhesions, ligation of a concurrent inguinal hernia, and by trimming any restricting cremasteric fibres. A Dartos pouch is then fashioned through a transverse scrotal incision and the mobilized testis is buttonholed through the Dartos to lie within the pouch, ensuring the testicular sinus remains in the lateral position. The appendix testis is removed and the testis is then anchored with a suture through the tunica albuginea to prevent torsion and displacement. Testicular atrophy is a recognized surgical complication and occurs in 5%. It can be avoided by meticulous dissection, respect for the cord's vascular supply and preventing fixation under tension.

1. *'High' retroperitoneal approach.* This approach is often advocated for the high testis. It maintains the integrity of the superficial inguinal ring and allows a more proximal dissection to be carried out. Staged operations are required for the very high testis.

2. *Fowler–Stephens.* This procedure involves proximal ligation of the testicular artery to increase cord length further. This relies on the assumption that the artery to the vas and other collaterals will be sufficient to supply the testis, which should be established by temporary clamping of the testicular artery.

3. *Silber–Kelly.* This procedure involves testicular artery and vein division with direct microvascular anastomosis to the internal epigastric vessels.

The impalpable testis

Testes can sometimes be identified pre-operatively by ultrasound, CT scan or MRI. Testicular venography demonstrates the absence of a normal venous plexus and thereby identifies the congenitally absent group (4% of impalpable testis are congenitally absent). Surgical exploration can reveal a blind-ending vas or a streak gonad, and laparoscopy can reveal a true intra-abdominal testis. Finally, PET scanning for testosterone has been used to locate testosterone-producing tissue.

Hormone therapy   Human chorionic gonadotrophin (HCG) or luteinizing hormone–releasing hormone (LHRH) can encourage a retractile testis to lower by relaxation of the cremaster muscle. This is ineffective, however, for a true undescended testicle.

Further reading

Hutson JM. Undescended testis. *Surgery*, 1992; 78–80.

Related topics of interest

Common paediatric conditions (p. 98)
Inguinal hernia (p. 176)
Testicular tumours (p. 292)

UPPER GASTROINTESTINAL HAEMORRHAGE

Seventy to eighty per cent of upper gastrointestinal bleeds stop spontaneously. Any trial of new therapeutic techniques must therefore improve on this to demonstrate any benefit. The aim is to stop continuing haemorrhage and decrease the risk of a rebleed. Peptic ulceration is the leading cause. The percentage of variceal bleeders increases in inner city areas. Upper gastrointestinal haemorrhage frequently occurs in hospital patients being treated for unrelated conditions. Of these, 25% bleed from acute erosive gastritis and 50% from peptic ulcers.

Cause	Incidence (%)
Duodenal ulcer	20
Gastric ulcer	20
Acute erosive gastritis	20
Oesophageal varices	20
Mallory–Weiss tear	10
Oesophagitis, duodenitis, tumour, other	10

Haemetemesis of fresh blood indicates a fast rate of bleeding. Melaena usually indicates an upper gastrointestinal cause. Bloody stools occur as the only feature of bleeding in 10% of patients.

Resuscitation

Resuscitation proceeds with diagnosis. The features of alcoholic liver disease should be sought (spider naevi, palmar erythema, ascites, hepatosplenomegaly, jaundice) although over 20% of patients with known varices bleed from a peptic ulcer. Patients are often elderly and tolerate blood loss poorly. Blood is taken for FBC, cross-match and clotting studies, and if liver disease is suspected vitamin K is administered and FFP requested. Thrombocytopenia is corrected with platelet transfusions. The preferred replacement fluid is blood. Crystalloids and colloids disturb fluid balance in patients prone to ascites and displace part of the remaining circulating blood. Orogastric or nasogastric aspiration of stomach contents allows gastric contraction and reduces the chances of aspiration. The absence of blood in the aspirate does not exclude an upper gastrointestinal cause. Head down and semi-prone positioning protects against an aspiration pneumonia which is the commonest cause of death in these patients.

Endoscopy

Emergency endoscopy is both therapeutic and diagnostic. Performed early it identifies the cause of bleeding in 90% of cases. Orogastric evacuation of retained blood with lavage greatly aids visibility. The diagnostic yield decreases with time following the initial bleed. Emergency endoscopy should therefore be mandatory. Rapid exsanguination calls for an immediate operation without prior endoscopy. In most of these cases, the bleeding lesion is obvious and appropriate surgery can be instituted. Emergency endoscopy establishes a diagnosis which will allow the surgeon to plan an operative approach. It will also suggest supportive measures for those conditions for which conservative management is settled on (Mallory–Weiss tear, erosive gastritis) and those in which surgery is usually inappropriate (varices). Endoscopic manoeuvres like injection sclerotherapy for varices and injection treatment for peptic ulcers can be performed at the same time.

Pharmacology

There is no evidence that any pharmacological intervention can alter the clinical course once bleeding starts. Antacids, H2 antagonists, proton pump inhibitors, vasopressin and somatostatin are ineffective in arresting haemorrhage from a spurting vessel or a ruptured varix. Haemoglobin is an effective natural buffer which can neutralize gastric pH without the need of additional anti-acid therapy. The time-honoured conservative treatment for upper gastrointestinal bleeding was bed rest and the antacid effect of a full diet.

Peptic ulcer

Peptic ulcer disease is decreasing but the number of operations for bleeding ulcers remains unchanged. Widespread H2 receptor antagonist use appears to have had little success in decreasing the incidence of bleeding peptic ulcers. Rebleeding can be predicted by the endoscopic findings and several clinical factors. A visible vessel indicates an early rebleeding rate of over 50%.

Endoscopic	Clinical
Visible vessel	Shock (systolic <90 mmHg)
Clot in ulcer base	Haemoglobin < 8 g/dl
Black/red spots	Haematemesis
Left gastric artery location	Age >60 years
Gastroduodenal artery location	

Endoscopic therapy can effectively reduce the incidence of rebleeding and allow an elective operation, with its reduced mortality, to take place. It is not yet known whether endoscopic therapy will be a true substitute for operation. A visible vessel (which is really a protruding clot overlying a rent in a non-protruding vessel) is seen in 45% of cases of ulcer haemorrhage but is present in 85% of deaths due to this condition. Surgery for bleeding peptic ulcer usually involves a duodenotomy and underrunning of the bleeding vessel. The ulcer, if possible, is excluded from the gastro-intestinal tract by suturing the mucosa over the ulcer.

Oesophageal varices

Ninety per cent of variceal bleeding occurs within 2 cm of the gastro-oesophageal junction. Evidence of a recent bleed is seen by finding a transparent fibrinous clot on the surface of a varix. Long-term survival is dependent on the severity of the liver disease (Child's classification). The therapeutic armamentarium is considered below.

1. Intravariceal sclerotherapy. This is the method of choice for acute bleeding control and future prophylaxis. Ethanolamine oleate is injected directly into the varix. Several courses of treatment are usually required.

2. Vasopressin/somatostatin. These both lower portal pressure and are useful in the acute situation.

3. Sengstaken–Blakemore tube. Balloon tamponade of the varices by a gastric balloon, filled with 200 ml of saline, pressed firmly up against the diaphragm is only a temporizing manoeuvre prior to definitive sclerotherapy. The oesophageal balloon, if required, is attached to a mercury manometer and inflated to not more than mean arterial pressure. It should be deflated every 2 hours to prevent iatrogenic ulceration.

4. Portal/systemic shunts. Mesocaval or splenorenal shunts decrease portal pressure. The more proximal the shunt, the more effective it is, but this is paralleled by a progressive increase in hepatic encephalopathy. Shunts are considered after two failed sessions of sclerotherapy.

5. Transjugular intrahepatic portasystemic anastomosis (TIPS). Portasystemic shunts may be performed intrahepatically under radiological control to lower portal venous pressure.

6. Major surgery. Oesophageal transection and reanastomosis with a stapler through a small gastrostomy is combined with a devascularization procedure. Its indications are rare as the operation carries a high mortality.

Acute erosive gastritis

This is caused by stress conditions like burns (Curling's ulcer), head injury (Cushing's ulcer), major trauma, sepsis, MOF or by the ingestion of injurious substances like alcohol or NSAIDs. Haemorrhage from the latter group can be arrested with a platelet transfusion in occasional cases. Endoscopic appearances are of multiple brown-coloured areas the size and shape of tea leaves. Pharmacological suppression of acid secretion or the use of sucralfate is the mainstay of therapy. A total gastrectomy is rarely indicated.

Mallory–Weiss tear

These are found at the gastro-oesophageal junction on the lesser curve in 80% of cases. The cause is usually violent vomiting after the consumption of a large meal with alcohol. In 90% of cases bleeding stops spontaneously. Endoscopic electrocoagulation or operative underrunning is indicated in resistant cases.

Aorto-enteric fistula

Almost all occur in the first few centimetres of jejunum. They should be considered in all patients with an aortic graft. There is usually a history of a minor haematemesis (herald bleed). Treatment involves graft removal with either extra-anatomical bypass or *in-situ* replacement with a rifampicin-bonded graft.

Gastric leiomyoma

This is the commonest tumour to cause a major upper gastrointestinal bleed. They are recognized by endoscopy as a yellowish polyp with an ulcer crater on the surface. Treatment by local excision is curative. Gastric carcinomas, in contrast, ooze slowly causing anaemia.

Further reading

Northfield T, Kirkham J. Towards endoscopic therapy for bleeding peptic ulcers: targets and weapons, trials and costs. *Current Practice in Surgery*, 1990; **5**: 8–20.
Steffes C, Fromm D. The current diagnosis and management of upper gastrointestinal bleeding. *Advances in Surgery*, 1992; **25**: 331–61.

Related topics of interest

Blood transfusion (p. 55)
Peptic ulceration (p. 236)

URINARY CALCULI

The last century has seen a rising incidence of renal calculi and a falling incidence of bladder calculi. Renal calculi are associated with an increase in dietary protein, dehydration and high temperature climates whereas bladder calculi occur in non-industrialized and developing nations.

Renal calculi

Types

Renal calculi are of various types.

Stone composition	Incidence (%)	Characteristics
Calcium oxylate	75	Hard, irregular, brittle
Triple phosphate	17.5	White, soft, infected
Uric acid	7.0	Yellow, radiolucent
Cystine, pure oxylate	0.5	Underlying genetic disorder

Aetiology

The vast majority of patients harbouring calculi have no detectable anatomical, biochemical or metabolic abnormality causal to stone formation. Impairment of renal drainage from a congenital abnormality (horseshoe kidney, megaureter, hydronephrosis, vesicoureteric reflux) encourages stones to form. Randall's plaques (areas of calcification on the renal papillae) and Carr's concretions (aggregations of microscopic calculi on the papillae) both occur in normal kidneys and their part in forming calculi is questionable.

Calcium oxylate

Calcium oxylate stones are laminated and have areas of black discoloration on and within them from altered blood. 'Envelope' crystals can be identified in the urine in many patients but their presence is not pathological. Hypercalciuria is the commonest detectable metabolic abnormality. It may be:

1. *Dietary* from excessive calcium intake. Protein and phosphates encourage calcium absorption.

2. *Absorptive* from increased 1,25-dihydroxycholecalciferol production secondary to hyperphosphataemia.

3. *Resorptive* from periods of immobilization or from primary hyperparathyroidism. The latter is found in only 2% of stone formers.

4. *Tubular* from secondary hyperparathyroidism.

5. *Idiopathic.* Idiopathic hypercalciuria forms the largest group. Thiazide diuretics impair calcium excretion at the renal tubular level and oral sodium cellulose phosphate combines with intestinal calcium to prevent its absorption. Both of these treatment methods may control hypercalciuria.

Triple phosphate

Triple phosphate stones (calcium, magnesium, ammonium) are invariably associated with infected urine. Infection makes urine alkaline which encourages the precipitation of calcium salts. *Proteus* splits urea into ammonia which thereby increases the local ammonia concentration. These stones grow rapidly in alkaline urine and are responsible for staghorn calculi. Pyrophosphate is a specific inhibitor of crystallization and is found in reduced urinary concentrations in patients with triple phosphate stones. Irradication of infection and urinary acidification help to prevent future stone formation.

Uric acid

Twenty-five per cent of all patients with gout develop uric acid stones. In most patients the urinary pH is low, uric acid secretion is increased and a specific inhibitor of crystallization, acidic mucopolysaccharide, is often found in reduced urinary concentration. Specific medical therapy usually consists of reducing dietary purine intake, alkalinizing the urine with 3–6 g per day of sodium bicarbonate and the addition of allopurinol at 200–400 mg per day.

Cystine

Cystine stones form in patients who are deficient in resorbing cystine, ornithine, arginine and lysine (COAL) from their renal tubules. The defect is autosomal recessive. The presence of cystine crystals in the urine is pathological. Urinary alkalization with sodium bicarbonate and oral penicillamine are effective in dissolving these stones.

Pure oxylate

Pure oxylate stones are due to a genetic failure of glycosylase or hydroxypyruvate to metabolize oxylates. Hyperoxaluria can also be secondary to the short bowel syndrome or the malabsorption syndrome.

Presentation

Presentation is usually as an incidental finding on a KUB (supine plain abdominal radiograph to include the kidneys and the bladder) or as an emergency with ureteric colic. The pain of ureteric colic is severe, exclusively unilateral, arises in the loin, and radiates into the groin, testis or tip of the penis. A writhing foetal posture with vomiting is typical. The renal area or right iliac fossa may be tender but haematuria is almost always present on urine testing. An elevated temperature implies superadded infection (pylonephrosis). An infected obstructed kidney must be decompressed with some urgency to prevent that kidney from failing. Focal interstitial nephritis is present to varying degrees on all kidneys harbouring calculi. Rarely, a stone may impact a calyx (hydrocalycosis), become secondarily infected (pyocalycosis) and rupture to form a perinephric abscess. Differential diagnosis of acute renal colic includes rupture of an AAA, a prolapsed intravertebral disc, Münchausen's syndrome and analgesia abuse.

Investigations

An emergency IVU is essential to make a diagnosis before the spontaneous undetected passage of a stone. The establishment of a diagnosis may also avoid an unnessesary cystoscopy for haematuria. A control, immediate, 5 min and 20 min (pre- and post-micturition) film sequence is requested. Prompt, bilateral, symmetrical excretion of contrast usually excludes stone disease. Abnormal radiographic features typical of calculi include: increasing nephrogram density, columnization of contrast and a filling defect/opacity along the line of the ureter. The intense contrast diuresis may cause an exacerbation of the pain which aids in confirming the suspicion of a stone. Delayed films may be helpful in localizing a calculus (10% of renal calculi are radiolucent). Plasma calcium, phosphate and uric acid estimations, with a 24-hour urine collection for composition, should be requested as a metabolic screen. A dynamic renal scan will indicate the extent and distribution of renal impairment.

Management

The principle of management is to correct the underlying metabolic defect (70% of patients will develop a recurrence within 10 years) and remove the offending stone. Avoidance of periods of dehydration, with an overall increase in fluid intake, and reduction in the consumption of protein-rich and calcium-containing foods are good general measures. A forced diuresis is not indicated as it may exacerbate renal failure if a kidney is obstructed. Symptomless stones are monitored radiologically on a yearly basis.

| **Natural history** | Stone size, site and shape determine the natural history. Those calculi less than 5 mm in size and within 5 cm of the vesicoureteric junction have a 90% chance of passing spontaneously. |

Minimally invasive techniques

Extracorporeal shock wave lithotripsy (ESWL), percutaneous nephrolithotomy (PCN) and ureteroscopy are techniques used to deal with obstinate stones. Open stone surgery occurs now for only 1% of all complicated stones.

1. Extracorporeal shock wave lithotripsy. This technique was developed by the Dornier Aircraft Company in Münich in 1981. The patient is anaesthetized and placed into a waterbath to transmit the shock waves. These are produced by a huge spark plug and focused by an ellipsoid reflector on to the stone which is located by biplanar X-rays. Second-generation machines like the Wolf are less powerful and require several more treatment sessions, but they can be performed as an outpatient procedure without anaesthetic. With this design, 2000 piezo-electric crystals are focused within a reflector and activated by an electric discharge. The Wolf uses ultrasound to localize the stone.

2. Percutaneous nephrolithotomy. This technique consists of a fine needle puncture of the kidney under radiological control and then the passage of graded plastic dilators over the wire until a nephroscope can be passed into the renal pelvis. The stone can be removed intact or piecemeal following crushing or destruction by an ultrasonic or electrohydraulic disintegration probe.

3. Ureteroscopy. This is a fine-bore fibreoptic scope that allows direct visualization of the ureter along its length from either direction (bladder or renal). It allows baskets to be passed to entrap lower third stones, and allows for middle or upper third stones to be pushed back into the kidney for PCN (push–pull) or ESWL (push–bang). A double J stent is usually passed alongside a ureteric stone to aid ESWL and provide continuous drainage.

Bladder calculi

Aetiology

Children of India, Thailand, Egypt and Turkey are the main groups of patients who develop bladder calculi. They are mostly composed of uric acid and are believed to be caused by episodes of severe dehydration. Adults can develop the calculi from outflow obstruction, chronic infection, a foreign body or an upper tract stone which has fallen into the bladder. A poorly differentiated bladder carcinoma may occasionally calcify and cause confusion.

Treatment Treatment involves correction of the underlying abnormality. Electrohydrolic lithotripsy is used for irradicating the smaller stones and an open operation is used for removing the larger ones (greater than 5 cm in diameter). A careful cystoscopy should be made following stone removal because an occult squamous bladder carcinoma is often associated.

Further reading

Tolley DA. The kidneys and ureter. In: Burnand KG, Young AE (eds) *The New Aird's Companion in Surgical Studies*. Edinburgh: Churchill Livingstone, 1992; 1233–85.
Wickham JEA. The management of renal calculous disease. *Recent Advances in Surgery*, 1988; **13**: 211–17.

Related topics of interest

URINARY OUTFLOW OBSTRUCTION

The urinary outflow tract commences at the bladder reservoir and ends at the urethral meatus. Outflow obstruction is usually distinguished from inflow restriction by the presence of a full bladder.

Causes

Urethral stricture and prostatic enlargement are the commonest causes and will be discussed in detail. Other causes can be classified as:

1. Intraluminal. Bladder tumours, calculi, blood clot and urethral tumours occasionally occur.

2. Neurological. Central lumbar disc prolapse, spinal cord injury and various drugs which act upon the autonomic nervous system can precipitate outflow obstruction by interfering with the sphincter and detrusor coordination of micturition.

3. Gynaecological. A variety of gynaecological conditions may lead to retention: ovarian cyst, gravid uterus or following pelvic surgery (hysterectomy and Caesarean section).

4. Congenital. Congenital urethral valves consist of two oblique membranes situated in the prostatic urethra at the level of the verumontanum. It can be diagnosed *in utero* by foetal ultrasound if a dilated bladder, hydroureter and hydronephrosis are imaged. Descending urethrography reveals the abnormality after birth. They can be removed by ureteroscopic valvotomy. Congenital mid-bulbar stenosis and a double ventral ureter are rare causes of outflow obstruction.

Consequences

Chronic outflow obstruction leads to detrusor hypertrophy and a gradual increase in intraluminal pressure necessary for micturition. The detrusor muscle becomes unstable and responds by contraction to even minor stimuli such as a UTI. This irritability results in the early symptoms of frequency and urgency. With the progression of time, trabeculation leads to sacculation and then to diverticulae which may become infected. Bladder capacity and the post-voiding residual volume increase with the development of bladder atony until finally overflow incontinence ensues. If the voiding pressure exceeds 40 cm of water, upper tract dilatation starts. Urine stagnation encourages infection, calculus formation, squamous metaplasia and bladder carcinoma. Renal failure with uraemia, hyperkalaemia, acidosis and an elevated creatinine is a late manifestation.

Urethral stricture

'Once a urethral stricture always a urethral stricture'. This adage still holds true. Pharaohs even took dilators with them to their burial chambers for the 'after life'. The causes are numerous.

Insult	Urethral site	Mechanism
Catheter	Penoscrotal junction	Pressure necrosis
		Paraurethral gland sepsis
Perineal injury	Bulbar	Crush injury
Pelvic fracture	Membranous	Prostatic displacement
		Sheer injury
Infection	Throughout	Gonorrhoea
		Chlamydia
BXO	Meatal	Fibrosis
Chemotherapy	Throughout	Chemical urethritis
Instrumentation	Throughout	Iatrogenic
		Masterbation

Presentation   Presentation is usually with a gradual deterioration in stream (straining may cause slight improvement) and post-micturitional dribbling.

Catheterization   Catheterization is the commonest cause. Prevention is best by using the smallest catheter that will do the job so that the paraurethral glands are free to discharge their secretions and provide lubrication rather than obstruct and become infected. Sialastic catheters cause less tissue reaction and are therefore preferred to latex. Increased use of suprapubic catheters should reduce this complication.

Perineal injury   A fall astride a bicycle cross-bar will cause the perineal injury. Meatal blood, a perineal haematoma and acute retention are presenting features. Urine may extravasate within the confines of Scarpa's and Colles' fascia and, if infected, may lead to ventral skin necrosis in a swimming trunk distribution. Management includes suprapubic catheterization with a check urethroscopy at 10 days. Most injuries will have healed by this time.

Pelvic fracture	Pelvic fractures are of three types.
	1. Central pubic displacement. The pubic rami are fractured and the prostate is driven posteriorly.
	2. Vertical sheer. With this injury, half of the pelvis is driven superiorly.
	3. Complete pelvic crush. Here, injury to the rectum occurs. Diagnosis is established with an ascending contrast urethrogram. Retention is relieved with a suprapubic catheter. Partial tears may be managed conservatively with a urethrotomy at a later date for any residual stricture. Direct early repair over a fine silicone catheter with prostatic reduction is the preferred management for complete tears. An external pelvic fixator will help to curtail the pelvic haemorrhage and support the prostate gland. If not, the prostate can be mobilized through a Pfannenstiel incision. With extensive injury, involving the rectum, faecal and urinary diversion procedures are required.
Surgery	Internal optical urethrotomy has replaced graded Bougie dilatation because the latter causes extensive spiral tears which heal by fibrosis rather than a discrete nick with minimal tissue damage. Extensive or resistant strictures are dealt with by a urethroplasty. Penile (anterior) or scrotal (posterior) skin is elevated on an island of subcutaneous tissue, inverted and sutured directly over the opened stricture. Pre-operative follicle electrolysis is needed to prevent the distressing complication of urethral hair growth.

Benign prostatic hyperplasia

Benign prostatic hyperplasia affects mainly the inner 'cranial' zone of the prostate whereas carcinomas develop usually within the outer zone. Prostatic size is not closely related to the degree of obstruction.

Diagnosis	Presentation is usually over many months with nocturia, increase in frequency, hesitation, post-micturitional dribbling and deterioration of stream (not usually improved by straining). Examination may reveal a palpable bladder, wet trousers and, on a rectal examination, an enlarged prostate. Essential investigations include an MSU, a KUB radiograph and an ultrasound of the upper tracts and bladder to detect evidence of chronic obstruction (upper tract

dilatation, increased bladder wall thickness and bladder size, a post-voiding residual volume). Prostatic specific antigen (PSA) estimations, if elevated, diagnose carcinoma with great accuracy.

Retention

Acute on chronic retention is the usual emergency presentation. Chronic retention is painless and associated with outflow incontinence and renal impairment. Therapy involves aseptic catheterization for pain and relief of post-renal failure. The residual volume is recorded. Intravenous fluids are usually given to combat the post-obstruction diuresis which can be fatal if patients are sent home from casualty without adequate fluid replacement regimens.

Indications for prostatectomy

The essential indications for prostatectomy are evidence of advanced disease, renal impairment and a poor stream. It is not indicated for mild nocturia and frequency because the prostate may be the only barrier preventing the effects of detrusor instability, and its removal may lead to incontinence. Simple measures to lessen nocturia like the avoidance of bed-time drinks (especially alcohol, coffee), treating anxiety, diagnosing and treating cardiac failure, and urinating prior to going to bed are usually all that is required. If doubt arises, voiding pressures and urodynamic studies are performed. Renal function, fluid balance and sepsis control are all optimized before any surgical intervention.

Transurethral resection of the prostate

Prostatic resection with a semi-circular diathermy loop (TURP) is the standard treatment in most cases. This is performed during continuous isotonic irrigation with non-electrolyte 2% glycine. The bladder neck and prostate are resected down to the level of the verumontanum thereby avoiding the external sphincter. A large catheter is placed at the end of the procedure with continous saline irrigation until the prostatic oozing diminishes. Patients are warned of the complication of retrograde ejaculation. Lengthy operations (>1 hour) result in significant irrigation fluid absorption with a risk of the TURP syndrome (hypotension, hyponatraemia and convulsions). Such large prostates are best removed by an open retropubic prostatectomy (Millin) where the adenoma is shelled out through a Pfannenstiel incision.

Advances

Intraurethral stenting and prostatic hyperthermia are research tools and have not yet found universal acceptance.

Bladder neck hypertrophy

Bladder neck hypertrophy involves the circular muscle of the internal sphincter. This condition starts in the 30s and presents with the symptoms of prostatism. Improvement with an alpha–blocker (phenoxybenzamine) can differentiate the condition from benign prostatic hyperplasia (BPH). An endoscopic bladder neck incision (BNI) is all that is required for treatment.

Further reading

Beynon LL. The prostate. In: Burnand KG, Young AE (eds) *The New Aird's Companion in Surgical Studies.* Edinburgh: Churchill Livingstone, 1992, 1319–31.
Blandy JP. *Lecture Notes on Urology.* Oxford: Blackwell Scientific Publications, 1989.

Related topics of interest

Carcinoma of the prostate (p. 79)
Penile conditions and scrotal swellings (p. 254)

VARICOSE VEINS

Varicose veins are defined by the World Health Organization as saccular dilatations of veins that are often tortuous. This excludes dilatations of small intradermal veins and tortuous dilated veins that are secondary to thrombophlebitis or arteriovenous fistula.

Epidemiology

Approximately 2% of Western populations have primary varicose veins, women 3–4 times more frequently than men. Varicose veins are less common in Eastern populations, particularly Africans and Indians. The prevalence of varicose veins increases with age with a peak frequency between 50 and 60 years of age. Pregnancy predisposes with an incidence between 8 and 20%, second and subsequent pregnancies compounding the risk. The rising levels of progesterone encountered during pregnancy encourage smooth muscle relaxation and venous distension, possibly resulting in the development of varicose veins. Compression of the iliac veins by the gravid uterus may also be important. Occupations involving prolonged periods of standing probably predispose. Heredity is an important factor with many patients having at least one parent affected. The mode of inheritance is, however, unclear and is probably polygenetic. Varicose veins are a human condition, being unreported in any animal species, including those who are bipedal.

Secondary varicose veins are caused by post-thrombotic damage, pelvic tumours, acquired arteriovenous fistulae and congenital venous anomalies including the Klippel–Trenaunay syndrome, Parkes–Weber syndrome and congenital valvular agenesis.

Aetiology

The principal aetiological theories advanced are valvular deficiency, defective vein wall structure and arteriovenous fistulae, the last of which has now largely be discounted. Trendelenberg proposed that a valve protects the vein wall from the venous pressure above it and that commonly the valve at the saphenofemoral junction becomes incompetent. He suggested that ligation and division of the valve at this point would restore the vein to its former dimension and abolish varices. The fact that saphenofemoral ligation fails to prevent the development of new varicose veins and that tributary veins can become varicose before the long saphenous suggests that valvular incompetence may be a secondary phenomenon. Evidence for there being a primary vein wall structural defect includes the early dilatation of the vein wall downstream to the valve and histological features of the vein wall, and the histochemical features of reduced collagen and increased muscle and hexosamine content of varicose veins.

Clinical features

The long saphenous venous system is most commonly affected, but the stem vein itself is frequently spared, the tributaries showing the most pronounced varicosis. The short saphenous vein is less commonly affected.

The commonest symptoms are unsightliness and mild aching. Mild ankle oedema is also common. More severe leg pain, which may accompany other conditions such as peripheral vascular disease and osteoarthritis is not usually caused by varicose veins. Complications include haemorrhage, superficial thrombophlebitis and the calf pump failure syndrome (pigmentation, eczema, lipoderma-tosclerosis, ulceration). Any history of DVT, PE, or associated events must be elicited and any previous treatment for varicose veins should be recorded.

Examination of the legs for varicose veins first involves a thorough inspection of the legs for the site of all major varicosities, the presence of a saphena varix, ankle oedema, signs of calf pump failure, angiomata, arterial insufficiency, joint disease, and previous trauma or surgery to the leg. It is important to distinguish long saphenous, short saphenous and communicating vein incompetence. The cough impulse test indicates the presence of valvular incompetence in the vein under examination and the percussion test is useful for demonstrating the origin of a varicose vein. Palpation for fascial defects indicating incompetent communicating veins is frequently performed but can be unreliable. The tourniquet test is extremely useful in determining the system of origin of varicose veins. When performed carefully it frequently obviates the need for further investigation.

Investigations

Where there is continuing doubt about the presence of superficial venous reflux, a hand-held Doppler probe is of considerable benefit. Duplex ultrasound (with or without colour flow facility) is also useful for demonstrating reflux, for identifying the saphenopopliteal junction and for imaging the deep and perforating veins. Where there is the possibility of previous DVT, ascending phlebography is mandatory to demonstrate post-thrombotic damage and to exclude deep vein obstruction. Where this is present, it must be assumed that any varicose veins must be secondary to the obstruction and should not be removed. Where the short saphenous vein is varicose it is important to identify the site of the saphenopopliteal junction as this is very variable. A short saphenous varicogram is the most convenient method and has the advantage over ultrasonography of providing an easily interpretable permanent record that can be referred to in the operating theatre. Where there is doubt about the distribution and connections of varicose veins, a varicogram is of great benefit. Where there are indications of calf pump failure further imaging tests and tests of calf pump function are necessary.

Treatment

The indications for treatment of varicose veins include the relief of symptoms, the relief and prevention of complications, correction of unacceptable cosmetic appearance and the development of the calf pump failure syndrome. The results of treatment are very variable and the chances of recurrence at 5 years are 8–50%. Patients should be warned appropriately before being offered treatment. Approximately 30% of patients attending a varicose vein clinic will not require treatment. It is generally assumed that untreated varicose veins will continue to enlarge and involve other adjacent veins in the varicose process.

The principles of treatment include the reduction of transmural venous pressure gradient (elastic compression stockings), disconnection of superficial veins from the deep veins at sites of valvular incompetence (saphenofemoral, saphenopopliteal, communicating vein ligation) and abolition of visible varices (obliteration or excision).

Patients who are unsuitable for surgery and pregnant women can be treated satisfactorily using class I or II graduated compression stockings. Below knee stockings are usually adequate and should be worn at all times other than in bed. Patients should be supplied with two pairs which should be replaced every 6 months.

Injection sclerotherapy has been used to treat all forms of varicose vein but in the UK is employed mainly for the obliteration of tributary vein varicosities with sapheno-femoral or saphenopopliteal incompetence being treated surgically. Contraindications include oral contraception, pregnancy, a history of severe allergy, and foot veins (because of the risk of intra-arterial injection). The technique depends on the induction of a chemical inflammation in the vein endothelium following injection of a sclerosant agent. The detergent sodium tetradecyl sulphate remains the most popular agent in use although newer agents including

Aethoxysclerol and Sclerovein are also being used. The sterile inflammation provoked by these agents causes vein wall adherence and obliteration. It is vital that the sclerosant is only injected into the vein lumen. Extraluminal sclerosant induces a brisk tissue reaction resulting in the formation of indolent ulcers that are painful, slow to heal and frequently leave residual pigmentation. Other complications include vasovagal attacks, allergic reactions, DVT and intra-arterial injection. Following injection, compression bandages are applied for a variable period (3–6 weeks) although the role and importance of this in producing variceal obliteration is unclear. Patients are encouraged to walk as much as possible during this period and to avoid standing for prolonged periods.

Surgical treatment is preferable if there is clear saphenofemoral or saphenopopliteal incompetence, if the varices are large and if there is communicating vein incompetence. Most surgical procedures in common use are best performed under general anaesthesia. Many healthy patients can be treated as day cases, but patients requiring extensive bilateral surgery with recurrent or communicating vein disease may require longer admission. Saphenofemoral ligation is performed where the saphenofemoral junction is incompetent and there are long saphenous system varicosities. Before ligation, the femoral vein must be clearly identified and all tributaries should be ligated and divided. Stripping of the long saphenous vein is advisable as the recurrence rate is lower than achieved by saphenofemoral ligation alone. The vein should be stripped to just below the knee, but no further to avoid damage to the saphenous nerve. This procedure is usually performed with local avulsions of the most prominent varicosities performed through small incisions placed in the direction of Langer's lines. Saphenopopliteal ligation is performed with the patient prone and with the aid of a saphenogram or duplex ultrasound scan to demonstrate the position of the junction. This vein is also usually stripped.

Ligation of the communicating veins is best performed using subfascial exposure and ligation. Having demonstrated the presence of incompetent communicating veins by clinical examination and/or by phlebography a long axial incision is made 2 cm posterior to the medial border of the tibia. The deep fascia is divided and the communicating veins sought and divided following ligation. Endoscopic division of communicating veins has recently been described.

Considerable care and skill is required for the optimum treatment of many patients with varicose veins, although frequently this is left to the most junior members of the surgical team.

Further reading

Bergan JJ, Yao JST (eds) *Surgery of the Veins*. Orlando: Grune and Stratton, 1985.
Browse NL, Burnand KG, Lea Thomas M. *Diseases of the Veins: Pathology, Diagnosis and Treatment*. London: Edward Arnold, 1988.

Related topics of interest

VASCULAR IMAGING AND INVESTIGATION

Arterial

Clinical examination

Inspection may reveal pulsatile aneurysms. The extremities may be pallid and cool to the touch, particularly on elevation, in chronic arterial insufficiency, with cyanosis of the foot on dependency (Buerger's sign). The presence of fixed mottling of the skin, arterial ulceration, pregangrenous dusky discoloration or frank gangrene amounts to critical ischaemia, and the limb will be lost unless urgent revascularization is undertaken.

A pulse will not be palpated distal to an arterial occlusion or a tight stenosis, which can be differentiated from an occlusion by the presence of a bruit. A clear distribution of the patent, stenotic and occluded segments of the arteries of a limb may thus be obtained clinically.

Non-invasive tests

1. *Doppler ultrasound and pressures.* The patency of an artery or graft is confirmed with an audible Doppler signal. Low amplitude prolonged signals indicate reduced flow, suggesting filling from collaterals in the presence of a proximal arterial occlusion, or reduced flow distal to a stenosis. A high amplitude abrupt signal suggests non-compliant calcified arteries.

A proximal sphygmomanometer cuff gradually inflated until the Doppler signal disappears reveals the pressure in the artery. The brachial systolic pressure is also assessed. The ratio of the best pedal measurement on either foot to the brachial pressure is the ankle–brachial pressure index (ABPI). Generally, normal arterial ABPI range from 0.9 to greater than 1.0, and critically ischaemic limbs have an ABPI of less than 0.5.

ABPI is important in the assessment of effects of surgery or angioplasty. It is useful to confirm vascular disease not evident in the quiescent patient by measuring ABPI under resting and exercise conditions.

2. *Duplex scanning.* The combination of B-mode and Doppler ultrasound is duplex scanning. It is used in the assessment of carotid stenoses, arterial graft surveillance, and in the localization of peripheral arterial disease. In the carotid artery, the ultrasound detects plaques, and their

content may be deduced from the appearance. The Doppler principle allows the velocity and flow to be calculated. This is used to calculate the percentage stenosis of an artery.

3. Radiology. CT and ultrasound scans are invaluable in the assessment of aneurysms, gauging their diameter accurately, and indicating the presence of mural thrombus. Magnetic resonance angiography (MRA) can image the arterial tree in a totally non-invasive fashion.

Invasive tests

1. Contrast angiography. Views of both legs plus the aorta can be obtained by direct needle puncture of the aorta (translumbar aortography) or by a transfemoral catheter advanced proximally. Direct arterial puncture carries complications, including dissection of the artery, distal embolization of thrombus or atheromatous debris, arterial thrombosis, and haemorrhage, which may be life-threatening if it occurs in the retroperitoneum.

2. Digital subtraction arteriography (DSA). DSA provides better resolution films than conventional contrast angiography. DSA can be achieved through the intravenous (i.v. DSA) or intra-arterial (i.a. DSA) route. In i.v. DSA, the aorta and its branches are well visualized, as are the femoral and popliteal arteries. The crural arteries cannot be visualized beyond their origin with clarity. An i.a. DSA will show vessels down to the foot with great clarity. Thus, for patients with aorto-iliac or carotid artery disease, i.v. DSA is usually sufficient, but those with critical ischaemia, who have distal arterial disease by implication, will need an i.a. DSA. Care should be taken in patients with renal failure, as large boluses of intravascular contrast are nephrotoxic, and i.v. DSA should be avoided.

Venous

Clinical examination

Visible varicosities will be seen in the back of the calf in short and the thigh and anterior and medial lower leg in long saphenous incompetence. These must be confirmed by tourniquet tests. Gentle palpation in the popliteal fossa with the patient standing with the knee slightly flexed will demonstrate an enlarged and incompetent short saphenous vein.

Incompetent communicating veins may be seen on the medial aspect of the leg. These may be primarily incompetent, or a manifestation of deep venous insufficiency. Other stigmata of deep venous insufficiency are swelling, dermatoliposclerosis (induration and pigmentation of the skin), eczema, and venous ulceration. Some may develop pale scarring of the skin with punctate or reticular red vascular tufts (atrophie blanche).

Non-invasive tests

1. Duplex scanning. This has become the optimal non-invasive method of assessment of the venous system of the lower limb. Sources of superficial venous incompetence and the presence of incompetent perforating veins are confirmed. The deep veins are assessed with regard to patency and the presence of venous reflux. This may be due to primary valvular incompetence, but it is usually due to post-thrombotic damage to the venous valves.

2. Venous function tests. The filling and emptying of the veins of a limb change the limb volume. This can be measured by venous plethysmography. These tests include foot volumetry by water displacement, and strain-gauge plethysmography, air-, photo- or impedance-plethysmography, depending on the physical method of determining venous filling of a limb. Light reflection rheography works along the same principles as photoplethysmography, using infrared light to penetrate the dermis of the skin of the leg, recording the amount reflected back, which is in proportion to the filling of the dermal vessels. Dermal capillary flow can be measured by laser Doppler fluximetry.

Invasive tests

1. Varicography. The injection of varicosities enables visualization of the source of varicose vein filling. This is particularly useful in recurrent varicose veins when the source is difficult to determine clinically.

2. Ascending phlebography. This is the optimal method of assessing the anatomy of the deep venous system, particularly in the detection of postphlebitic deep vein damage. It is useful in detecting incompetent perforating veins, but not all may be detected.

3. Descending phlebography. Deep venous reflux may be assessed by descending phlebography. Reflux is classed according to Kistner's grading 0–IV. Grade I is reflux into the superficial femoral vein and is deemed normal, and grade IV is gross reflux down to the calf veins.

Lymphatic

Clinical examination

Lymphoedema results in swelling of the lower limb, which can range from as little as mild swelling of the dorsum of the foot to gross swelling of the entire limb. There is usually squaring of the toes. In advanced cases, the skin develops filiform and nodular excrescences. Classically, chronic lymphoedema is said not to pit with pressure, though this is not true in all cases. Lymphoedema due to lymphatic obstruction at the level of the groin nodes with patient lymphatics distally may produce swelling of the thigh and leg with sparing of the foot. This is important to detect clinically and to confirm by special investigations, as this may be amenable to surgical bypass using an entero-mesenteric bridge.

Invasive tests

1. Isotope lymphography. This provides rapid confirmation of a clinical diagnosis of lymphoedema. A reduced isotope uptake in the lymph vessels and nodes of the groin confirm lymphoedema, and additionally an obstructive pattern may be discerned. A higher uptake than the normal range may be indicative of a venous cause for swelling.

2. Contrast lymphography. This is performed under general anaesthesia. Dorsal pedal lymphatics are dissected and cannulated using an operating microscope, and lipid-soluble contrast is slowly infused. It is time-consuming and expensive, and cannot be used to confirm all cases of suspected lymphoedema. It should be used only when there is clinical and isotopic evidence of proximal lymphatic obstruction.

Further reading

Beard JD, Scott DJA. Investigation of chronic lower limb ischaemia. *Hospital Update*, 1991; **June**: 496–506.
Nicolaides AN. Assessment of leg ischaemia. *British Medical Journal*, 1991; **303**: 1323–6.

Related topics of interest

VASCULAR MALFORMATIONS AND TUMOURS

Malformations

These may have arterial, venous or lymphatic elements, or they may be mixed. The majority are congenital, in which case they are hamartomatous in origin and not neoplastic. Acquired vascular malformations are usually traumatic in origin.

Arterial

1. Congenital arteriovenous malformations (fistulae). These are rare, and can arise in any part of the body but are more frequent on the head and neck and in the upper limb. They vary in size, and may be very unsightly and distressing. An appreciable increase in size may occur at the time of puberty. The swelling caused by the malformation is usually warm, soft and pulsatile, with a palpable thrill and a bruit. Occlusion of the fistula by compression may result in a bradycardia from the transiently reduced venous return (Branham's sign). There is often an erythematous hue of the overlying skin. Tissues distal to an arteriovenous fistula may become ischaemic as a result of the 'steal' of oxygenated blood, and ulceration or haemorrhage may occur.

The diagnosis can be confirmed by arteriography, which might enable therapeutic embolization of the feeding vessels. This is a risky undertaking which may lead to further ischaemia of the distal tissues, or inadvertent embolization into vital structures. Simple ligation of the feeding vessels is rarely successful in controlling the malformation. Excision of an arteriovenous malformation is hazardous as blood loss may be enormous. Quilting sutures may be successful in reducing the size of a malformation.

2. Parkes–Weber syndrome. This comprises multiple deep arteriovenous fistulae resulting in a generally swollen and often lengthened limb which is warm to the touch, and mildly red in colour. Bruits and thrills are rare because the fistulae are small. The diagnosis is confirmed by angiography. Symptoms may be controlled by repeated angiography and embolization, which reduces the shunting of arterial blood to the venous system and thus prevents or delays the onset of high output cardiac failure, which is a serious complication.

Venous

1. Venous angioma. These malformations vary widely in appearance, and may occur virtually anywhere. If superficial, they may present as a bulky, blue-coloured, compressible mass. Deeper angiomas may be painful, and manifest only by diffuse swelling with a hint of blue discoloration. Frequently, the abnormality extends further than can be appreciated by external examination. CT scan after injection of contrast or magnetic resonance venography will demonstrate the true extent, and involvement of muscle groups and joints may be identified. Excision can result in symptomatic or cosmetic improvement, although lesions are rarely completely excised.

2. Klippel–Trenaunay syndrome. This condition is essentially a triad of venous, bone and lymphatic congenital anomalies. The lower limb is most commonly affected, followed by the arm then the pelvis. The overriding abnormality is usually venous, although the extent of venous, bone and lymphatic involvement varies widely. The affected limb is swollen, and often longer, with an extensive cutaneous venous haemangioma following a metameric distribution. There are usually grossly dilated and incompetent superficial varicosities. Support hosiery remains the most effective and simple treatment. Deep venous abnormalities may be present, and this must be excluded by phlebography should surgery be planned for symptomatic superficial varicosities.

Lymphatic

1. Cystic hygroma. This is a bulky swelling present in the root of the neck at birth. It is soft and cystic on examination, and transilluminates. The management is conservative as resolution often occurs by the age of four. Aspiration and injection with sclerosants may be required for recalcitrant lesions.

2. Lymphangioma circumscripta. This is a cutaneous lesion comprising multiple, small, cutaneous vesicles in very close approximation to each other. They are usually colourless but are occasionally blood-filled. They contain lymph, and may be a manifestation of an underlying chronic lymphatic abnormality. They may cause troublesome seepage of fluid, and may act as a source of infection. Excision of a patch of vesicles is unlikely to prevent recurrence, though symptoms may be temporarily relieved.

3. Haemolymphangioma. This is a diffuse congenital abnormality of the lymphatics, usually affecting a limb, and most commonly the leg. The abnormality is present in the subcutaneous tissues, but may also involve deeper structures. The limb is swollen, indurated and discoloured, and some degree of disability usually results. Because of the diffuse nature of the abnormality, excision is not feasible although reduction of limb volume may be of help.

Tumours

Glomus tumour

These are benign vascular tumours that typically occur on extremities. They arise from the dermal glomus apparatus, a vascular organ that has a role in temperature regulation. The majority affect upper limb, and 50% occur on the finger, one-third of which are sub-ungual. They present as exquisitely painful and tender lesions. Pain may result from very minor disturbances, particularly changes in temperature and on pressure. They are often purple or red in colour, though they may appear colourless if sub-ungual. Although they are often very small, often only millimetres in diameter, they may be localized on examination by their intense point tenderness. Treatment is by excision.

Carotid body tumour

These are also known as chemodectomas. They are rare tumours arising from the chemoreceptor cells of the carotid body. Exceptionally, they may arise from chemoreceptor tissue at other sites. They are highly vascular. Ten per cent are bilateral. They affect males and females equally and at all ages, although the peak incidence is at 50. They present as a painless, often long-standing mass below the angle of the jaw, which will be compressible with gentle sustained pressure, and refills when pressure is released (the 'sign of emptying' of a vascular mass). The diagnosis is confirmed by intravenous digital subtraction angiogram (DSA), which shows characteristic splaying of the carotid bifurcation, or by CT scan. Macroscopically they appear as featureless oval masses, leading to the description 'potato tumour' although on cut section they are red or brown.

The treatment is by excision by an experienced vascular surgeon, as the internal carotid artery may need to be shunted or even resected and grafted, though the latter is unusual. Their behaviour is unpredictable, with the majority not recurring following excision, though a proportion will have frank evidence of malignancy with local invasion. If left unresected, 10–20% will develop metastases. Radiotherapy may be of use in the elderly or unfit patient, or in the treatment of local recurrence.

Glomus jugulare tumour

These are similar to chemodectomas but arise in the jugular bulb in association with the ninth, tenth and eleventh cranial nerves. They are slow growing but locally invasive. Presentation is with pulsatile tinnitus, or as a lump anterior to the mastoid process. Surgical excision is a major undertaking that risks facial and other cranial nerve palsies, and radiotherapy is an alternative option.

Haemangioendothelioma

These are purple nodular subcutaneous tumours which usually occur on extremities, most often on fingers or toes. They are histologically benign, but are prone to local recurrence. They may be treated by repeated resection or amputation of the affected digit.

Kaposi's sarcoma

This is a malignant tumour arising from vascular tissue that is also termed haemangiosarcoma. It sporadically arises in middle-aged Mediterranean and African populations and in Eastern European Jews. Men are mostly affected. It is frequently found on the leg and trunk and is commonly multiple. It appears as a red or bluish usually painless papule. The incidence of this has risen greatly with the increase in HIV infection, which predisposes to the appearance of Kaposi's sarcoma in the skin and throughout the intestinal tract. It responds initially to cytotoxic chemotherapy and radiotherapy, but spreads readily to the liver and lungs, carrying a dismal prognosis.

Angiosarcoma

Sarcomatous change is a very rare complication in a long-standing angioma. Rapid enlargement and induration of the lesion will occur. Primary angiosarcoma also occurs in the liver in children and young adults.

Venous leiomyosarcoma

Leiomyosarcoma may arise from the vena cava, and more rarely from the iliac or femoral veins. The sarcoma invades locally and may present with pain. There may be symptoms from venous obstruction. These tumours should be treated by excision and interposition grafting as necessary. Further local control may be achieved by radiotherapy. However local recurrence is usual, and the prognosis is poor.

Lymphangiosarcoma

This is a rare primary malignancy arising from lymphatic vessels. It may occur in long-standing lymphoedematous limbs, in which case it is known as Stuart–Treeves syndrome. Rapid growth is characteristic, and the prognosis is poor.

Further reading

Allison DJ, Kennedy A. Peripheral arteriovenous malformations. *British Medical Journal*, 1991; **303**: 1191–4.

Halliday AW, Mansfield AO. Congenital arteriovenous malformations. *British Journal of Surgery*, 1993; **80**: 2–3.

Related topics of interest

VASCULAR TRAUMA

Mechanism of injury

Urban, terrorist and military violence involving blunt and penetrating arterial and venous injuries is increasingly common. Road traffic accidents may also result in penetrating injuries but commonly cause fractures and dislocations that damage adjacent vessels. Low velocity penetrating injuries (pistols, knives) produce localized, direct injury to vessels. High velocity injuries (high velocity rifles) produce a shock wave effect resulting in widespread tissue destruction. Secondary missiles (bullet or bone fragments) can produce further damage. Iatrogenic injuries occur with the increasing use of invasive or minimally invasive procedures. Vessels may also be injured by chemical agents and by cold.

Types of vessel injury

- Contusion.
- Puncture.
- Laceration.
- Partial division.
- Transection.

Effects of vessel injury

- Haemorrhage. Primary, reactionary or secondary. Revealed or concealed.
- Occlusion. Thrombosis, dissection, external compression, spasm.
- False aneurysm.
- Traumatic arteriovenous fistula.

Clinical assessment

The history of injury is usually clear. External haemorrhage or expanding haematoma are usually evident. Weak or absent distal pulses are an important sign but distal ischaemia is uncommon in isolated arterial injuries and pulses are present in 20% of patients with arterial wounds. Duplex ultrasound and/or arteriography may be helpful but should not delay the control of severe haemorrhage.

1. Indications for surgical exploration
- Weak or absent distal pulse.
- Persistent arterial bleeding.
- Large expanding haematoma.
- Ischaemia.
- Bruit.

Treatment

1. Principles of repair. Major vascular injuries in a haemodynamically unstable patient require immediate operation. Direct pressure should be used to control bleeding initially, whilst intravenous access is gained for the infusion of electrolyte solutions until blood is available. Vertical incisions enable easy extension if necessary and reduce the likelihood of injury to adjacent neurovascular structures. Control proximal and distal to the site of injury will allow control where a large haematoma obscures the site of injury. In major vessel transection a heparin-bonded shunt may be used to re-establish arterial and/or venous continuity whilst adjacent fractures are stabilized, or more life-threatening injuries are repaired. Careful embolectomy proximal and distal to the site of injury should be performed before the repair is completed. Ultrasound or arteriography should be used to confirm distal patency if there is any doubt. Systemic anticoagulants are best avoided in patients with multiple injuries. Where synthetic grafts are necessary, aspirin should be used. Small and medium-sized veins can safely be ligated but axial outflow veins should be repaired and continuity established to prevent subsequent thrombosis with swelling and aching. Reperfusion injury may occur after revascularization of an ischaemic limb and fasciotomy may be necessary.

2. *Techniques of repair*
- Simple suture – for small holes.
- Transverse suture – for small tears.
- Patch repair – where direct closure would cause stenosis. A segment of autologous internal iliac artery can be used for aortic tears.
- End to end anastomosis–for complete transection or where excision of a short segment of damaged vessel is necessary.
- Interposition graft – where there is significant loss of vessel length. Use autogenous vein if possible.

Iatrogenic injury

1. *Ligation.* Unexpected arterial injury at operation may result in ligation of a major artery. Removal of the ligature (or repair of the artery where appropriate) should be undertaken rather than relying on collateral circulation.

2. *Compression from plasters and splints.* These problems should be prevented by adequate padding, splinting and monitoring of the limb.

3. *Arterial puncture.* Cardiac catheterization via femoral or brachial arteries results in sporadic arterial injuries which

can be minimized by careful dissection, compression and suture where necessary. Distal ischaemia is usually caused by thrombosis or dissection and is treated by exploration, embolectomy/thrombectomy and repair of the damaged segment by patch or interposition graft.

4. Intra-arterial injection. Barbiturates, sodium tetradecyl sulphate and substances used by drug abusers inadvertently injected into an artery may cause thrombosis and distal ischaemia. A dextran infusion should be started immediately the injury is recognized. Systemic anticoagulants, sympathetic block, prostaglandin infusion and thrombolysis should also be considered.

Venous injury

Damage to major veins frequently accompanies arterial injury. Data from recent military and civilian conflicts have demonstrated enhanced limb salvage and function where concomitant venous injuries are repaired rather than ligated. Venous injury is usually caused by penetrating trauma, although hepatic vein injuries result from blunt shearing forces. Injuries to major thoracic, abdominal and pelvic veins carry a high mortality. Repair of venous limb injuries should only be undertaken in haemodynamically stable patients. Anticoagulation or the construction of a temporary arteriovenous fistula may be necessary to maintain patency.

Frostbite

Frostbite affects the distal extremities not adequately protected from cold. The fingers and toes redden at about 15°C because of a relative oxygen surplus. Below 10°C the skin becomes painful and hypersensitive. At 2.5°C the skin becomes anaesthetic and ice crystals form. Tissue destruction occurs between −4 and −10°C. Slowing of blood flow leads to thrombosis and gangrene. Pain and swelling occur as the tissues rewarm and blisters form as plasma seeps out of the damaged microcirculation. The use of properly insulated garments together with movement and, if necessary, enforced exercise will usually prevent frostbite. Rapid whole body rewarming in a whirlpool at 37–40°C is the preferred treatment. Dextran, heparin or thrombolysis may be required to treat thrombosis. The place of hyperbaric oxygen is unclear. Local amputations should be performed when demarcation lines have become evident.

Immersion foot

Explorers and vagrants are prone to this condition which occurs in those wearing constrictive footwear in cold, wet environments. The extremities become numb causing the sensation of walking on cotton wool. Feelings of cramp and constriction occur and the skin becomes inflamed, then pale blue and finally black. The footwear should be removed and the feet gently rewarmed, but kept dry. The feet should be elevated until the swelling has resolved. Smoking should be prohibited and sympathectomy may be of benefit. Local amputation may be necessary, but should be delayed until demarcation of dead tissue has occurred.

Further reading

Browse NL, Burnand KG, Lea Thomas M. *Diseases of the Veins: Pathology, Diagnosis and Treatment*. London: Edward Arnold, 1988; 643–59.
Burnand KG. The arteries. In: Burnand KG, Young AE (eds) *The New Aird's Companion in Surgical Studies*. Edinburgh: Churchill Livingstone, 1992; 301–84.

Related topics of interest

VASOMOTOR AND VASCULITIC CONDITIONS

The vasospastic conditions affect the small arteries of the extremities causing local ischaemia, ulceration and sometimes gangrene. They may be primary or secondary. The arteritic conditions are characterized by an inflammatory infiltrate of the arterial wall (lymphocytes, plasma cells and histiocytes) causing luminal narrowing or obliteration. Different patterns of ischaemia result depending on the size and distribution of the vessels affected. The vasculitic conditions, systemic lupus erythematosus (SLE), scleroderma and polyarteritis nodosa (PAN) are not widely encountered in surgical practice and are not discussed.

Vasomotor conditions

Raynaud's disease

Attacks of bilateral digital ischaemia occur comprising a blanching phase (white), caused by arterial spasm, a cyanotic phase (blue) and a reactive hyperaemia phase (red). Cold or emotion are the precipitating causes and the condition is generally most severe during winter months. Young women (12–45 years) are most commonly affected (M:F = 1:4). The hands are usually involved, but feet are affected in 40% of cases. In severe cases, trophic changes including ulceration and gangrene may occur. The ischaemia is caused by spasm of the digital arteries, but the cause is unknown.

The diagnosis is made by exclusion of factors implicated in (secondary) Raynaud's phenomenon. Patients should be advised to avoid getting their hands and feet cold, and to avoid smoking and beta-blockers. Calcium antagonists (nifeepine), serotonin receptor antagonists (ketanserin), α-adrenoceptor blockers (prazosin), methyldopa, prostaglandin analogues and transdermal glyceryl trinitrate have been tried with varying success. Prostaglandin infusions and plasmapheresis are sometimes required. Surgical thoracodorsal sympathectomy is effective initially, but symptoms generally recur within 6 months. Occasionally, local deridement or amputation is required. The Raynaud's Association is able to supply patients with useful practical information and self-help sheers.

Raynaud's phenomenon

This term is used where the features of Raynaud's disease are secondary to another condition.

- Connective tissue disorders: scleroderma SLE, dermatomyositis, PAN, rheumatoid arthritis.
- Arterial disease: atherosclerosis, arteritis, cervical rib.

- Physical: neurovascular compression, vibration-induced white finger, frost bite.
- Haematological abnormalities: cryoglobulinaemia, cold agglutinins, polycythaemia, thrombocythaemia.
- Drugs: beta-blockers, sympathomimetics, nicotine, ergot, oral contraceptive, cytotoxics.

Acrocyanosis

There is a generalized cyanosis of the hands (and sometimes feet) which is exacerbated by exposure to cold. Women are principally affected. The vasospasm affects smaller arteries and arterioles than are affected in Raynaud's disease, and the stagnant hypoxia that occurs in the capillary bed causes the marked cyanosis. Trophic changes do not occur. Avoidance of cold is the main treatment, drugs and sympathectomy giving only marginal relief.

Livedo reticularis

Men and women of all ages are affected. Cyanotic mottling of the skin occurs, especially of the leg and foot. Spasm of the arterioles and dilatation of the capillaries and venules causes local stagnation of blood resulting in a reticular pattern. There is a perivascular infiltrate of inflammatory cells. Ulceration may occur which is painful and indolent. Some variants of livedo are associated with SLE, anticardiolipin antibody, PAN and syphilis.

Erythrocyanosis (pernio)

This condition typically affects obese young women. The legs develop dusky erythematous patches just above the ankles, although the skin over the triceps may also be affected. The erythematous patches may become indurated and nodular ('chilblains'). Ulceration may occur. Histologically these lesions show fat necrosis and scanty giant cells. Treatment is by cold avoidance and weight loss.

Erythromelalgia

Erythema and a burning pain of the extremities occur in this condition which may be primary or associated with gout, SLE, rheumatoid arthritis, PAN, vascular disease, diabetes mellitus, neurological conditions and vasoactive drugs. Symptoms are exacerbated by warmth and limb dependency, and relieved by cooling and rest. The cause is unknown, but a platelet-mediated arteriolar inflammation has been proposed following the marked response to aspirin obtained in some cases.

Hyperhydrosis

Excessive sweating of the hands and sometimes feet and axillae occurs in this condition. Sweating may be so severe as to make letter writing and other manual and social pastimes virtually impossible. Sweating can be reduced by regular application of aluminium chloride hexahydrate or 2% glycopyrolate. More permanent relief can be obtained by excision of axillary skin. Thoracoscopic sympathectomy provides effective and permanent relief of palmar sweating, but compensatory hyperhydrosis of the trunk ususaly occurs. Lumbar sympathectomy is similarly effective for plantar sweating.

Vasculitic conditions

Buerger's disease

This condition is also known as thromboangiitis obliterans and typically affects male smokers between 20 and 45 years. The distal, medium-sized arteries of the upper and lower limbs are obliterated by a transmural round cell infiltration and intimal proliferation which lead to luminal thrombosis. Depositions of collagen are often found around the vessels. Patients present with chronic low-grade digital infection, indolent ulceration or gangrene. The principal trunk arteries are usually intact, but the foot pulses are frequently missing. The condition must be differentiated from diabetic arterial disease, atherosclerosis and embolic ischaemia. Arteriography shows a typical distal distribution of occlusive disease with collateral vessel formation and intact proximal arteries.

Patients must be strongly advised to stop smoking to avoid progressive ischaemia and amputation. Sympathectomy is effective at relieving rest pain and healing ulceration. Arterial bypass is usually impractical and patients who do not stop smoking frequently require distal amputations. Prostaglandin infusions sometimes provide short-term relief.

Temporal arteritis

This condition usually affects men and women over 60 years and frequently starts with a fever and myalgia. A frontal headache develops and the region of the affected temporal artery becomes tender. The superficial temporal artery may be thickened and palpable. The retinal artery and its branches may become involved and, if left untreated, occlusion resulting in blindness may develop.

The diagnosis is usually confirmed by a high ESR, associated polymyalgia rheumatica and a temporal artery biopsy which shows round cell infiltration and scattered giant cells. Treatment with high-dose steroids to prevent blindness should not be delayed.

Takayasu's disease   This arteritis typically affects the large vessels of the aortic arch, but may also affect the thoracic and abdominal aorta. Symptoms include transient ischaemic attack, stroke and arm claudication. An upper limb or/and carotid pulse may disappear and there is often a difference in blood pressure measured in each arm. A course of steroids may kerb the disease process. Surgical bypass to revascularize the ischaemic territory yields good results and the disease process often resolves itself over several years.

Further reading

Burnand KG. The arteries. In: Burnand KG, Young AE (eds) *The New Aird's Companion in Surgical Studies*. Edinburgh: Churchill Livingstone, 1992; 301–84.

Duprez DA. Secondary vasospastic disorders. In: Clement DL, Shepherd JT (eds) *Vascular Diseases in the Limbs*. St Louis: Mosby Year Book, 1993; 169–86.

Shepherd RFJ, Shepherd JT. Primary Raynaud's disease. In: Clement DL, Shepherd JT (eds) *Vascular Diseases in the Limbs*. St Louis: Mosby Year Book, 1993; 153–68.

Related topics of interest

WOUNDS: HEALING AND CLOSURE

Normal healing

Coagulative and substrate phases

Wounds fill with blood, the coagulation cascade is activated and platelets degranulate, releasing transforming growth factor-ß and platelet-derived growth factor from their α-granules. These are potent regulators of subsequent events. The fibrin clot loosely seals the wound edges, and acts as a matrix for the adhesion of migrating cells. Local vessels leak protein rich fluid into the matrix.

Inflammatory phase

Vessels contract under the influence of locally produced histamine. Platelet plugs are formed to occlude open vessels, and the coagulation cascade is initiated. Within hours of wounding neutrophils enter the wound matrix. They phagocytose contaminating bacteria and debris for the first few days until circulating monocytes enter the wound matrix.

Synthesis phase

Migrating monocytes enter the wound under chemotaxis by growth factors. These become activated macrophages which also phagocytose debris, produce more growth factors, and recycle the provisional wound matrix, releasing degradation products that are also chemotactic.

Remodelling phase

Stimulated by transforming growth factor-β, fibroblasts migrate into the provisional wound matrix producing the collagen and glycoproteins that form the definitive extracellular matrix. Endothelial buds sprout from capillaries forming capillary loops. Basic fibroblast growth factor is a major stimulant of this process of angiogenesis. The new vessels are visible macroscopically as red, friable granulation tissue which bleeds easily on contact, and this is a hallmark of a healthy wound.

Maturation phase

The matrix undergoes organization into mature fibrous tissue. Specialized myofibroblasts contract the wound. Continuous collagen deposition and degradation by matrix proteinases allow connective tissue deposition in bundles. This strengthens the wound, though only reaching about 80% of the strength of unwounded skin. This fibroplasia results in a scar. The underlying fibrous scar tissue eventually loses its vascularity and changes in colour from red to white.

Epithelialization

During the last two phases of wound healing, or as the principal event if there is only a superficial wound, epithelialization of the exposed new dermis occurs from the wound edges. This is under control of local growth factors, such as basic fibroblast growth factor-7 (known as keratinocyte growth factor) and epidermal growth factor. Keratinocytes migrate through and attach to a wound matrix, as well as dividing and encroaching from the wound edge.

Wound contamination

Wounds can be classified according to their degree of or potential for being contaminated. This is of practical importance, as it will have a bearing on the treatment and closure of a wound.

1. Infected wound. A frankly infected wound bears the hallmarks of acute inflammation (tumor, calor, dolor, and rubor, the signs of Celsus) and there may be cellulitis in the surrounding tissues. There may be pus in the wound, necrotic tissue in the wound base, and if the infecting organisms include anaerobes, there may be an offensive odour. Surgical wounds are said to be infected or 'dirty' if the operative field contains pus or faecal contamination.

2. Contaminated wound. A wound that has been exposed to a source of bacteria is a contaminated wound. These clearly have the potential to become infected. Surgical wounds are contaminated if surgery is being undertaken on an infected viscus, or there is a breach in the sterility of the operation, such as spillage of faeces during a colonic resection. Traumatic wounds are usually considered contaminated, a good example being stab wounds.

3. Clean wounds. These are wounds that are sterile from start to finish, and are usually only encountered in surgical procedures on non-infected sites. An example is an elective cholecystectomy. Clean wounds made at operation can be classified as 'clean-contaminated' if a source of bacteria is operated upon during the course of the procedure, but potential for contamination is limited by meticulous surgical technique.

Healing by primary intention

If wounds are closed by means of sutures, then healing is said to occur by primary intention.

1. Primary closure. If a wound is closed at the time of surgery, or following trauma, this is called primary closure.

This must only be performed on wounds that are clean and healthy. Unhealthy tissue at a wound edge, whether it is devitalized following trauma, or old scar tissue from previous surgery, must be debrided. Sutures in the scalp or face should be removed after 4 days. Those in the leg or back may need to be left for 2 weeks, and those closing a laparotomy wound should be left for 10 days. Most other sutures can be removed after 1 week.

2. *Delayed primary closure.* Sometimes a wound is contaminated and yet controlled closure by sutures is desirable. The wound may be treated with antiseptic dressing and sutures placed after 3 or 4 days, by which time the wound should be free of potentially infecting organisms. This is delayed primary closure.

Healing by secondary intention

If wounds are left alone to heal, healing is said to occur by granulation or secondary intention. Grossly contaminated or infected wounds are debrided and left to granulate. Wounds following the excision of pilonidal disease in the natal cleft or excision of axillary or groin skin for hidradenitis or hyperhidrosis may heal satisfactorily in this way. The process is that of normal wound healing, but this takes longer than in wounds that have been closed. Prominent scars may result.

Disorders of healing

Various medical conditions may inhibit normal wound healing. Treatment with steroids, diabetes mellitus, uraemia, carcinomatosis, jaundice, vitamin deficiency particularly vitamin C, trace metal deficiency, for example zinc, have all been incriminated.

If a wound fails to heal, it becomes chronic. Some chronic wounds have a clear aetiology; for example, the majority of chronic leg ulcers are arterial, venous (or mixed) or are secondary to rheumatoid or other connective tissue, autoimmune, or vasculitic disease. Treatment should be aimed at dealing with the underlying cause. Venous ulcers require compression, arterial ulcers may need vascular reconstruction, and steroids may be required if there is a vasculitis.

Disorders of scarring

1. *Hypertrophic scarring.* Scarring always results in full-thickness wounds. The degree of scarring may vary, however. Some scars become hypertrophic, resulting in unsightly and disorganized scars within 3 months of wounding. These are common, and the changes do not

extend beyond the confines of the scar. The best form of treatment is avoidance, and this may be achieved by recognition of the potential for scarring. Burn wounds frequently become hypertrophic, and elasticated compression stockings worn following treatment reduce the likelihood of this.

2. *Keloid scarring.* This results in a mass of fibrous tissue at the site of a wound (though some appear to arise spontaneously), which continues to expand and apparently involve skin beyond the confines of the original wound. These are more common in African people, and in the young.

    Keloids often recur after excision. The development of keloid scarring may be inhibited by radiotherapy or intralesional triamcinolone injection. Removal of an established keloid scar may require reconstructive surgery.

Further reading

Forrester JC. Wounds and their management. In: Cuschieri A, Giles GR, Moosa AR (eds) *Essential Surgical Practice.* London: Wright, 1988.
Kingsnorth AN, Slavin J. Peptide growth factors and wound healing. *British Journal of Surgery,* 1991; **78**: 1286–90.

Related topics of interest

Burns (p. 64)
Sepsis in the surgical patient (p. 272)
Suture materials (p. 290)

INDEX